Coronary Artery Surgery

Editor: Felix Unger

With 135 Figures

Springer-Verlag
Berlin Heidelberg New York Tokyo 1984

Universitäts-Professor Dr. med. Felix Unger

Universitäts-Klinik für Chirurgie
Anichstr. 35, 6020 Innsbruck/Austria

ISBN-13: 978-3-540-13264-6 e-ISBN-13: 978-3-642-69638-1
DOI: 10.1007/978-3-642-69638-1

Library of Congress Cataloging in Publication Data.
Main entry under title: Coronary artery surgery. Proceedings of a joint workshop between the European Society of Cardiology and the European Society of Cardiovascular Surgery, held Oct. 14–15, 1983, in Innsbruck. Includes bibliographies and index. 1. Aortocoronary bypass-Congresses. 2. Coronary heart disease Surgery-Congresses. I. Unger, Felix, 1946. II. European Society of Cardiology. III. European Society of Cardiovascular Surgery. (DNLM: 1. Aortocoronary Bypass-congresses. 2. Coronary Vessels-surgery-congresses. WG 300 C8212 1983). RD598.C6674 1984 617'.412 84-10674

2127/3020–543210

Introduction

The joint workshop between the European Society of Cardiology and the European Society of Cardiovascular Surgery, held October 14–15, 1983 in Innsbruck, Austria, was a unique event. The idea originated in Atlanta, 1982, with C. Hahn and was supported by V. Björk and N. Browse. H. Denolin and F. Loogen brought added impact from the European Society of Cardiology. The joint workshop specifically emphasized new trends and controversies in coronary artery surgery. The contributions appearing in this edition were selected by a scientific committee: H. Denolin, H. Kraft-Kinz, F. Unger, F. Loop, L. Cohn, F. Loogen, P. Lichtlen, T. Killip, and F. Kaindl.

The specific aim was to evaluate controversial review points in coronary artery surgery. These were covered in six discussions and in nine forums with slide presentations. The topics were:

1. Indications for coronary artery surgery
2. Graft patency and long-term results
3. New operative techniques
4. Myocardial preservation and anesthetic management
5. Combined procedures
6. Long-term follow-up

Coronary artery surgery is a model for comprehensive cardiology, whereby surgery serves as a link between diagnosis and rehabilitation. Because coronary artery surgery has become a routine procedure with standardized techniques, the demand is increasing dramatically as reflected by enormous waiting lists.

Hospital mortality can be kept under 1%, so that the value of this operation can also be discussed with regard to its social and economic aspects. In the majority of cases, patients improve and finally return to work, finding life most enjoyable again.

As more diagnostic procedures are performed, the incidence of operation will increase, so that the designing of new cardiovascular centers is desirable. This workshop has stimulated the creation of a working group on operative cardiology, sponsored by the European Society of Cardiology and the European Society of Cardiovascular Surgery to evaluate and define the different demands and developments of the future.

I am very grateful to Springer for making possible the publication of this workshop in this fine edition.

Innsbruck, January 1984 — Felix Unger

Participants

R. Achatzy, Münster, FRG
P. C. Adams, Newcastle upon Tyne, UK
F. Akhras, London, UK
G. Alber, Traunstein, FRG
K. G. M. Alberti, Newcastle upon Tyne, UK
J. A. Alexander, Gainesville, USA
O. Alfieri, Utrecht, Netherlands
E. Anyanwu, Münster, FRG
N. Arunachalam, Liverpool
E. Astorri, Parma, Italy
D. Banzer, Berlin, FRG
G. Bastianen, Utrecht, Netherlands
E. Baudet, Bordeaux, France
H. Berggren, Göteborg, Sweden
E. Berglin, Göteborg, Sweden
T. Bianchi, Bergamo, Italy
W. Bircks, Düsseldorf, FRG
D. Birnbaum, Berlin, FRG
N. Bleese, Hamburg, FRG
M. Borggrefe, Düsseldorf, FRG
E. Bos, Rotterdam, Netherlands
V. Braimbridge, London, UK
W. Brands, Utrecht, Netherlands
G. Breithardt, Düsseldorf, FRG
A. H. Brown, Newcastle upon Tyne, UK
P. Brücke, Linz, Austria
E. S. Bücherl, Berlin, FRG
F. Burgarella, S. Pellegrino, Italy
M. Busi, Parma, Italy
T. Bwakura, Münster, FRG
R. W. F. Campbell, Newcastle upon Tyne, UK
S. Caparrotti, Utrecht, Netherlands
M. Chello, Naples, Italy
M. Chimienti, Pavia, Italy
J. Cleary, London, UK
C. R. Conti, Gainesville, USA
G. A. Contini, Parma, Italy
F. Coraim, Vienna, Austria
H. Dalichan, Cologne, FRG
S. Dalla Volta, Padova, Italy
C. Dal Palù, Padova, Italy
J. Defauw, Utrecht, Netherlands
R. De Geest, Utrecht, Netherlands
C. Del Naja, Naples, Italy
M. Deutsch, Vienna, Austria
F. Di Lello, Naples, Italy
R. A. E. Dion, Utrecht, Netherlands
H. Dittrich, Münster, FRG
R. v. Domburg, Rotterdam, Netherlands
V. Dor, Nice, France
V. Döring, Hamburg, FRG
C. Dorste, Bad Krozingen, FRG
R. Ekroth, Göteborg, Sweden
M. J. Elliot, Newcastle upon Tyne, UK
J. von der Emde, Erlangen, FRG
J. Ernst, Utrecht, Netherlands
E. Eschenbruch, Innsbruck, Austria
B. Fabri, Liverpool, UK
R. S. Faro, Gainesville, USA
M. Feis, Utrecht, Netherlands
R. L. Feldman, Gainesville, USA
P. D. Ferretti, Parma, Italy
G. Fraedrich, Gießen, FRG
L. Fridrich, Grimmenstein, Austria
C. Gagliardi, Naples, Italy

V. Gallucci, Padova, Italy
A. Gassner, Grimmenstein, Austria
T. Gherli, Utrecht, Netherlands
E. Godehardt, Cologne, FRG
N. Goebel, Zurich, Switzerland
C. Goggi, Pavia, Italy
H. Gohlke, Bad Krozingen, FRG
H. Greve, Münster, FRG
C. Griffiths, Newcastle upon Tyne, UK
F. Gschnitzer, Innsbruck, Austria
R. W. Hacker, Erlangen, FRG
C. Hahn, Genolier, Switzerland
W. Haider, Vienna, Austria
P. Hairston, Charleston, USA
M. M. P. Haalebos, Rotterdam, Netherlands
A. Hannekum, Cologne, FRG
N. van Hemel, Utrecht, Netherlands
F. W. Hehrlein, Gießen, FRG
B. Herse, Cologne, FRG
C. J. Hilton, Newcastle upon Tyne, UK
J. F. Hitchcock, Utrecht, Netherlands
M. P. Holden, Newcastle upon Tyne, UK
R. A. Horney, Charleston, USA
P. G. Hugenholtz, Rotterdam, Netherlands
W. Hügel, Cologne, FRG
J. Ikwueke, London, UK
M. Inberg, Turku, Finland
G. Invernizzi, Bergamo, Italy
D. Iorio, Naples, Italy
G. Jackson, London, UK
G. Jambroes, Utrecht, Netherlands
V. Jelesijevic, Münster, FRG
R. Jenni, Innsbruck, Austria
D. G. Julian, Newcastle upon Tyne, UK
F. Kaindl, Vienna, Austria
P. Kalmar, Hamburg, FRG
M. Kaltenbach, Frankfurt, FRG
H. Kassal, Vienna, Austria
J. Keates, London, UK
B. Kemkes, Munich, FRG
W. J. Keon, Ottawa, Canada
D. Kettler, Göttingen, FRG
T. Killip, Detroit, USA
J. Kitchen, Newcastle upon Tyne, UK
W. Klinner, Munich, FRG
P. Knaepen, Utrecht, Netherlands
E. Knapp, Innsbruck, Austria
D. G. Knauf, Gainesville, USA
M. Kölbel, Gießen, FRG
H.-J. Krebber, Hamburg, FRG
E. R. Krefting, Münster, FRG
K. Laird-Meeter, Rotterdam, Netherlands
C. Liassides, London, UK
F. Loogen, Düsseldorf, FRG
J. Lubsen, Rotterdam, Netherlands
C. Maduro, Minneapolis, USA
A. R. Marchese, Naples, Italy
J. Marks, Minneapolis, USA
L. Martinelli, Pavia, Italy
D. Mathey, Hamburg, FRG
C. K. McKnight, Newcastle upon Tyne, UK
G. Minzioni, Pavia, Italy
J. E. Molina, Minneapolis, USA
A. Moritz, Vienna, Austria
V. Mühlberger, Innsbruck, Austria
J. Mulch, Gießen, FRG
E. P. Nicolaides, London, UK
M. Nijsen-Karelse, Utrecht, Netherlands
J. Ostermeyer, Düsseldorf, FRG
D. Pantaleo, Naples, Italy
C. P. Parali, Münster, FRG
G. Pauser, Vienna, Austria
C. J. Pepine, Gainesville, USA
D. T. Pearson, Newcastle upon Tyne, UK

N. Pflüger, Zurich, Switzerland
M. Pichler, Grimmenstein, Austria
R. Pigato, Padova, Italy
P. Pothen, Padova, Italy
W. H. Prioleau, Charleston, USA
A. Rashid, Liverpool, UK
B. Reichart, Munich, FRG
D. S. Reid, Newcastle upon Tyne, UK
E. Restori, Parma, Italy
B. Rigler, Graz, Austria
T. Rigo, Padova, Italy
A. J. Roberts, Gainesville, USA
P. Rocco, Naples, Italy
G. Rodewald, Hamburg, FRG
H. Roskamm, Bad Krozingen, FRG
M. Rothlin, Zurich, Switzerland
J. Salerno, Pavia, Italy
W. Sandtner, Vienna, Austria
A. Santana, Freiburg, FRG
M. R. Sastry, Liverpool, UK
A. Schaepkens van Riempst, Utrecht, Netherlands
H. Scharfetter, Innsbruck, Austria
H. H. Scheld, Gießen, FRG
R. Schistek, Innsbruck, Austria
V. Schlosser, Freiburg, FRG
M. Schmuziger, Bad Krozingen, FRG
A. Schreuders, Utrecht, Netherlands
W. Schütz, Vienna, Austria
F. Sebening, Munich, FRG
M. Semsroth, Vienna, Austria
A. Senning, Zurich, Switzerland
J. Slany, Vienna, Austria
N. Spampinato, Naples, Italy
K. Speiser, Zurich, Switzerland
G. Spillner, Freiburg, FRG
W. Steinbrunn, Innsbruck, Austria
F. Stellwag, Vienna, Austria
P. Stürzenhofecker, Innsbruck, Austria
L. B. Tecchia, Naples, Italy
A. Thevenet, Montpellier, France
M. Torka, Erlangen, FRG
P. Überfuhr, Munich, FRG
G. Ugolotti, Parma, Italy
F. Unger, Innsbruck, Austria
J. Upward, London, UK
B. Urbanyi, Freiburg, FRG
C. Valfré, Padova, Italy
R. J. Vecht, London, UK
F. Vermeulen, Utrecht, Netherlands
H. O. Vetter, Munich, FRG
M. Vigano, Pavia, Italy
L. D. Voegele, Charleston, USA
A. Waldenström, Göteborg, Sweden
A. Welz, Munich, FRG
G. William-Olsson, Göteborg, Sweden
B. Wimmer, Freiburg, FRG
K. Wink, Freiburg, FRG
E. Wolner, Vienna, Austria
M. Zembala, Utrecht, Netherlands

Contents

I Prospectives in Coronary Artery Surgery

Opening address: New Trends in Cardiology
F. Loogen (Düsseldorf, FRG) 1

Adress: Trends in Coronary Entry Surgery
C. Hahn (Genolier, Switzerland) 4

Prognosis in Ischemic Heart Disease
T. Killip (Detroit, USA) 6

II Indications for Coronary Artery Surgery

Anatomical and Tactical Considerations for Peripheral Revascularization in Patients with Diffuse Triple-Vessel Disease
M. Schmuziger, E. Eschenbruch, and P. Stürzenhofecker (Bad Krozingen, FRG) 14

Myocardial Revascularization for Early Postinfarction Angina
T. Bianchi, G. Invernizzi, and F. Burgarella (Bergamo, Italy) 18

Single Lesion of Proximal LAD in Young Patients: Medical Therapy, SVG, IMA Graft, PTCA?
N. Spampinato, F. Di Lello, M. Chello, D. Iorio, A. R. Marchese, and L. B. Tecchia (Naples, Italy) 22

Reoperation for Coronary Artery Disease
W. J. Keon (Ottawa, Canada) 27

Cardiac Transplantation: An Approach to End-Stage Coronary Heart Disease
A. Welz, B. Reichart, P. Überfuhr, B. Kemkes, and W. Klinner (Munich, FRG) 35

III Operative Techniques

Coronary Endarterectomy Associated with Aortocoronary Bypass
A. Thevenet and E. Baudet (Montpellier, France) 40

Selective Treatment of Diffuse Coronary Artery Disease by a Combination of Coronary Artery Bypass Grafting and Transluminal Balloon-Catheter Dilatation
A. J. Roberts, D. G. Knauf, J. A. Alexander, R. S. Faro, R. L. Feldman, C. R. Conti, and C. J. Pepine (Gainsville, USA) 44

The Technique of Subcutaneous Vein Harvest
A. Rashid, B. Fabri, M. R. Sastry, N. Arunachalam, and J. B. Meade (Liverpool, UK) 51

Flow in Saphenous Vein Bypass Grafts
W. H. Prioleau Jr., R. A. Horney, L. D. Voegele, and P. Hairston (Charleston, S. C., USA) 55

A New Method of Assessing Myocardial Ischemic Injury During Cardiac Operations: Electron Probe X-Ray Microanalysis
E. Anyanwu, E. R. Krefting, and H. Dittrich (Münster, FRG) 58

Direct Revascularization of the Septal Arteries: Preliminary Report on 112 Patients
S. Caparrotti, O. Alfieri, W. Brands, J. Defauw, R. De Geest, P. Knaepen, F. Vermeulen, and M. Zembala (Utrecht, the Netherlands) 68

IV Anaesthetic Management in Coronary Artery Surgery

The Use of Timolol in Reducing the Incidence of Supraventricular Arrhythmias After Coronary Artery Bypass Surgery
R. J. Vecht, J. Ikwueke, E. P. Nicolaides, C. Liassiades, and J. Cleary (London, UK) 72

Effect of the Bypass Pump Priming Fluid on the Metabolic Response to Open-Heart Surgery
C. K. McKnight, M. J. Elliott, D. T. Pearson, M. P. Holden, and K. G. M. M. Alberti (Newcastle Upon Tyne, UK) 76

Hemodynamic Results with Hemofiltration in Postoperative Cardiac Surgical Patients
F. Coraim, H. Kassal, G. Pauser, F. Stellwag, and E. Wolner (Vienna, Austria) . 80

V Myocardial Protection

Myocardial Preservation by Preoperative of High Amounts of Insulin Administration
W. Haider, W. Schütz, A. Moritz, W. Sandtner, M. Semsroth, and J. Slany (Vienna, Austria) 90

Myocardial Preservation in Emergency Coronary Surgery
N. Bleese, V. Döring, P. Kalmar, H.-J. Krebber, D. Mathey, and G. Rodewald (Hamburg-Eppendorf, FRG) 95

Thermographic Evaluation of Cardioplegia Diffusion in Coronary Patients
C. Gagliardi, D. Pantaleo, C. del Naja, P. Rocco, and N. Spampinato
(Naples, Italy) 100

Magnesium Augmentation During Reperfusion for the Reduction of
Postischaemic Myocardial Damage
A. H. Brown and J. Kitchen (Newcastle-Upon-Tyne, UK) 106

Calcium Flux Across the Myocardial Cellular Membrane During
Cardioplegic Cardiac Arrest
E. Anyanwu, E. R. Krefting, C. P. Parali, T. Bwakura, and H. Dittrich
(Münster, FRG) 112

Intracoronary Nifedipine in Patients Suspected of Perioperative Coronary
Spasm
R. A. E. Dion, M. Nijsen-Karelse, G. Jambroes, G. Bastianen, and
J. F. Hitchcock (Utrecht, the Netherlands) 119

Myocardial Protection with Cardioplegia in Patients with Severe CAD
J. Mulch, H. H. Scheld, H. Kölbel, G. Fraedrich, and F. W. Hehrlein
(Gießen, Bad Nauheim, FRG) 126

Enhanced Myocardial Protection by Means of Maintained β Blockade and
Preoperative Carbohydrate Infusion
H. Berggren, E. Berglin, R. Ekroth, A. Waldenström, and G. William-Olsson
(Göteborg, Sweden) 131

Establishing Safe Parameters for the Administration of Clear Cardioplegia
in Humans
J. E. Molina, C. Maduro, and J. Marks (Minneapolis, USA) 134

VI Left Ventricular Aneurysmectomy

Patient Selection for Left Ventricular Aneurysmectomy
A. Hannekum, H. Dalichau, B. Herse, and W. Hügel (Cologne, FRG) 139

False Aneurysm of the Left Ventricle After Myocardial Infarction
N. Goebel, R. Jenni, W. Steinbrunn, M. Turina, M. Rothlin, and A. Senning
(Zurich, Switzerland) 145

Clinical Experience in 445 Resections of Ventricular Aneurysms
R. Achatzy, E. Anyanwu, F. Klinke, V. Jelesijevic, H. Greve and H. Dittrich
(Münster, FRG) 149

Left Ventricular Aneurysmectomy Combined with Encircling Endocardial
Ventriculotomy for Treatment of Recurrent Sustained Ventricular
Tachycardio (VT)
J. Ostermeyer, G. Breithardt, M. Borggrefe, E. Godehardt, and W. Bircks
(Düsseldorf, FRG) 153

Surgical Treatment of Ventricular Tachycardias with Partial Endocardial Ventriculotomy
M. Vigano, L. Martinelli, G. Minzioni, C. Goggi, J. Salerno, and M. Chimienti (Pavia, Italy) 157

Ventricular Arrhythmias Before and After Aortocoronary Bypass Surgery
P. Pothen, R. Pigato, T. Rigo, C. Valfrè, V. Gallucci, and C. Dal Palù (Padova, Italy) 162

Endocardial Resection for Ventricular Tachycardia and Ventricular Fibrillation
C. J. Hilton, R. W. F. Campbell, D. S. Reid, P. C. Adams, C. Griffiths, and D. G. Julian (Newcastle-Upon-Tyne, UK) 166

Hemodynamic and Angiographic Results After Left Ventricular Aneurysmectomy
V. Mühlberger, E. Knapp, R. Schistek, H. Scharfetter, and F. Unger (Innsbruck, Austria) 171

Combined Procedures with Aortocoronary Bypass Surgery
H. O. Vetter, B. Reichart, B. M. Kemkes, and W. Klinner (Munich, FRG) . . . 176

Encircling Endocardial Ventriculotomy Versus Endocardial Resection for the Treatment of Drug-Refractory. Ischemic Ventricular Tachycardia
J. Defauw, S. Caparrotti, N. van Hemel, and F. Vermeulen (Utrecht, The Netherlands) 181

VII Graft Patency and Long Term Follow up

Changes in the Native Vessels After Aortocoronary Bypass Surgery
N. Goebel, N. Pfluger, K. Speiser, M. Turina, and M. Rothlin (Zurich, Switzerland) 187

Variables Influencing Patency of Coronary Artery Bypass Grafts
M. Torka and R. W. Hacker (Erlangen, Nürnberg, FRG) 191

Evaluation of Aortocoronary Graft Patency with Computed Tomography
B. Urbanyi, B. Wimmer, K. Wink, A. Santana, G. Spillner, and V. Schlosser (Freiburg, FRG) 197

Early Exercise Testing and Coronary Bypass Surgery Post-infarction
F. Akhras, J. Upward, J. Keates, and G. Jackson (London, UK) 201

Short-Term Radionuclide Study of Ventricular Function After Coronary Bypass Surgery
E. Astorri, M. Busi, G. A. Contini, G. Ugolotti, E. Restori and P. P. Ferretti (Parma, Italy) 206

Stress-Radionuclide Ventriculography in the Evaluation of CABG Patients
L. Fridrich, A. Gaszner, and M. Pichler (Grimmenstein, Austria) 211

Long-Term Results of Aortocoronary Bypass Surgery
H. Roskamm, M. Schmuziger, H. Gohlke, and C. Dorste (Bad Krozingen, FRG) 216

Influence of Residual Disease on Late Survival After Coronary Artery Bypass Surgery
R. W. Hacker and M. Torka (Erlangen, Nürnberg, FRG) 220

Survival in 1041 Patients with Consecutive Aortocoronary Bypass Operations
K. Laird-Meeter, M. M. P. Haalebos, R. v. Domburg, J. Lubsen, E. Bos, and P. G. Hugenholtz (Rotterdam, The Netherlands) 225

Long-Term Follow-up of Reoperation After Coronary Bypass Surgery
R. A. E. Dion, M. Feis, G. Jambroes, T. Gherli, and J. F. Hitchcock (Utrecht, The Netherlands) 230

Long-Term Results After Early Revascularization for Impending Infarction
F. Vermeulen, O. Alfieri, J. Defauw, J. Ernst, R. De Geest, P. Knaepen, A. Schaepkens van Riempst, and A. Schreuders (Utrecht, the Netherlands) . . 235

Imaging of Coronary Grafts Without Catheterization of Coronary Ostia
D. Birnbaum and D. Banzer (Berlin, FRG) 240

Opening Address: New Trends in Cardiology

F. Loogen

First of all I should like to thank cordially the European Society of Cardiovascular Surgery, together with the President of the workshop, Prof. Unger, for the invitation to this meeting. It is a great pleasure and honor for me to give the opening address.

As far as I know, this is the first time that the two European Societies have held a joint session. That is also a contribution to the "new trends" in cardiology.

The topic of the current meeting is "new trends and controversies in coronary artery surgery." I am not daring enough to make up my mind on new developments in cardiosurgery, so you will surely understand that I'll say nothing about the topics "new operative techniques in coronary artery surgery" and "anesthetic management in coronary artery surgery."

There are however several new procedures in cardiology involving cardiologists as well as cardiosurgeons. Without any doubt, these new methods have enlarged the therapeutic range within recent years; however, they have also created new problems. Let me go a bit more into two new procedures: (1) thrombolysis of acute myocardial infarction and (2) percutaneous transluminal coronary angioplasty (PTCA).

Thrombolytic therapy of acute myocardial infarction with systemic administration of streptokinase was introduced 20 years ago. The breakthrough, however, came only in 1978 when Rentrop introduced into clinical practice the concept of limiting infarct size by intracoronary infusion of streptokinase, and when Schröder and coworkers showed at the same time that a coronary thrombus can also be lysed by systemic administration of streptokinase. In 1977, Grüntzig introduced percutaneous transluminal coronary angioplasty (PTCA).

Both the streptokinase therapy and PTCA became rapidly known worldwide and are commonly applied today.

It is easily understood that European cardiologists are proud that these methods have been developed in Europe and from here have made their way around the world, i.e., also to the United States. This means that we could reciprocate a little for all the borrowing we have done from our American colleagues in recent decades. Unfortunately, with the export of these methods, we also lost their inaugurators to the United States.

Undoubtedly, streptokinase therapy is able to dissolve thrombus formations and can rebuild coronary flow. Undoubted, too, is the fact that PTCA is able to dilate a coronary stenosis or even remove it. I will not exaggerate the initial successes such as the frequency of lysis with the intracoronary or systemic application of streptokinase or the rates for successful PTCA. You all know the figures. They differ from group to group depending on facility with the methods, choice of patients, and treatment after intervention.

You know however that each coin has two sides; the other side is the numerous questions and problems brought up by the new treatment methods:

1. Can jeopardized myocardium in acute myocardial infarction be saved by thrombolysis?
2. Is the prognosis of these patients improved?
3. What kind of treatment is preferable – intracoronary or intravenous administration?
4. Should a bypass procedure be done after recanalization?
5. Should PTCA be done after recanalization?

Recanalization of an occluded vessel does not mean that the jeopardized myocardium has been saved. To evaluate the effect of recanalization on the extent of myocardial necrosis and on limiting infarct size, several methods have been applied on which numerous articles have been published.

The results of the different studies are not identical; in several cases they even contradict each other. This means that conclusive answers to the above-mentioned questions cannot be given. Whether and in how far jeopardized myocardium can be saved by thrombolysis is still unknown. Improvement in left ventricular function is mostly shown when reperfusion takes place within the first 3 h after the onset of symptoms.

With regard to the prognoses of the patients, it can be determined that the mortality of patients with successful lysis is about 7%, according to the registry of the European Society of Cardiology. This rate is identical to that of patients with uncomplicated myocardial infarction treated conventionally. In patients with unsuccessful lysis, mortality is about 20%. These two groups, however, cannot be compared to each other. As there are still no definite results from randomized studies with and without thrombolytic therapy, no final statement can be made about whether or not the rate of acute mortality is improved by this treatment. For the same reason, there are also no reliable results with regard to long-term prognosis.

No definite results are yet available from the groups applying the intravenous thrombolysis method.

In the choice of therapeutic procedure, knowledge of the advantages and disadvantages of each procedure is of importance. The advantages of intracoronary therapy are as follows:

1. A correct diagnosis by coronary angiography is possible.
2. The rate of recanalization is higher than with i.v. administration.
3. Additional therapeutic interventions, e.g., PTCA or bypass surgery, can be performed immediately.

The disadvantages of intracoronary therapy are:

1. It can be performed only in hospitals with catheter laboratories.
2. There is a greater delay before starting intracoronary therapy as compared to intravenous treatment.
3. It must be performed in collaboration with a coronary surgical unit.

The advantages of intravenous therapy are:

1. Treatment can be started immediately after diagnosis.
2. No special equipment is necessary.
3. Treatment can be performed in almost any hospital, even without a coronary surgical unit.

The disadvantages of intravenous therapy are:

1. Correct localization of the thrombus is not possible.
2. The rate of recanalization is lower than with intracoronary administration.
3. No additional therapeutic intervention (PTCA, bypass surgery) is possible.

After considering the advantages and disadvantages of either method, several groups started to combine the advantages of both methods. Upon the patient's admission to the hospital treatment is started intravenously, followed by coronary angiography and intracoronary infusion if necessary.

Preliminary results show a higher rate of recanalization than with either method alone. Furthermore, in these patients left ventricular function seems to be improved significantly as compared to patients with recanalization after intracoronary infusion alone.

In about 30% of patients reinfarction may occur after successful thrombolysis while the patient is still in the hospital. In order to prevent this, in many centers, an angioplasty or bypass procedure is performed. I do not want to address the problems involved in this approach. They will be discussed in some papers at this workshop. Perhaps we will hear some new aspects besides the well-known opinions.

Please allow me some remarks in regard to PTCA. As mentioned, coronary stenoses can be dilated in a high percentage of cases. In around 10% of the dilatation procedure is not successful; in 15%–40% recurrence of the stenosis, which can be accompanied in up to 10% by infarction or in some instances by sudden death, may occur in spite of successful dilatation. The high rate of recurrence, which is similar after repeat PTCA, and the above-mentioned rates of complications demand strict indications and careful selection of patients.

The dilatation of so-called mild stenoses has been disappointing. In many patients it was observed that recurrence of the stenosis exceeded the original degree of luminal narrowing. Therefore, it is questionable whether there is any indication at all for the dilatation of mild stenoses, either when isolated or in combination with other more severe stenoses.

There is no doubt that PTCA is less harmful, more easily performed, and less expensive than surgery. However, careful studies on the long-term results of PTCA are still necessary to provide reliable data.

In this short report only a few examples of new developments in cardiology are considered. Looking through the list of speakers in this workshop I'm sure that we will have occasion to discuss some of the above-mentioned questions and problems. Perhaps we will see more reliable data concerning long-term treatment results.

Address: Trends in Coronary Entry Surgery

C. Hahn

Every step in cardiac surgery was in the past considered a provocation to the art and science of cardiology. This did not happen everywhere, but there were many places where the general opinion was to try to refrain from the natural aggressiveness of surgery. I was lucky enough to work in close collaboration with medical specialists who could be convinced as long as we could show them facts. But generally speaking, the youthfulness of open-heart operations – first used in cases of congenital malformation with or without cyanosis, then in valvular surgery – was widely debated, as were the types of valve replacement and all techniques of valvular repairs developed during these past 35 years. It was even worse when we started, 16 years ago, to do coronary bypass procedures for myocardial revascularization. Being a pioneer in this field in Europe, I had the privilege to work mainly with Dutch and German cardiologists who had such a scientific education and a sense of their own limits that they accepted the advances in surgical procedures as progress which could help their patients. When I started my training in cardiac surgery in Leiden, 25 years ago, I understood from the medical environment in which I was living, that surgery was only one type of treatment which had to be used in the proper way at the proper time when it was absolutely necessary. We never got the idea that there was competition between surgical and medical therapy. Despite or because of that, it took a lot of energy to build the actual modern cardiac surgery, especially in a conservative country like mine.

In fact, we found here as well as in other countries (especially in French-speaking areas), a lot of resistance from the medical side; partly due to a general tendency of surgeons to claim their methods were innocuous the risks low, and the results excellent. This was not always in accordance with the truth. We can easily understand that the short period of time during which the surgeon takes care of the patient is probably one of the good reasons why the cardiologists cannot accept our new conceptions. In fact, cardiologists are faced with the long-term problems before and after surgery; they know much more about the different types of complications that can come out of surgery than we do. Nevertheless, it was not long ago when some cardiologists were explaining to an audience of surgeons what they would have to do in some instances: where to cut, how to cut, which type of valve they wanted or did not want, how many bypasses would be necessary on which arteries, or whether it was wise to resect an associated aneurysm of the left ventricle. The brains guiding the hands!

But now the time of "robot" surgeons is ended. Every cardiac surgeon knows enough of the basis of cardiology to understand what is going on, what must be done, what is helpful or not, which kind of risk can be acceptable, how to improve this risk in his own team, what can be accepted as a result of an operation, and how this short period of sudden hemodynamic change resulting from the surgical procedure can be integrated in the general treatment controlled by the cardiologists. In chronic progressive diseases nothing can cure, neither the medical nor the surgical treatments, but a good combination and coordination of both can surely give the patient the best chance of a better and longer life.

Cardiology is progressing because of cardiac surgery, and vice versa. They are two poles of the same approach. The time of cockfighting is over. Working together, we know when surgery is unnecessary, the medical measures as a whole being perfectly able to control the situation and to achieve our goals. We know too when a potentially dangerous situation can be controlled rapidly with the appropriate type of surgery.

In my opinion, what is done in our institution must be applied on a more general level. This is why we started a year ago to discuss with Felix Unger the possibility of a workshop on coronary artery surgery in Innsbruck, organized under the auspices of both the European Society of Cardiology and the European Society of Cardiovascular Surgery (the European chapter of the ISCVS), with the best specialists coming from all over the world. It is not the first time that medical and surgical specialists have shared their experiences, but it is probably the first time that the two societies have combined to enable a good organizing committee to put together an excellent program. Despite the tremendous role of computerization in a lot of situations, for example in the randomized studies, I got the feeling that we were speaking about patients and not about electronic substitutes. That is probably what was most enjoyable in this meeting: to have the firm impression that the patients were really present with their problems and their dignity.

Prognosis in Ischemic Heart Disease

T. Killip

Old lessons must be relearned. That the incidence and severity of disease have varied through the ages is well known. In the sixteenth century, syphilis was an aggressive and often fatal infection. Scarlet fever carried a high mortality and was a dreaded disease 150 years ago. Both the severity and frequency of tuberculosis began to decline even before Koch discovered the bacillus. The severity and case fatality rate in rheumatic heart disease has been declining for at least 100 years.

Careful study of the natural history of a disease is critical to the cautious evaluation of new therapy. In the United States, the death rate from all causes has been falling for at least the past 2 decades. A major contribution to this change has been an apparent precipitant decline in the fatality of coronary artery disease and other forms of vascular disease. In some high risk groups, such as black females, where the incidence of hypertension and cerebral complications has been extraordinarily high, the decline in mortality from cardiovascular causes is truly dramatic.

The following proposition is advanced: For the first time in history man has entered an era, beginning perhaps in the middle of the 1970s, when what the doctor does really makes a difference. Doctoring influences not only how a patient feels, but how long he lives. It will take another decade or two to prove (or fail to prove) this thesis. However, evidence is accumulating. Two examples from the field of infectious disease are pertinent. If the mortality from tuberculosis in New York City is closely examined, the curve shows a continual decline beginning in the early part of the twentieth century with two break points preceding significant decreases. One occurs in 1948 coincident with the introduction of streptomycin; the second in 1952 when isoniazid appeared. Similarly, data on the incidence of rheumatic fever show a decrease in 1945 when penicillin became available for civilian use.

In the United States, the age-adjusted mortality rates for coronary artery disease show a change in slope in 1967 when three interesting events occurred: the publication of a report by the Surgeon General of the United States on the dangers of smoking, the introduction of the first effective anti-hypertension agents, and the decision of the American Heart Association to emphasize the prudent dient and modification of risk factors. The influence of these apparently unrelated factors on mortality is speculative [1].

It can now be stated with reasonable certainty that modification of risk factors and specific forms of treatment in coronary artery disease favorably alter prognosis. Thus, cessation of smoking, treatment of hypertension (probably), maintenance of ideal body weight, vigorous exercise, and effective use of beta adrenergic blockers following myocardial infarction have been documented to have a favorable influence of prognosis in selected patient populations. It is likely that the effectiveness of coronary care, the widespread availability of resuscitation in the civilian population, and the influence of coronary artery bypass surgery in selected groups also contribute in a small way to the improved outlook.

Thus it is increasingly evident that a critical evaluation of the effect of coronary artery bypass surgery on longevity requires close analysis of the natural history of coronary artery disease in the current era. In this report, data will be presented from a variety of the studies which have been performed in the coronary artery surgery study (CASS) sponsored by the National Institutes of Health in the United States [2]. CASS consists of (1) a *registry* of clinical data, including survival, for all consecutive patients undergoing coronary arteriography for suspected coronary artery disease at 15 cooperating sites in the United States and Canada; and (2) a *randomized trial* of 780 patients with less than severe angina pectoris (Canadian Heart Association class II) or asymptomatic postmyocardial infarction assigned to medical or surgical therapy and followed for 5 years.

All patients entering the CASS underwent clinical evaluation followed by ventriculography and coronary arteriography. Data were recorded and analyzed according to a standard protocol and entered into the computer file at the coordinating center. The large number of patients followed closely for 5 years or more in the CASS registry represent a unique resource for study of the natural history and response to treatment of coronary artery disease in the current era. For example, CASS has recently reported 12 cases of total occlusion of the left main coronary artery, a decidedly uncommon occurrence [3].

Complications of coronary arteriography have been reported from the CASS experience by Davis et al. using data on 7553 consecutive patients undergoing diagnostic study in 13 cooperative clinics [4]. Mortality in the first 48 h after study was 2/1000 cases, and the rate of myocardial infarction 2.5/1000 cases. Left main disease increased the risk of death during coronary angiography by almost sevenfold. Other factors increasing risk included unstable angina, congestive heart failure, presence of multiple premature contractions, and hypertension. Since the clinics in

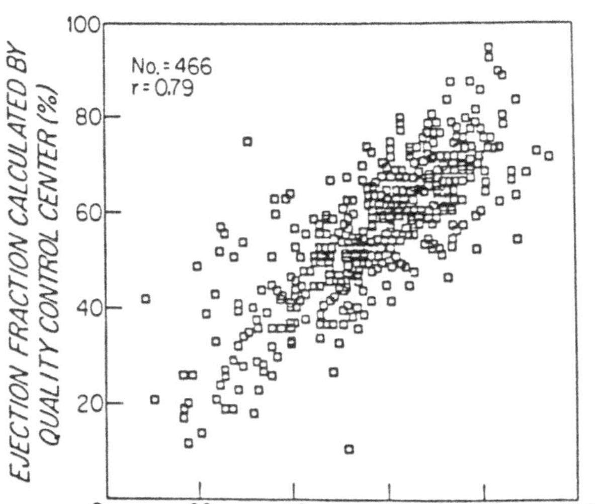

Fig. 1. Observer variability of angiographic interpretation in CASS. Calculation of ejection fraction (EF) from standard formula. *Ordinate:* EF calculated by quality control center. *Abscissia:* EF calculated by local site. Correlation coefficient is 0.79 but note wide range for many of the determinations. (Wexler et al. [5])

CASS are widespread nationally and vary in their clientele and practice, we believe this report of complications represents the current "state of the art" in North America.

While angiography provides objective evidence of the extent of coronary artery disease and the level of ventricular function, it is important for the physician to be aware of both technical problems and observer variability. In CASS an angiography committee met regularly to review quality of films and to agree on anatomical nomenclature. Technical discussions and development of optimal standards led to a dramatic improvement in quality of the films in the first 2 or 3 years of the study. This occurred despite the fact that many of the investigators were of national or international renown and had had long experience in the field.

Observer variation is a well-known problem contributing to diagnostic error in the analysis of the chest X-ray and the electrocardiogram. The same problem is an important variable contributing to difficulties of interpretation both for the coronary arteriogram and the left ventriculogram [15]. Although the correlation coefficients are respectable when local site interpretation is compared to that of a quality control group, the range of variation for important diagnostic determinants is troublesome (Fig. 1). While the angiogram is an "objective" anatomical depiction of cardiac circulation, the image on film is influenced by many physical factors and is ultimately interpreted by a fallible angiographer. The wise physician takes these factors into account when utilizing the angiographic interpretation in patient management.

An important question in the management of patients with coronary artery disease is the relationship between symptoms and extent of disease. This question was examined in several thousand patients with definite angina, probable angina, or nonspecific chest pain, as determined by the physician's analysis of the complaint [6]. Subjects with unstable angina or myocardial infarction were excluded from the study. The data revealed that age, sex, and character of chest pain were important determinants of the extent of disease found on angiography. Thus, coronary artery disease was present in patients with definite angina, probable angina, or nonspecific chest pain in 93%, 66%, and 14% respectively in men; and in 72%, 36%, and 6% respectively in women.

In men with nonspecific chest pain, the incidence of coronary artery disease rises sharply beyond age 65, suggesting that in this group the disease is probably asymptomatic but its extent and incidence are age-related. Left main coronary artery disease occurred in less than 2% of men with nonspecific chest pain and in less than 1% of women in the same category. These data lend weight to the ability of the physician to diagnose the presence of significant coronary disease on the presence of symptoms reflecting myocardial ischemia.

Operative mortality during coronary artery bypass grafting has steadily improved during the past decade. In a CASS study of more than 6500 patients, mortality for all operated patients was 2.9% with the following variations: elective operation 1.7%; urgent or emergency operation, 4.1%; age <60, 1.4%; age >60, 4.2%; men, 1.8%; women, 4.5% [7]. Discriminant analysis identified the following factors in order of importance as significantly contributing to operative mortality: age, presence of left main coronary artery disease with $\geqslant 90\%$ obstruction, sex, left ventricular wall motion score, left ventricular end-diastolic pressure, and presence of rales preoperatively [7, 8].

The reason that operative mortality for coronary bypass grafting in women is higher than in men is not clear. The data suggest but do not prove that an important factor may be size. Women, of course, tend to be smaller than men, and the coronary arteries are significantly smaller implying a greater technical problem in the performance of some of the anastomoses.

Another aspect of CASS was the ability to compare the operative results among various centers. Among the 15 cooperating clinical centers in the United States and Canada, all of whom had a large cumulative operative experience, CASS observed more than a twenty fold variation in mortality [7]. There was also a wide range of difference in severity of illness, which contributed importantly to the variation in operative mortality. The data show that the CASS centers performed bypass surgery at an acceptable level of risk.

The patients with left main disease represent a special subset. By definition, they have at least two-vessel disease and most have three vessels involved. The VA study found a significant improvement in mortality with bypass surgery in this group. The European Cooperative Study showed marked differences in survival, but the results were not significantly different, probably because of the small numbers and a consequent type II error.

Patients with left main disease were not randomized in CASS, but large numbers were followed in the registry [9]. In 1492 patients with left main disease (defined as $\geqslant 50\%$ luminal stenosis) for whom treatment was defined by the physician and patient choice, three-year cumulative survival was 91% in the surgical group and 69% for those treated medically. This was, of course, not a randomized study but represents the result of the clinical choices made in individual cases.

A statistical technique termed the Cox Proportional Hazards Model was utilized to analyze the importance of various clinical factors for subsequent mortality. Independent predictors of mortality so identified in patients with left main stenosis are, in order of selection: left ventricular score (an index of segmental wall motion abnormality), congestive heart failure, age, percent left main stenosis, presence of hypertension, and coronary circulation dominance.

Cause of death of patients with left main disease is of some interest (Table 1). The incidence of sudden death was sharply reduced in the surgical patients, whereas the percentage of noncardiac death, mostly due to malignancy, was higher than in the medical group.

In other studies investigators from CASS reviewed the operative risk factors in patients with left main disease [10]. Operative mortality was 4.2% overall. Noteworthy was the fact that 7 of the 15 participating centers had an operative mortality of

Table 1. Causes of death in patients with left main disease from the CASS registry: medical vs surgical treatment

Death	*Medical* (%)	*Surgical* (%)
Sudden	31	17
Other cardiac	66	65
Noncardiac	3	18

left main disease of <3%. Variables associated with an increased risk included age, being female, duration and severity of angina, urgency of operation, severity of disease, presence of left dominance, and degree of impairment of left ventricular function.

Analysis of the effects of surgical therapy compared to medical therapy on survival can best be obtained from a randomized trial. Two such trials have been reported to date: the U.S. Veterans Administration study and the European cooperative study in coronary artery bypass surgery. The CASS Randomized Trial will announce five-year follow-up results in the fall of 1983.

It remains useful, however, to evaluate the results of medical therapy from a large data bank such as the CASS registry. These observational results are important because surgical results are often reported in comparison to historical controls or patients not operated upon for a variety of reasons from the same institution.

Clinical reports suggest that the outlook for patients with angina pectoris under medical therapy had not changed, until recently, for many years. It appears that about 10 years ago the survival of medically treated patients with angina pectoris probably began to change significantly. A wide variety of factors have been at work, such as the recognition of the importance of risk factors and their treatment, treatment of hypertension, dietary manipulation, changes in eating and exercise habits of the middleclass population, introduction of beta blockers as prophylactic therapy, and many other as yet unknown factors.

Earlier reports of survival and angina pectoris were remarkably similar. Thus Richards et al. reported a 25-year follow-up of 250 patients with typical clinical angina in 1956 and documented an annual mortality of 4% [11]. Data from the Framingham study by Kannel et al. and by Frank et al. from a New York group practice in 1971 and 1973 showed exactly the same mortality, namely 4% per year [12, 13]. Frank, as others had before him, identified important risk factors which increased mortality, including presence of hypertension or an abnormal electrocardiogram.

During the past several years the data suggest a significant improvement in outcome from medical management in ischemic heart disease. Although there are important differences in patient selection, the annual medical mortality in the VA bypass study reported in 1978 was 4.2% [14]. Annual medical mortality in the European cooperative study reported in 1982 was 3.3% [15]. The data from CASS to be reported in the fall of this year are likely show even lower figures.

Figure 2 displays data from medically treated patients in the CASS registry [16]. As been observed by others, mortality is directly related to the number of vessels diseased. Note, however, that even in three-vessel disease, the CASS registry shows a mortality of less than 7% per year. It is important to note that in the patients studied in the registry, treatment, and especially the decision not to undergo surgical bypass, was a choice made by the physician and the patient. The reasons for a particular choice of treatment are not available. Severity of symptoms, exercise tolerance, operability, presence of other conditions, and the desires of the patient were certainly important factors.

CASS registry data emphasize the importance of left ventricular function in determining survival in patients with coronary artery disease. Data on ejection fraction are shown in Fig. 3. Similar curves could be drawn for an index of the degree of wall motion abnormality, the left ventricular score developed by CASS. It is clear

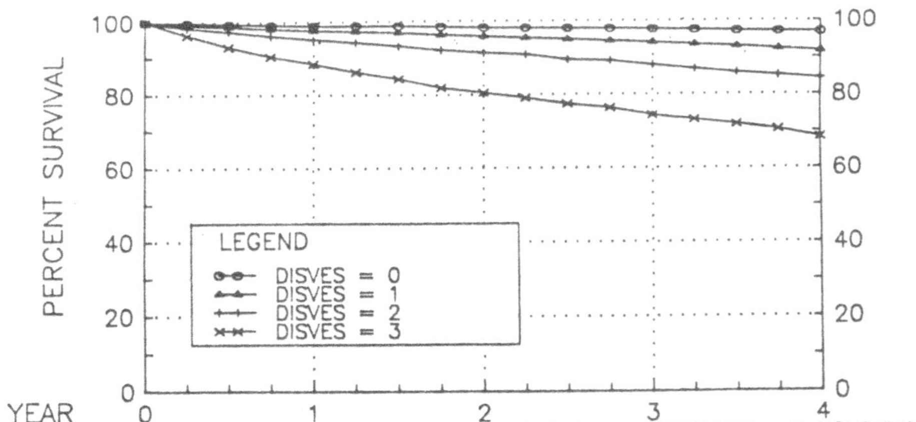

YEAR	0		1		2		3		4	
	N	%SURVIVAL	N	%SURVIVAL	N	%SURVIVAL	N	%SURVIVAL	N	%SURVIVAL
—o—	5804	100	5695	99	5429	98	4529	98	3081	97
—▲—	4138	100	2716	97	2521	96	2026	94	1301	92
—+—	4482	100	1943	95	1743	91	1370	88	850	84
—×—	5629	100	1576	88	1301	80	1004	74	614	68

P < .0001

Fig. 2. Survival of patients with coronary artery disease in CASS registry treated medically by physician and patient choice, by number of diseased vessels *(DISVES)*. Control population *(0 DISVES)* are CASS patients without significant coronary artery disease at angiography. Note excellent survival with medical therapy. Survival is directly related to extent of disease. Number of patients and percent survival are listed below for zero-, one-, two-, and three-vessel disease. (Mock et al. [16])

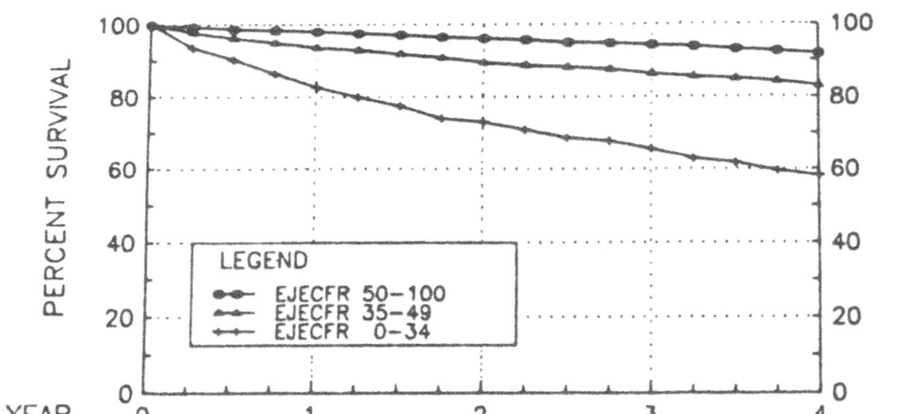

YEAR	0		1		2		3		4	
	N	%SURVIVAL	N	%SURVIVAL	N	%SURVIVAL	N	%SURVIVAL	N	%SURVIVAL
—●—	6791	100	3081	98	2802	96	2232	94	1403	92
—▲—	1977	100	988	94	893	89	702	86	416	83
—+—	909	100	513	83	410	73	318	66	183	58

P < .0001

Fig. 3. Survival of patients with coronary artery disease in CASS registry treated medically by physician and patient choice, by ejection fraction *(EJECFR)*. Survival is directly related to degree of preservation of ventricular function, as measured by ejection fraction. Number of patients and percent survival for each category of ejection fraction are listed below. (Mock et al. [16])

that left ventricular function has an important influence on survival, especially in patients with more advanced coronary artery disease.

The data from CASS show that medical survival in nonrandomized patients with anatomically proven coronary artery disease is considerably better than has been reported earlier by others [16, 17]. It is my opinion, one that cannot be proved at the present time, that current medical management has a significant and favorable impact on survival in coronary artery disease. There are many other factors that are also operative, of course. The relatively good outlook for many of the medically treated patients with established coronary artery disease, especially those with good left ventricular function, must be taken into account in evaluating uncontrolled reports of new forms of therapy, including surgical management.

We now return to the thesis stated earlier. A wide variety of factors influence the natural history of disease. As with so many other conditions, the prognosis of coronary artery disease is changing. The prognosis has improved, due in some part, but not exclusively, to medical management. The changing outlook is a factor which must be considered in evaluating the effectiveness of bypass grafting and makes the use of historical controls fraught with difficulty.

References

1. Havlik RJ, Feinleib M (eds) (1979) Proceedings of the conference on the decline in coronary heart disease mortality. National Heart, Lung and Blood Institute. Public Health Service, National Institutes of Health, Publication No 79-1610
2. Principal Investigators of CASS and their Associates, Killip T (ed) Fisher LD, Mock MB (associate eds) (1981) National heart , lung and blood institute, coronary artery surgery study (CASS). Circulation 63 (Suppl 2): 1-81
3. Zimmern SH, Rogers WJ, Bream PR et al. (1982) Total occlusion of the left main coronary artery: the coronary artery surgery study (CASS) experience. Am J Cardiol 49: 2003-2010
4. Davis K, Kennedy JW, Kemp H, Judkins MP, Gosselin AJ, Killip T (1979) Complications of coronary arteriography from the collaborative study of coronary artery surgery (CASS). Circulation 59: 1105-1112
5. Wexler LF, Lesperance J, Ryan TJ et al. (1982) Interobserver variability in interpreting contrast left ventriculograms (CASS). Cathet Cardiovasc Diagn 8: 341-355
6. Vliestra RE, Kronmal RA, Frye RL et al. (1982) Factors affecting the extent and severity of coronary artery disease in patients enrolled in the coronary artery surgery study. Arteriosclerosis 2 (3): 208-215
7. Kennedy JW, Kaiser GC, Fisher LD et al. (1980) Multivariate discriminant analysis of the clinical and angiographic predictors of operative mortality from the collaborative study in coronary artery surgery (CASS). J Thorac Cardiovasc Surg 80 (6): 876-877
8. Kennedy JW, Kaiser GC, Fisher LD et al. (1981) Clinical and angiographic predictors of operative mortality from the collaborative study in coronary artery surgery (CASS). Circulation 63 (4): 793-802
9. Chaitman BR, Fisher LD, Bourassa MG et al. (1981) Effect of coronary bypass surgery on survival patterns in subsets of patients with left main coronary artery disease. Am J Cardiol 48: 765-777
10. Chaitman BR, Rogers WJ, Davis K et al. (1980) Operative risk factors in patients with left main coronary artery disease. N Engl J Med 303: 953-957
11. Richards DW, Bland EF, White PD (1956) A completed 25-year follow-up study of 456 patients with angina pectoris. J Chron Dis 4: 423-433
12. Kannel WB, Feinleib M (1972) Natural history of angina pectoris in the Framingham study: prognosis and survival. Am J Cardiol 29: 154-163

13. Frank CW, Weinblatt E, Shapiro S (1973) Angina pectoris in men. Circulation 47: 507–509
14. Read RC, Murphy ML, Hultgren HN, Takaro T (1978) Survival of men treated for chronic stable angina pectoris. J Thorac Cardiovasc Surg 75: 1
15. European Coronary Surgery Study Group (1982) Long-term results of prospective randomized study of coronary artery bypass surgery in stable angina pectoris. Lancet 2: 1173
16. Mock MB, Ringqvist I, Fisher LD et al. (1982) Survival of medically treated patients in the coronary artery surgery study (CASS) registry. Circulation 66: 562
17. Gersh BJ, Kronmal RA, Frye RL et al. (1983) Coronary arteriography and coronary artery bypass surgery. Morbidity and mortality in patients 65 years or older. Circulation 67: 484

Anatomical and Tactical Considerations for Peripheral Revascularization in Patients with Diffuse Triple-Vessel Disease

M. Schmuziger, E. Eschenbruch, and P. Stürzenhofecker, M. D.

Long-term follow-up of coronary bypass patients demonstrates better subjective and objective improvement in work parameters and better prognosis for completely revascularized patients compared to those who have had incomplete revascularization (because of bypass graft closure or where incomplete revascularization was done originally) [1, 2].

In proximal localized stenoses of the three major coronary arteries, complete revascularization can usually be accomplished with three or four single grafts.

When all three coronary arteries are diffusely diseased with proximal and distal stenoses, either complete revascularization must be abandoned or the number of peripheral anastomoses increased. With the single-graft technique, a large number of peripheral anastomoses is associated with diminished flow in individual grafts, which means a higher risk of graft occlusion [3].

Endarterectomy is a possible alternative to multiple grafts for complete revascularization of diffusely diseased vessels. Unfortunately, coronary angiography in over 150 patients in our clinic demonstrated very good results in only slightly more than one-third of all endarterectomies. Our experience is that an open bypass graft does not necessarily imply a good result [4, 5, 6].

The introduction by Bigelow [7] of the sequential graft technique during the early 1970s provided a possible solution to the problem. This technique appears to have many advantages:

- It is possible to supply more coronary vessels using less vein material.
- Through multiple peripheral anastomoses the flow-through and long-term patencyrate of single-vein grafts can be increased. (Although it has been argued that there is increased risk of closure of the low-flow distal tip of a sequential graft, this is not necessarily the case).
- Side-to-side anastomoses can often be placed on only moderately diseased coronary artery segments, with concomitant improvement in long-term results.
- Because only two or three proximal anastomoses must be performed, large myocardial areas can be quickly and completely revascularized.
- A peripherally anastomosed sequential graft functions during surgery as a "large

Table 1. Patency rates for single and sequential grafts

	Patency rate (%)
Single grafts	82.2
Jump grafts (two anast.)	85.7
Sequential grafts (three to five anast.)	96.3

n, 161 patients with 381 sequential and 248 single anastomoses

Table 2. Patency rates for different graft positions

Flow capacity end-to-side	Patency rate (%)
< side-to-side	68.0
≅ side-to-side	84.0
> side-to-side	90.3

n, 161 patients with 381 sequential and 248 single anastomoses

collateral," and also delivers cardioplegia solution in a homogeneous distribution.

We retrospectively examined follow-up angiograms of 161 patients who had been operated between 1978 and 1980, in whom both single grafts and sequential grafts with two, three, or more anastomoses had been performed. In this series the patency-rate was better for sequential grafts than for single-vein grafts (Table 1).

The data also confirmed our hypothesis that the best results are obtained if the artery with the largest flow capacity is placed in the most distal position (Table 2).

Considering the great variability of coronary artery anatomy, the best graft pathway had to be found.

Anatomically, coronary arteries with branches to the septum have a higher flow capacity than vessels which only supply the left ventricular free wall. Although the left anterior descending (LAD) and posterior descending arteries usually provide the mayor septal blood supply, important septal branches may arise from the acute marginal branch of the right coronary artery or posterolateral branches of the left circumflex artery.

There are, therefore, two vessel regions with high flow capacities as potential distal anastomotic sites for sequential grafts: (1) the anterior wall septal vessel, and (2) the posterior wall septal vessel.

From either of these high-flow capacity vessels, the anterolateral, lateral, and posterolateral supply areas must be sequentially joined with side-to-side anastomoses.

Our experience has been that the optimal graft pathway usually begins with a posterior wall end-to-side anastomosis to the middle one-third of the posterior descending artery, then side-to-side anastomoses to the posterolateral branches of the right and left circumflex arteries parallel to the atrioventricular sulcus in the transverse sinus, with proximal anastomoses to the right convex side of the aorta (Fig. 1).

Anterior wall revascularization begins with distal anastomoses to the LAD, then side-to-side anastomosis to one or more anterolateral branches or occasionally even a marginal circumflex branch. Although this bypass can also be led through the transverse sinus, there is the disadvantage that the length determination for the proximal portion can be difficult (Fig. 2).

The advantages of the transverse sinus pathway are substantial:

- Grafts led through the sinus have a nearly straight path, thus graft stability is increased.
- If reoperation is required, the anterior aorta remains free for graft implantation.
- The often heavily postoperatively scarred anterior mediastinum is avoided and closure of the pericardium can be done without danger of graft compression.

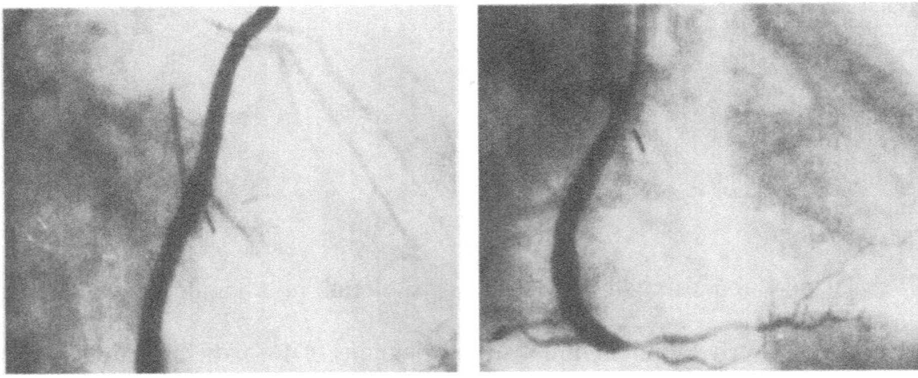

Fig. 1. Optimal graft pathway through the transverse sinus

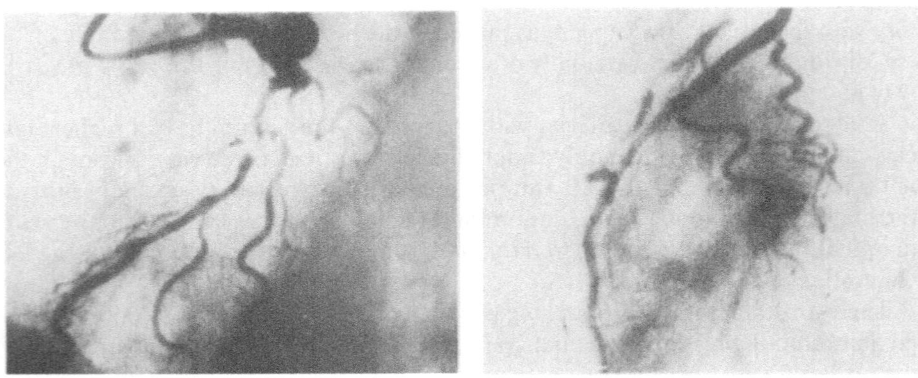

Fig. 2. Anterior wall revascularization

The transverse sinus approach can almost never be used during reoperation because of scarred tissue in this area. Although difficult bleeding problems may result from the transverse sinus route, routine use of the procedure allows one to deal rapidly with this.

Other graft pathways may be used if anatomical variations require. If there is a shortage of vein material, it is possible to revascularize the entire heart with one "snakegraft."

We believe it is technically important that all side-to-side anastomoses should be made in a "diamond-shape" manner and that whenever possible grafts be led over areas of minimal cardiac movement.

Follow-up coronary angiography has not been routinely performed at our rehabilitation center since July 1982. Therefore our follow-up of the sequential bypass technique is limited to 156 patients who had routine restudy between October 1980 and July 1982. These patients had diffuse three-vessel disease and more than five peripheral anastomoses. Follow-up angiography was performed 8 weeks postoperatively.

Table 3. Follow-up of sequential bypass technique by means of postoperative angiographic control in 156 of the 237 patients with five or more peripheral anastomoses

	All anastomoses $n = 906$	Sequential anastomoses $n = 863$
Patency rate (%)	85.43	86.00
Mean no. of anast./pt.	5.81	5.53
Mean patent anast./pt.	4.96	4.76

There were a mean 5.53 sequential anastomoses per patient. Patency rate was 86%, therefore, there were 4.7 patent anastomoses per patient. Two-thirds of these patients had all peripheral anastomoses open and could be considered totally revascularized (Table 3).

Thus multiple peripheral revascularization with sequential grafts appears to be worthwhile.

References

1. Gohlke H, Gohlke-Bärwolf C, Samek L, Stürzenhofecker P, Schmuziger M, Roskamm H (1983) Serial exercise testing up to 6 years after coronary bypass surgery: behaviour of experience parameters in groups with different degrees of revascularization determined by postoperative angiography. Am J Cardiol 51: 1301–1306
2. Roskamm H, Schmuziger M, Stürzenhofecker P, Petersen J, Görnandt L, Reichelt M, Huesmann A, Betz P, Spinder M, Heidecker K, Weisswange A, Gohlke-Bärwolf C, Gohlke H, Samek L, Schnellbacher K, Bubenheimer P (1981) Bestimmt die Vollständigkeit der Revaskularisation die funktionelle Verbesserung und die Überlebensdaten koronaroperierter Patienten? Ergebnisse von 1000 konsekutiv operierten Patienten. Z Kardiol 70: 590–599
3. Roth JA, Cukingnan RA, Brown BG, Gocka E, Carey JS (1979) Factors influencing patency of saphenous vein grafts. Ann Thorac Surg 28 (2): 176–183
4. Eschenbruch EM, Görnandt L, Tollenaere P, Schmuziger M (1982) Klinische und angiographische Befunde nach instrumenteller Endarteriektomie der Arteria coronaria dextra. Presented at the 11th Jahrestagung der Deutschen Gesellschaft für Thorax-, Herz- und Gefäßchirurgie, 18–20 February 1982, Bad Nauheim
5. Schmuziger M, Hahn C, Görnandt L, Kröner U, Eschenbruch EM (1981). Instrumental endarterectomy of the right and left coronary artery and its angiographic results. Presented at the 15th world congress of the International Cardiovascular Society, 6–10 September 1981, Athen
6. Eschenbruch EM, Schmuziger M, Tollenaere P, Görnandt L, Hahn C (1980) Endarterectomy of the left coronary artery (LCA) as a supplementary surgical means of myocardial revascularization with aortocoronary vein bypass procedure. Thorac Cardiovasc Surg 28 (4): 280–284
7. Bartley TD, Bigelow JC, Scott Page U (1972) Aortocoronary bypass grafting with multiple sequential anastomoses to a single vein. Arch Surg 105: 915–917

Myocardial Revascularization for Early Postinfarction Angina

T. Bianchi, G. Invernizzi, and F. Burgarella

In spite of earlier controversies [3, 7] aortocoronary bypass (ACBP) procedures have recently been performed with good operative and late results [1, 8] for treatment of acute myocardial infarction (AMI) and its early ischemic and nonischemic complications. Early postinfarction angina (EPIA) seems an important incremental risk factor for recurrent AMI and late mortality [10], and surgical treatment of patients whose symptoms do not respond to medical treatment has been advocated [6]. On the other hand ACBP seems to be of little benefit for coronary patients who do not actually experience angina [4]. The question arises as to whether those patients with EPIA completely relieved by full medical treatment should or should not undergo ACBP. Comparison of late results of a medical and a surgical group should help in answering this question.

Methods

In a series of patients undergoing a standard rehabilitation program after AMI between October 1977 and March 1982, the occurrence of EPIA was checked by clinical examination, spiroergometric, and dynamic ECG tests. Patients without angina with ECG patterns indicating ischemia were excluded from this study. All patients with EPIA initially received full medical treatment for at least 2 months. If symptoms could be controlled, the patients were dismissed from the center and followed up 6 months from the first occurrence of EPIA. Patients with persistent unrelieved symptoms underwent coronary arteriography and, when indicated, ACBP. They were rehabilitated, and also followed up 6 months after the onset of EPIA. Both medical and surgical groups of patients were thereafter followed for a mean time of 26.2 ± 15.7 months. Clinical evaluation of all survivors was made in May 1983. Symptomatic patients also repeated ergometric and dynamic ECG tests. Statistical analysis of the results includes calculation of mean plus or minus standard deviation, 70% confidence limits of proportions, and Yates-corrected chi-square tests (significant level $\leqslant 0.05$).

Results

Among 476 rehabilitated patients, 110 (23.1%) cases of EPIA were observed, the symptoms arising from 11 to 60 (mean 27.8 ± 12.5) days after AMI. Their ages ranged from 32.1 to 74.2 (mean 57.6 ± 10) years. The absolute prevalence for sex, age, and type of angina is summarized in Table 1. The outcome of the whole series is presented in Table 2. Eleven patients (10%) whose angina was initially controlled by medical therapy died within 6 months: four sudden deaths, six progressive left ventricular (LV) failures and one recurrent AMI. Twenty asymptomatic survivors were

Table 1. Early postinfarction angina: absolute prevalence for sex, age, and type of angina

Angina type	< 50 years			> 50 years			Total		
	M	F	T	M	F	T	M	F	T
R	18	2	20	30	12	42	48	14	62
E	13	0	13	28	7	35	41	7	48
T	31	2	33	58	19	77	89	21	110

Mean interval from infarction, 27.8 ± 1.5 days; Mean age of patients, 57.5 ± 10 years; R, Angina at rest or mixed; E, Angina on effort; T, total; M, males; F, females

Table 2. Results of treatment

Infarct	EPIA	First 6 months	Patients in follow-up	Results
476	110	– 11 deaths – 4 sudden deaths (VF) – 6 left ventricular failures – 1 recurrent AMI		
		– 20 MT (lost to follow-up)		
		– 33 MT	41 MT	4 deaths: 3 sudden deaths 1 recurrent AMI 5 angina at rest 15 angina on effort* 3 left ventricular failure 11 asymptomatic
		(8 no indication for surgery)		
		– 46 coronary arteriography	38 ACBP	1 death (intraop. AMI) 1 angina on effort 36 asymptomatic

MT, Medical treatment; VF, ventricular fibrillation; *, 3 crossover to surgery

lost to follow-up. Thirty-three patients with controlled angina entered the medical follow-up group. Forty-six patients with uncontrolled angina underwent coronary arteriography 2.1 to 3.9 (mean 3.1 ± 0.5) months after the onset of EPIA. In eight cases surgical intervention was denied because of excessive (five cases) or insufficient (three cases) coronary pathology. They were returned to the medical group. Forty-one patients (37.3% of all EPIA), aged from 32.1 to 74.2 (mean 59.1 ± 11.2) years, therefore comprised the medical group. In four of them (9.5%) death was either sudden or from recurrent AMI. Three patients (7.3%) developed recurrent anginal pain so severe as to indicate surgery. They are not included in the surgical group. Three patients in the medical group (7.3%) had recurrent AMI, 20 (48.8%) developed recurrent angina (15 on effort and 5 at rest), and 3 (7.3%) episodic LV failure. Only 11 patients (26.8%) are asymptomatic.

Thirty-eight patients (34.5% of all those with EPIA) underwent ACBP 2.3 to 5.6 (mean 4.5 ± 1) months after the onset of EPIA, and form the surgical group. Their

Table 3. Composition of medical and surgical groups

Group	Age		Sex		Infarction		Angina	
	<50 Y	>50 Y	M	F	ant	inf	R	E
Medical (%)	24.2	40.3	32.6	57.1	30.9	43.6	27.2	38.7
Surgical (%)	45.4	28.6	35.9	23.8	36.4	30.9	38.7	29.2
P value[a]	0.07	0.12	0.63	0.03	0.55	0.16	0.18	0.05

%, percentage of total EPIA observed in the same subgroup; Y, years; M, males; F, females; R, angina at rest or mixed; E, angina on effort; Ant, anterior; Inf, inferior
[a]Calculated by the corrected chi-square method of Yates

Table 4. Results of follow-up in medical and surgical groups

Group		Deaths	Asympt.	Angina			LV failure	Rec. AMI
				R	E	T		
Medical	*N*	4	11	5	15	20*	3	3
(41 patients)	%	9.8	26.8	12.2	36.6	48.8	7.3	7.3
Surgical	*N*	1$	36	0	1	1	0	0
(38 patients)	%	2.6	94.7	0	2.6	2.6	0	0
P Value[a]		0.18	0	0.08	0.02	0.00001	0	0.08

[a]Calculated by the corrected chi-square method of Yates; *N* number of observed cases; *, 3 crossover to surgery; %, percentage; R, angina at rest or mixed; E, angina on effort; T, total; LV, left ventricular; $, intraoperative AMI; Rec. AMI, recurrent AMI

ages ranged from 34 to 74.1 (mean 54±8) years. One patient (2.6%) died from intraoperative AMI, and one had residual angina on effort. Thirty-six patients (94.8%) are asymptomatic. No late death, AMI, or LV failure was observed. Statistical analysis of the composition of the two groups of patients shows only a significant majority of females and patients with angina on effort in the medical group (Table 3). Analysis of the results at the end of follow-up shows a significantly higher percentage of angina, LV failure, and recurrent AMI in the medical group (Table 4).

Discussion

EPIA is usually defined as angina arising within 7 [6] to 30 [3] days from AMI. Our limit of 60 days covers the whole rehabilitation period, but 70% of our patients had symptoms within 30 days. In order to simplify the follow-up a restricted definition of EPIA was adopted, excluding patients with ischemic ECG patterns even though those patterns are also reported to be incremental risk factors for late mortality [10]. In order to standardize the onset of follow-up, we also excluded from the study patients who died within 6 months. The statistical analysis of our results is not perfect because the study is retrospective and the two series were not randomized or matched [5]. On the other hand, when dealing with critically evolving clinical situations it is difficult to create matched cohorts [2]. In our view, one advantage of this study is the fact that all consecutive patients were treated by the same surgical and rehabilitation centers, and the diagnosis was ascertained by both strict clinical examination and ECG tests. The five patients not controlled by medical therapy and not operated upon because of extensive coronary disease represent only 12.2% of the whole medical group. This is mostly composed of patients with controlled angina, and can therefore be assumed to form a "lower risk" subset. The surgical group, all composed of patients with intractable angina, represents a "higher risk" subset. The early and late surgical results were good in patients with intractable EPIA. In contrast, the results of medical treatment after initial control of angina were very poor. In our view, the probability is very high that early surgical treatment of "temporarily" asymptomatic EPIA patients improves the late prognosis. Conventionally the major indication for ACBP surgery has always been intractable anginal pain. Some cardiologists however advise surgery even for the asymptomatic patient with a "jeopardized" myocardium [9]. In our view the bad late results of the medical group support the hypothesis that, in spite of the initial improvement, such patients still have jeopardized myocardium and need an operation. We therefore now propose early coronary arteriography and surgery for all our patients with EPIA, regardless of their initial response to medical treatment.

References

1. Berg R, Selinger SL, Leonard JJ, Grunwald RP, O'Grady WP (1981) Immediate coronary artery bypass for acute evolving myocardial infarction (AEMI). J Thorac Cardiovasc Surg 81: 493–497
2. Daily PO (1983) Discussion on the paper of Nunley. J Thorac Cardiovasc Surg 85: 490
3. Favaloro RG (1975) Surgical treatment of acute coronary insufficiency. In: Second Henry Ford hospital international symposium on cardiac surgery. Appleton Century Crofts, New York, pp 571
4. Grondin CM, Kretz JG, Vouhe P, Tubau JF, Campeau L, Bourassa MG (1979) Prophylactic coronary artery grafting in patients with few or no symptoms. Ann Thorac Surg 18: 113–117
5. Killip T (1979) Changing medical and surgical therapy in coronary artery disease – need for prospective studies. In: Roskamm H, Schmutziger M (eds) Coronary heart surgery: a rehabilitation measure. Springer, Berlin Heidelberg New York, pp 2–9
6. Jones EL, Waites TF, Craver GM, Bradford JM, Douglas JS, King SB, Bone DK, Dorney ER, Clements SD, Thompkins T, Hatcher CR (1981) Coronary bypass for relief of persistent pain following acute myocardial infarction. Ann Thorac Surg 32: 33–43
7. McNamara J, Lacro R, Yee M, Smith G (1981) Hemorrhagic infarction in coronary reperfusion. J Thorac Cardiovasc Surg 81: 498–501
8. Nunley DL, Grunkemeier GL, Teply JF, Abbruzzese PA, Davis JS, Khonsari S, Starr A (1983) Coronary bypass operation following acute complicated myocardial infarction. J Thorac Cardiovasc Surg 85: 485–491
9. Sheldon WC (1982) Panel discussion. In: Bruschke AVG, Van Herpen G, Vermeulen FEE (eds) Coronary artery disease today. Excerpta Medica, Amsterdam, pp 427–439
10. Starling MR, Crawford MH, Kennedy GT, O'Rourke RA (1980) Exercise testing early after myocardial infarction: predictive value for subsequent unstable angina and death. Am J Cardiol 46: 909–914

Single Lesion of Proximal LAD in Young Patients: Medical Therapy, SVG, IMA Graft, PTCA?

N. Spampinato, F. Di Lello, M. Chello, D. Iorio, A. R. Marchese, and L. B. Tecchia

Introduction

Optimal therapy for proximal severe narrowing of the left anterior descending coronary artery (LAD) in young people has been for the last decade a matter of debate.

In the past years, for various reasons (medical and sometimes nonmedical – read: economical), single lesions of a coronary artery have been considered not worthy of surgical treatment and were relegated to medical treatment [1, 2, 3].

We have reviewed our experience on single LAD lesions in young patients to point out what the prognosis is for this type of patient in relation to the chosen therapy, considering that atherosclerotic disease is inevitably progressive and chronic, especially in young people.

Materials and Methods

We selected a group of 77 patients with severe angina, aged 28–45, who showed at coronary angiography a severe (90%–99%) stenosis of the proximal LAD. The follow-up covered from 1975 to 1982.

Twenty-two patients received full medical treatment (nitrates, Ca^{++}antagonists, beta-blockers, antiplatelet drugs etc.). Medical treatment for these patients was chosen mainly as a matter of personal decision on the part of the patient and in some cases of the referring cardiologist, following the trend of nonsurgical treatment of single-vessel coronary disease.

Thirty-four patients underwent saphenous vein graft coronary bypass (SVG); 11 had an internal mammary artery anastomosis (IMA graft), and, more recently, 10 underwent percutaneous transluminal coronary angioplasty (PTCA). All patients were operated on using standard techniques under cold potassium cardioplegia.

Distal saphenous vein graft anastomosis was performed with a running 7–0 polypropylene suture, while a running 6–0 polypropylene suture was used for the proximal anastomosis.

The IMA grafts were performed with the "pedicle" prepared using the Favaloro-Sewell technique. The distal anastomosis was made with 8–0 interrupted silk sutures. In one case in which the flow from the internal mammary artery did not seem satisfactory, the artery was transected at the origin and used as a free graft in aorto-coronary position. Proximal anastomosis in this case was performed with a running 7–0 polypropylene suture.

PTCA was usually performed during the first coronary angiography after consultation with the surgical team. Only in two cases, studied in other institutions, was PTCA performed during a second coronary angiography.

Results

Group A: Medical Treatment

Two patients (9%) died from acute myocardial infarction within 6–12 months. Four patients (18%) suffered acute myocardial infarctions, survived and later developed a left ventricular aneurysm: they are candidates for a left ventricular aneurysmectomy.

Five patients had persistent angina in spite of full medical therapy and made a crossover to surgery. Eleven patients are alive and well, but with activity restrictions not compatible with their age.

Group B: SVG

Operative mortality was zero. Complete follow-up has been obtained for up to 7 years (Fig. 1).

All patients are in NYHA, functional class I, except one who developed angina after about 7 years. Coronary angiography showed closure of the graft and progression of the disease to RCA and Cx (circumflex artery); the patient is scheduled for reoperation.

Group C: IMA Graft

Operative mortality was zero.

All patients are in excellent condition except one who developed angina 6 years after surgery. A repeat coronary angiography showed a beautiful patent IMA-LAD graft (Fig. 2) and a new 90% stenosis of a large obtuse marginal branch of the circumflex coronary artery (Fig. 3). The patient is now under medical treatment but his symptoms are not completely controlled. A reoperation is planned. We foresee technical problems for the second sternotomy because there is a risk of injuring the IMA graft during the operative dissection; a left thoracotomy might be a more suitable approach.

Group D: PTCA

All patients tolerated the procedure well without any problems whatsoever, and with complete immediate resolution of their symptoms (Fig. 4).

Follow-up, however, covers only 12 months, including some cases performed during the last year.

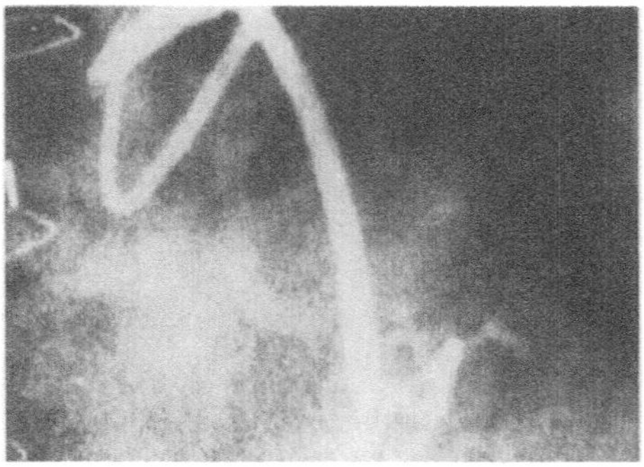

Fig. 1. Postoperative control of SVG to LAD. In spite of a good function, discrepancy of calibers between saphenous vein and coronary artery is evident

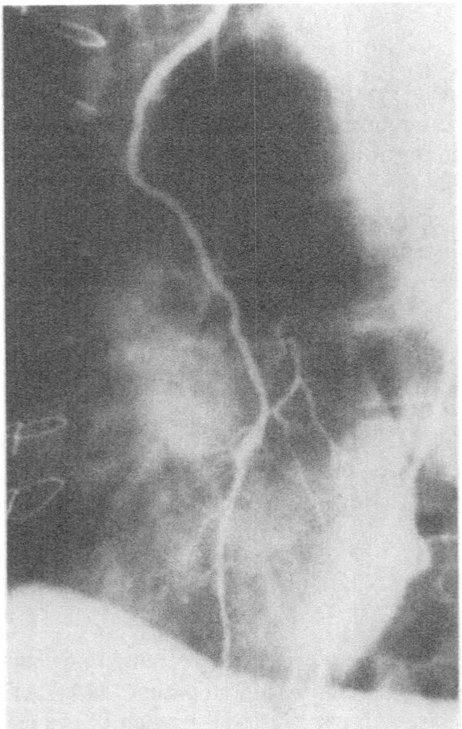

Fig. 2. Patent IMA to LAD graft – note the perfect matching of vessel calibers

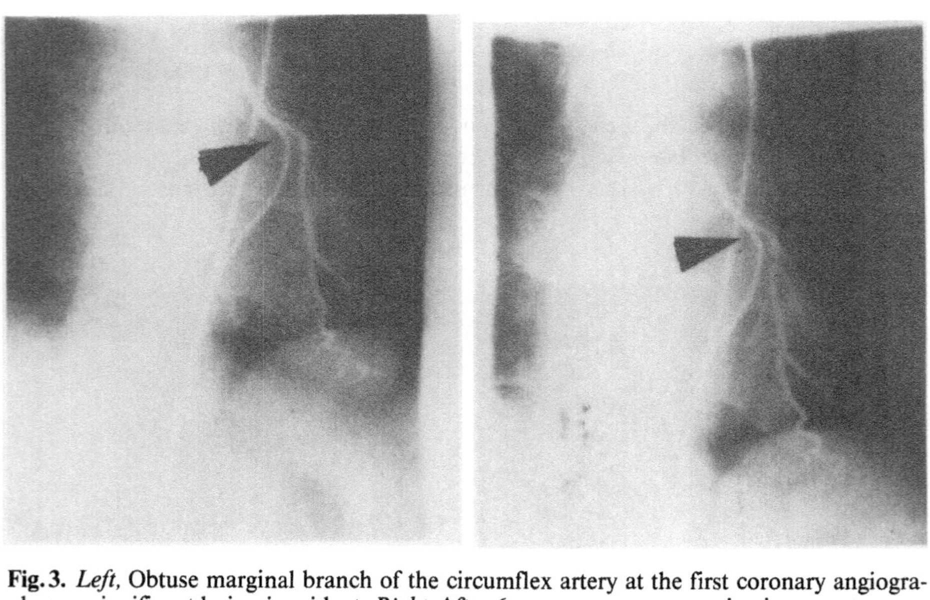

Fig. 3. *Left,* Obtuse marginal branch of the circumflex artery at the first coronary angiography: no significant lesion is evident. *Right,* After 6 years a severe narrowing is present

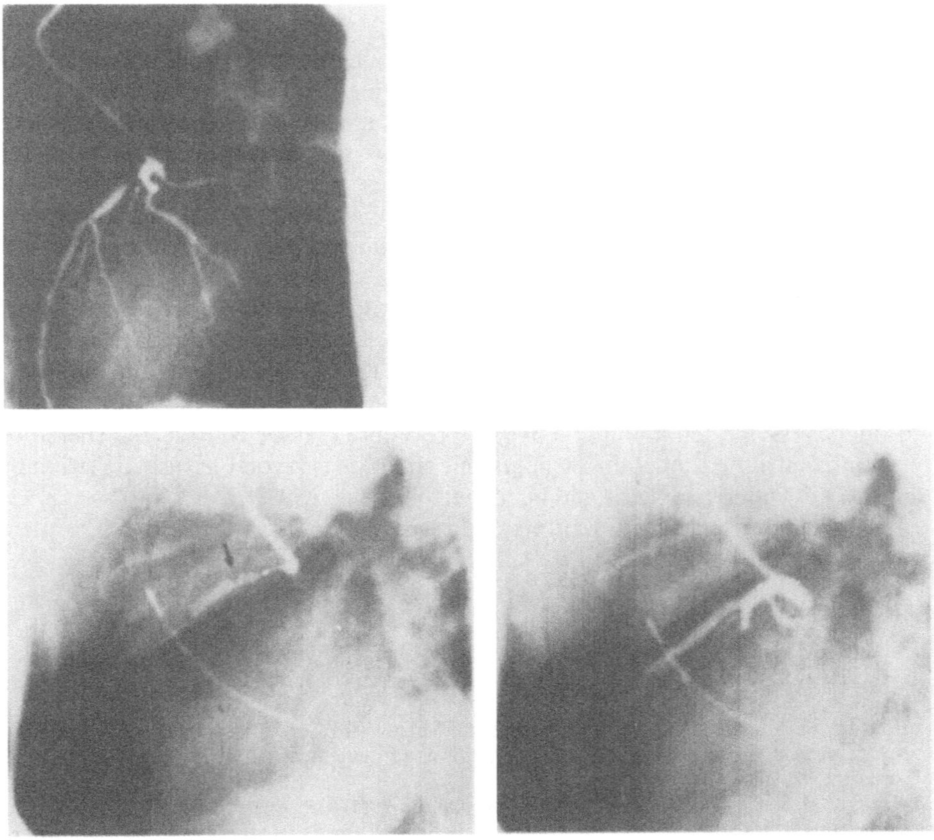

Fig. 4 a. Severe narrowing of proximal LAD; **b** the inflated ballon with the intention at the level of the plaque; **c** complete PTCA: the stenosis appears completely relieved

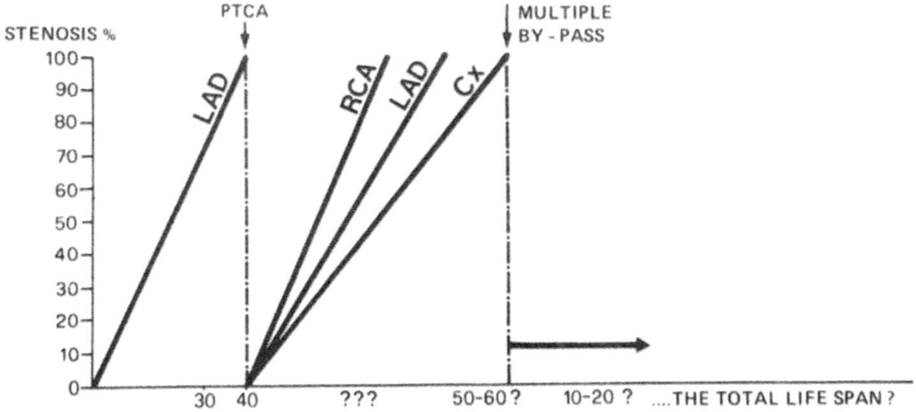

Fig. 5. Influence of PTCA or surgery on the patient's life span. So far PTCA seems to be a valuable alternative therapy, bringing the progression of the disease "back to zero"

Comments

Severe single lesions of the proximal LAD in young people should not be treated medically. The incidence of lethal or incapacitating myocardial infarction is unacceptable. SVG is a good alternative with no risk and satisfactory follow-up. However occlusion of the graft and progression of the disease in other coronary branches may occur.

IMA grafts give the best resultats: they almost never fail. In these patients, as for the SVG patients, progression of the disease in other coronary branches appears inevitable. Recently PTCA has been shown to be a very valuable procedure in these cases [4]. If the patient selection is accurate, results are consistently excellent and complications nonexistent. The advantage of this invasive but nonsurgical procedure is that it brings the disease "back to zero" (Fig. 5) for a certain time (months? years?). When the inevitable progression of the disease involves most of the major coronary vessels, then a multiple bypass procedure may be considered. Therefore we think that at present, if the angiographic situation is favorable, a single lesion of the LAD in young people should be treated electively with PTCA.

As an alternative an IMA graft may be advisable.

References

1. Califf RM, Tomabechi Y, Phillips HR, Lee KL, Behar VS, Peter RH, Kong Y, Pryor DB, Harrel FE Jr, Rosati RA (1982) Survival in single vessel coronary disease. Am J Cardiol 49: 1008
2. Phillips P, Borer JS, Goldstein J, Jacobstein J, Moses J, Fisher J (1982) Proximal left anterior descending coronary stenosis: the functional equivalent of triple vessel disease? Am J Cardiol 49: 957
3. Gohlke H, Samek L, Stürzenhofecker P, Roskamm H (1982) Does the degree of a proximal left anterior descending (LAD) stenosis influence prognosis in young patients after transmural anterior myocardial infarction (TAMI)? Am J Cardiol 49: 1019
4. Kent KM, Bentivoglio LG, Block PC, Cowley MJ, Dorros G, Gosselin AJ, Grüntzig A, Myler RK, Simpson J, Stertzer SH, Williams DO, Bourassa MG, Kelsey SF, Detre KM, Mullin S, Passamani E (1982) NHLBI percutaneous transluminal coronary angioplasty (PTCA) registry: four years experience. Am J Cardiol 49: 904

Reoperation for Coronary Artery Disease

W. J. Keon

Introduction

The progressive nature of coronary atherosclerosis together with the increasing number of primary operative procedures for coronary artery disease ultimately increases the number of patients who are candidates for reoperation. Therefore the rate of reoperation for coronary artery disease is on the rise. Irarrazaval et al. [1] report less than 1% of their caseload being reoperations in 1974 versus 3% in 1979, Loop [2] went from 3% in 1969 to 4.5% in 1979, and Schaff [3] reported a 6.2% reoperation rate in 1980. Angina has been reported to recur in patients postoperatively at rates of 3.5% to 7.2% per year [2–5]. Recurrent symptoms can be attributed to narrowing or occlusion of the vein graft, progression of disease in native arteries, diseased but unbypassed arteries at the time of initial operation, or a combination of these factors. During the early years of coronary artery bypass grafting (CABG) the incidence of graft patency was 65%–75% [6]. With further development of the technique and experience the patency rates are now 80%–85% at one year, with an annual attrition rate of 2% [7].

The original stenosis in a grafted artery may progress to complete occlusion distal to the graft site [8]. McLaughlin [9] reported, in a series of 100 patients undergoing postoperative angiograms 1–4 years after coronary revascularization, a 55% incidence of progression of lesions proximal to the graft insertion and 7% distal to the graft. In addition, disease progressed in 14% of vessels not grafted. Many of the patients with this type of disease and recurring chest pain are candidates for repeat coronary revascularization.

Although reoperation is technically more difficult, there have been reports showing a definite improvement in symptoms and acceptable mortality and morbidity. Consequently a number of indications for repeat surgery are now recognized. A summary of several recent publications is given in Table 1. The mean male/female ratio is nine: one, the mean age at reoperation is the early 50s and the time between operations ranges from 13 to 51 months. Most reoperations are performed 5 years postoperatively and the interval between the two surgeries appears to be increasing. The hospital mortality ranges from 0 [12, 13] up to 8% [14]. Loop [2], in an extensive report on 500 patients, links hospital mortality at reoperation to factors known to be related to hospital mortality at initial operation, that is, left main disease and incomplete revascularization. There was a trend towards increased mortality when based on NYHA (New York Heart Association) functional class although it was not statistically significant. Significant improvement in angina and overall functional status was reported by the majority of the authors.

Two major indications for reoperation are evolving; the first is progression of atherosclerosis or "new disease", including atherosclerosis affecting originally dis-

Table 1. Summary of publications on reoperation

Author (ref. #)	Year	*n*	M/F ratio	Mean age in years	Time between ORs	%Mortality Hosp.	%Mortality Late	Angina class	Angina postop	Reason for reoperation (number of pts) a gft. occ.	b new dis.	c incomp. 1st OR	a+b	a+c	b+c	Periop MI	Patency
Kobayashi (10)	78	79	56/23	53	3w-78 m mean 24 m	6	8	38% 33% 23% 6%	class I improved unchanged worse	31	12	6	14	13	3	4/79 5%	7/18 94%
Krause[a] (11)	78	79	69/10	53	2d-5yrs mean 13 m	1.3	3.8	54% 34% 12%	class I class II class III	57			21	–	7	7%@2nd OR 4.6% at 3rd OR	68%
Irarrazaval (1)	77	219	200/19	53	1w-169 m mean 38 m	3.7	4.1	65% 22% 10% 3%	class I class II class III class IV	46 a+b+c: 7 constrictive pericarditis –1	42	39	19	18	47	9%	84.4%
Qazi (12)	81	40	31/9	33–78 yrs.	N/A	0	2.3	22% 58% 14%	class I class II class III & IV	11	28	pericardial fibrosis – 1				N/A	N/A
Vouhe[b] (13)	78	43/46	40/3	N/A	13.5 m	0	2/36 5.6	76% 24%	class I class II	30	6	3	7	0	–	9.3%	70.9%
Norwood (14)	76	26	24/2	48.5	N/A	8%	4%	30% 18% 52%	class I class II class III & IV	12	5	–	9	–	–	11.5%	N/A
Reul (15)	79	168	149/19	51.4	N/A	4.8	10.6	25% 59% 16%	class I class II class III or IV	41	52	13	45	4	13	2%	N/A
Pucci (16)	82	34	29/5	52	N/A	2.9	0	42% 27% 31%	class I class II class III or IV	10	6	–	combined causes – 18			0	66% in class III & IV pts

Loop (2)	80	500	452/48	54	51 m	4	5.8	59.9% 29.3% 8.2% 2.7%	class I class II class III class IV	147	257	–	96	–	–	6.6%	LAD 93.2% Cy 84.6% R 65.4% total 78.8%
Schaff (3)	82	106	96/10	49	N/A	2.8	6.6	60%	class I & II at 5 yrs	31	10	5	29	5	19 a, b, c 7	9.4%	N/A
Hanna (17)	82	124	87/37	57	47 m	2.4	N/A		N/A	44	27	6	47	–	–	5.6%	N/A
Keon	–	183	166/17	48.8	36.2 m	7.6	7.1	62% 22% 13.8% 2.2%	class I class II class III class IV	71 technical errors: 2	19	–	97	–	–	7.1%	patent 68.4% comp. 5.8% occl. 25.8%

[a] 79 patients, 85 reops; [b] 43 patients, 46 reops
Abbreviations: Ref. #, reference number in bibliography; N, number of patients; OR's, operations; Hosp., hospital mortality, within 30 days of surgery; Gft. occ., Graft occlusion; New dis., new disease; Incomp. 1st OR, incomplete first operation; Periop M.I., perioperative myocardial infarction; class I–IV, NYHA classification of for angina; LAD, left anterior descending coronary artery; comp., compromised; occl., occluded; Cy ?; R ?

ease-free coronary arteries and progression of minimal or mild disease to severe stenosis or occlusion; the second comes under the broad heading, "occlusion of bypass grafts". This includes all grafts that are thrombosed or that have progressive atherosclerosis causing either stenosis or total occlusion. It also includes a few cases of graft occlusion caused by some technical difficulties such as kinking or tenting of a conduit. Frequently a combination of the two indications is present. A third indication for reoperation is "incomplete" first operation. These are patients who did not have all diseased vessels grafted at the first procedure. The incidence of this is decreasing because in most centres patients are receiving more coronary artery grafts per operation than they were in the early years when the procedure was in its developmental stages. The practice of most centres now is that all primary coronary vessels and any major secondary branches are grafted even if there is as much as a 30% or 40% proximal luminal narrowing. Indications for reoperation in our own experience are illustrated in Table 2.

Experience at the University of Ottawa Heart Institute

From 1969 to September 1981 we performed repeat surgery for coronary artery disease in 183 patients: 166 males (91%) and 17 females (9%). The mean age of these patients at second surgery was 48.8 years. Seven patients underwent surgery a third time. Seven patients had their first operation elsewhere, one having had his first two operations at another centre. Therefore we have performed 189 reoperations on 183 patients. The mean time between operations was 36.2 months.

Of the 189 reoperations, 162 patients presented with severe incapacitating angina. Routine postoperative angiography in 27 patients demonstrated abnormalities that necessitated reoperation. Table 2 presents a summary of our indications for reoperation. There were 71 patients requiring repeat surgery for occlusion or severe stenosis of grafts. Of these, 54 had angina. In the remaining 17 patients the stenosis or occlusion was discovered at routine postoperative angiography. The mean time between operations for this group of patients was 14.35 months. Nineteen patients, two without angina, required reoperation because of progression of disease in the native coronary vessels. The mean time between operations for this group of pat-

Table 2. Indications for reoperation

	Indication	*n* – with angina	*n* – without	Total	Mean time between operations (months)
A	Angiographic demonstration of tech. failure	0	2	2	1
B	Occl. or severe stenosis of gft	54	17	71	14.35
C	Progression of disease	17	2	19	55.31
D	B+C	91	6	97	49.9
	Total	162	27	189	36.2 months

ients was 55.31 months. These time intervals support the observations of Loop [2] that angina recurs earlier in the group who have graft closure and later in those who have progressive atherosclerosis in the native coronary arteries. Occlusion of one or more grafts plus progression of disease in the native circulation necessitated reoperation in 97 cases, 91 with angina, and the mean time between operations for this group of patients was 49.9 months.

The total number of patients with three-vessel disease at second surgery was 148, a 17% increase over first surgery. There were 33 patients with two-vessel disease, a decrease of 9.5% from first surgery, and two with single vessel disease, a decrease of 7.5%. At first surgery 16 patients (8.8%) had left main disease and at second surgery 23 patients (12.6%) had left main disease. Surgery was required on an emergency basis at first operation in 22 (12%) of the cases; 4 for acute myocardial infarction and 18 for unstable angina. At second surgery only nine (5%) were emergencies; four acute myocardial infarctions and five unstable anginas.

Results

The hospital mortality for reoperation in our institute is 14 (7.6%). The causes of death are shown in Table 3. The predominant cause was perioperative myocardial infarction in 11 patients, 2 complicated with low cardiac output and 1 with pulmonary emboli; in 4 cases the infarction was caused by atheroemboli from old CABG. Operative mortality was directly related to the number of diseased vessels (3 with left main stenosis) NYHA class, and left ventricular dysfunction. Hospital mortality rates for class IV ventricle was 43%, class III, 9%; class II, 8.8%; class I, 1.7%; and normal, 1.9%.

Of the 156 survivors, 138 (88%) were followed up for a mean of 22.8 months, range 1 month to 8 years. Using the NYHA classification system for angina, 117 patients (84.7%) had improved symptoms; 18 (12.1%) remained the same, 8 of which were asymptomatic prior to second surgery, and 3 (2.2%) had a worsening of their symptoms. The details of this are demonstrated in Table 1. A total of 85 (62%) of the patients were free from angina, 31 (22%) were class II, 19 (13.8%) were class III, and 3 (2.2%) were class IV. At follow-up the work status of 120 patients was known. Six patients were working more than preoperatively, 59 were working at the same level, and 5 were working less. There were 14 patients who were not working but were able to and 3 of these had taken early retirement. There were

Table 3. Causes of operative death

Cause	no. of deaths
MI: total	8
atheroemboli from CABG	4
MI + LCO	2
LCO	2
MI + Pulmonary emboli	1
Hemorrhage from transection of graft at reopening + LCO	1

MI, myocardial infarction; LCO, low cardiac output

16 patients who were unable to work due to their cardiac status. There was a group of 17 patients who had retired but remained active at a mean age of 61.5 years and a smaller group of 3 patients who were retired and quite sedentary with a mean age of 56.3 years. The late mortality was 13 (7.1%); the cause of death was unknown in five cases, myocardial infarction in two cases, congestive heart failure in two cases, and one each from arrhythmia, stroke, pericarditis, and left ventricular perforation at a subsequent thoracic operation.

Postoperative angiography was performed on 61 patients after second surgery (34%) and two patients after third surgery (29%). There were 46 patients who had angiography on a routine basis and who were asymptomatic at angiography at a mean of 11 months. These patients had 124 grafts and the patency rate was 79%, 5% of the grafts being patent but compromised. Angiograms were done on 15 patients with 39 bypass grafts at a mean time of 36 months. All of these 15 patients had angina; 7 class II, 6 class III, and 2 class IV. Their patency rate was considerably lower than those patients angiographed on a routine basis, that is, 59% with 8% of those grafts patent but compromised. Two of the 15 went on to third surgery and received five grafts, all of which were patent at early angiography. The overall patency rate of 69% plus 5% compromised is substantially lower than our total patency rate of 89% for 1400 grafts studied postoperatively.

Discussion

The number of reoperations for myocardial revascularization is increasing steadily. This is not unexpected since the total population from which candidates for reoperation are derived is cumulative.

The hazards of performing repeat revascularization are very real [1, 10–15]. Normally there is a higher operative mortality although this is not always the case. There is also the risk of damage to functioning grafts, the native coronary circulation, or the heart musculature itself. Various precautions such as deflation of the lungs, division of the sternum from the xiphisternal and upwards, gentle dissection of the heart from the undersurface of the sternum and retrograde dissection of the functioning grafts to their origin at the aorta can assist in reducing accidents. Loop [2] reports that reoperative risk in their centre is not related to primary adhesion formation and that the nature of the disease itself is to become more extensive with time and bring to reoperation patients with a higher prevalence of multi-vessel disease, left main coronary artery narrowing and deteriorated left ventricular function. This has been our experience and we have also identified these as major reoperative risk factors. Certainly the anticipation of technical problems at reoperation is not sufficient reason to deny a patient surgery, particularly if he or she is incapacitated by angina.

The morbidity surrounding reoperation, although higher than at first operation, is acceptable. The perioperative myocardial infarction rates are slightly higher [1, 2, 3, 14], although the introduction of cardioplegia and hypothermia have reduced the incidence of myocardial damage. The incidence of cerebrovascular complications [15] and significant bleeding [11] were slightly higher. This increase in bleeding lends credence to the clinical impression that adhesions are highly vascularized during the early postop period and hemostasis more difficult on early reoperation. Although the hospital mortality rate is higher than that at first surgery, it is a relatively safe procedure if the necessary precautions are taken. The implications of the current data available on reoperation are that through technical gains, introduction of cardioplegia, and increased operative experience the mortality and morbidity of reoperation have been reduced to an acceptable level.

Although functional results vary from centre to centre, the number of patients who experience improvement in symptoms and return to a productive lifestyle are considerable. Approximately 80% have a reduction in chest pain with substantial numbers of patients asymptomatic and others having only mild symptomatology. This clinical improvement correlates directly with angiographic evidence. The vein graft patency ranges from 66% to 94% depending on whether angiography was done on a routine basis or at recurrence of symptoms postoperatively 2. This is normally lower than the patency rate at the primary revascularization. Loop [2] reports that the internal mammary artery is a good a conduit as a saphenous vein in terms of patency and has the advantage of being suitable for distal anastomoses on vessels as small as 1 mm in diameter. The improvement in symptoms attests to the reasonable patency rates and the efficacy of performing this procedure for relief of pain.

At most institutions the primary indication for cardiac catheterization at reoperation is recurrent disabling angina.

Routine follow-up angiography may demonstrate evidence of a defective operation in an asymptomatic patient (2 of 183). Such a defect leaves the patient at serious risk of infarction which may or may not be fatal. We also believe that adequate assessment of the effect of initial revascularization on late mortality cannot be made unless the operation is satisfactory from a technical viewpoint and that the criteria defining "satisfactory technical operation" require further study.

Conclusions

Although reoperation is technically challenging, it can be performed without undue morbidity or mortality and is justified by the improved clinical conditions observed in previously symptomatic patients. Our results and those of others indicate that rehabilitation can be effective and a large majority of individuals returned to a productive lifestyle. Therefore, patients who have recurring angina after initial revascularization should be evaluated as possible candidates for reoperation. Routine follow-up angiography may also reveal surgically correctable stenoses in bypass grafts or native coronary arteries. If these stenoses represent a significant risk for major infarction and/or death they should be corrected by reoperation.

References

1. Irarrazaval MJ, Cosgrove DM, Loop FD, Enniz CL, Groves LK, Taylor PC (1977) Reoperations for myocardial revascularization. J Thorac Cardiovasc Surg 73: 181–188
2. Loop FD, Cosgrove DM, Kramer JR, Lytle BW, Taylor PC, Golding LAR, Groves LK (1981) Late clinical and arteriographic results in 500 coronary artery reoperations. J Thorac Cardiovasc Surg 81: 675–685
3. Schaff HV, Orszulak TA, Gersh BJ, Pichler JM, Puga FJ, Danielson GK, and Pluth JR (1983) The morbidity and mortality of reoperation for coronary artery disease and analy-

sis of late results with use of actuarial estimate of event-free interval. J Thorac Cardiovasc Surg 85: 508–515
4. Loop FD (1981) On reoperations. Ann Thorac Surg 32: 4–5
5. Cameron A, Kemp HG Jr, Shimomura S, Santilli E, Green GE, Hutchison JE III, Mekhjian HA (1979) Aortocoronary bypass surgery, a 7-year follow-up. Circulation 60 (Suppl 1): 9–13
6. Fuchs JCA (1981) Pathologic changes occurring in venous autografts. In: Sabiston DC Jr (ed) Textbook of surgery, 12th ed. Saunders, Philadelphia, pp 2312–2328
7. Vlodaver Z, Edwards JE (1973) Pathologic analysis in fatal cases following saphenous vein coronary arterial bypass. Chest 54: 555–561
8. Aldridge HE, Trimble AS (1971) Progression of proximal coronary artery lesions to total occlusion after aortocoronary saphenous vein bypass grafting. J Thorac Cardiovasc Surg 62: 7–12
9. McLaughlin PB, Berman ND, Morton BC, MgLaughlin N, Aldridge HE, Adelman AG, Goldman BS, Trimble AS, Morch JE (1975) Saphenous vein bypass grafting; change in native circulation and collaterals. Circulation 51/52 (Suppl 1): 66–71
10. Kobayashi T, Mendez AM, Zubiate P, Vanstram NR, Yokoyama T, Kay JH (1978) Repeat aortocoronary bypass grafting; early and late results. Chest 73: 446–449
11. Krause AH, Page US, Bigelow JC, Okies JE, Dunlap SF (1978) Reoperation in symptomatic patients after direct coronary artery revascularization. J Thorac Cardiovasc Surg 75: 499–504
12. Qazi A, Garcia JM, Mispireta LA, Corso PJ (1981) Reoperation for coronary artery disease. Ann Thorac Surg 32: 16–18
13. Vouhe P, Grondin CM (1977) Reoperation for coronary graft failure: clinical and angiographic results in 43 patients. Ann Thorac Surg 27: 328–334, Ann Thorac Surg 23: 9–13
14. Norwood WI, Cohn LH, Collins JJ Jr (1982)(J of Thoracic and Cardiovasc. Surgery 84, 211) Results of reoperation for recurrent angina pectoris.
15. Reul GJ, Cooley DA, Ott DA, Coelho A, Chepa L, Eterovic I (1982)(J Thoracic and Cardiovasc. Surgery 83, 374) Reoperation for recurrent coronary artery disease.
16. Pucci JJ, Walesby RK, Smith EEJ, Edmondson SS, Sapsford RN, Bentall HH, Cleland WP (1982) Reoperation for failed aortocoronary bypass. J Cardiovasc Surg 23: 453–457
17. Hanna ES, Ellerttson DG, Jones RJ, Crew JR (1982) Coronary artery revascularization: reoperations performed on 124 consecutive patients. Texas Heart Institute J 9: 293–297

Cardiac Transplantation: An Approach to End-Stage Coronary Heart Disease

A. Welz, B. Reichart, P. Überfuhr, B. Kemkes, and W. Klinner

Coronary heart disease is perhaps the most important fatal disease in industrialized countries. In our population it is the cause of nearly 50% of all deaths. Despite the advances in therapeutic methods there are still patients whose disease is no longer amenable to any conservative or conventional surgical therapy. After screening for the well-defined contraindications, these patients should be considered candidates for cardiac transplantation.

Patients

Between August 1981 and August 1983 five patients were given cardiac transplants for end-stage coronary heart disease (Table 1). The mean age at the time of the operation was 40 years, ranging from 32 to 45 years.

Table 1. Patients who had cardiac transplantation because of end-stage coronary heart disease

Patient	Age at operation	Sex	Time from onset of symptoms until operation (months)	Date of transplantation
1 (L)	32	M	14	August 1981
2 (G)	44	M	12	August 1982
3 (K)	37	M	9	December 1982
4 (V)	41	M	24	April 1983
5 (Sch)	45	M	24	July 1983

Table 2. Results of the preoperative heart catheterization in five patients who had cardiac transplantation for end-stage coronary heart disease

Patient	Ejection fraction (%)	Cardiac index (Liters/min per m²)	Mean left atrial pressure (mmHg)	Mean pulmonary artery pressure (mmHg)	Mean pulmonary vascular resistance (Wood units)
1 (L)	19	2.2	28	42	3.3
2 (G)	30	2.3	14	23	2.0
3 (K)	20	1.3	32	36	1.6
4 (V)	12	1.3	27	38	5
5 (Sch)	20	1.2	37	(79)	(20)
Mean values	20.2%	1.6 Liters/min per m^2	27.6 mmHg	34.7 mmHg ($n=4$)	2.9 units ($n=4$)

Table 3. Clinical diagnosis of myocardial infarction and results of coronary angiography with ventriculography

Patient	Clinically diagnosed myo. infarction	Coronary angiography			Left ventriculography			
		LAD	R. circ.	RCA	Apical	Anterior	Lateral	Inferior
1 (L)	anterior	no sig. stenosis	no sig. stenosis	no sig. stenosis	dys	dys	akin	norm
2 (G)	inferior	totally occluded	subtotal stenosis	totally occluded	akin	norm	norm	akin
3 (K)	anterior	subtotal stenosis	no sig. stenosis	totally occluded	norm	akin	norm	akin
4 (V)	anterior	subtotal stenosis	subtotal stenosis	totally occluded	dys	akin	akin	norm
5 (Sch)	anterior	subtotal stenosis	subtotal stenosis	no sig. stenosis	hyp	dys	hyp	dys

dys, dyskinesia; akin, akinesia; hyp, hypokinesia; norm, normokinesia; LAD, left anterior descending coronary artery; RCA, right coronary artery; R. circ, right circumflex artery

All patients had an extremely impaired left ventricular function (Table 2). The ejection fraction (EF) was 20.2% on the average, the cardiac index (CI) 1.6 liters/min per m^2. The pulmonary vascular resistance was slightly elevated in four patients. The high resistance calculated in patient 5 was due to a severe mitral incompetence.

In all cases the history revealed a clinically severe myocardial infarction (Table 3), and the left ventriculograph showed remarkable segmental contraction abnormalities. The anterolateroseptal infarction of patient 1 was treated by thrombolytic drugs. Accordingly, the coronary angiography showed no significant stenosis. Figure 1 shows crosssections through this heart. The myocardium of the whole anterolateral left ventricular wall and parts of the septum are replaced by fibrous tissue.

Surgical Technique

The operations were carried out according to the Lower-Shumway technique [7]. The donors were three men and two women with a mean age of 27.8 years, ranging from 20 to 37 years. The explanted hearts were transported in three cases by Learjet, helicopter, and ambulance from distant places to our department. The maximum total ischemic time of these grafts was 195 min.

Postoperative Treatment

Except in patient 1, who was treated until postoperative day 27 with azathioprine, prednisone, and antithymocyte globulin, cyclosporin A (CyA) was used from the outset as the main immunosuppressive drug. In the first two patients the Stanford regimen was adopted, beginning with 18 mg CyA/kg body weight preoperatively [8]. For patient 3 the CyA dosage was adjusted according to the preoperatively determined renal and hepatic function and the serum trough levels of CyA measured twice daily by radioimmunoassay [6]. Values between 100 and 300 ng/ml were considered to be therapeutic levels [1].

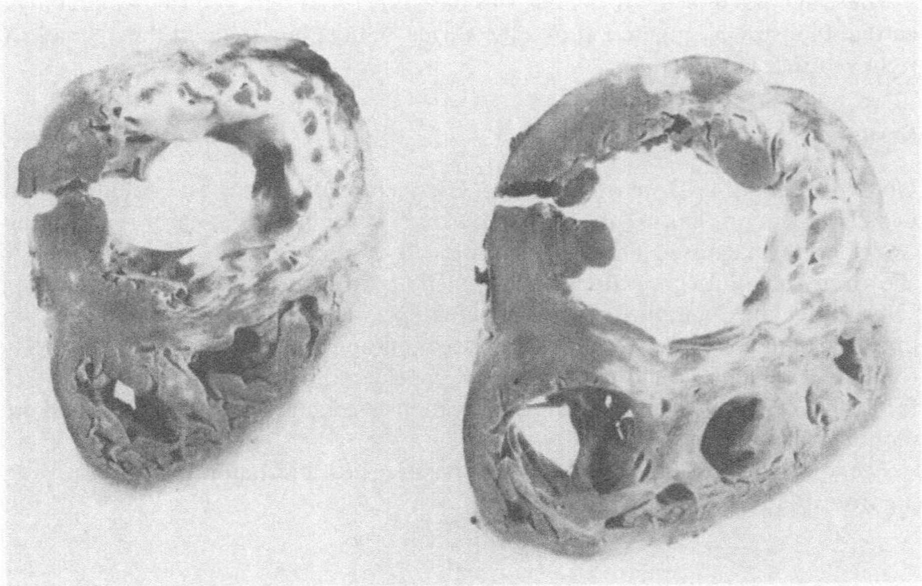

Fig. 1. Cross sections through the explanted heart of patient 1 (male, age 32 years). This patient survived a giant anterolateroseptal infarction. The myocardium of the whole left ventricular anterolateral wall together with parts of the interventricular septum is replaced by fibrous tissue.

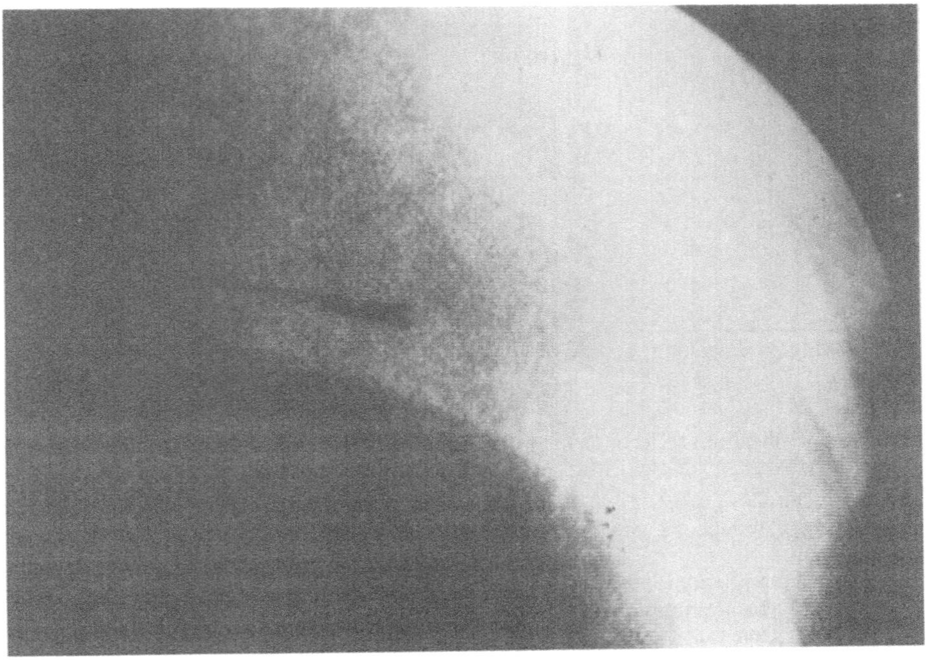

Fig. 2. Percutaneous endomyocardial biopsy. The Caves-Schultz bioptom in the apex of the right ventricle, branches opened.

The diagnosis of acute rejections was based on serial right ventricular endomyocardial biopsies [3]. Figure 2 shows the Caves-Schultz bioptome in the apex of the right ventricle [4].

Results

Up to September 1983 we performed 81 endomyocardial biopsies without any serious complication. During the first 60 postoperative days eight early rejection episodes were diagnosed (Table 4). Additionally there was one late rejection. As shown in Table 4, the rejections were treated according to the histological grading.

The infectious complications were three episodes of herpes simplex infection, one of legionellosis, and one of exacerbated pulmonary tuberculosis (Table 5). The four cases of oliguria and azotemia were considered to be due to nephrotoxic effects of CyA [2]. The neurological complications were one severe psychosis and one mononeuritis.

The total average duration of the postoperative hospitalization was 65 days, ranging from 36 to 86 days.

Table 4. Rejection episodes and therapies

Patient	Duration of the rejection episode (postop. days)	Staging of the rejection episode	Antirejection therapy	Total number of biopsies
1 (L)	6–15	II–III	6 g MPL i.v., prednisone↑, ATG↑	27
	22–34	II–III	3 g MPL i.v.	
2 (G)	39–52	II	7 g MPL i.v., prednisone↑, CyA↑	22
	80–89	I	prednisone↑, CyA↑	
3 (K)	12–19	II	5 g MPL i.v., prednisone↑	15
4 (V)	3– 7	I	3 g MPL i.v.	17
	10–14	I	3 g MPL i.v.	
	17–28	II–III	3 g MPL i.v.	
	31–71	II	9 g MPL i.v.	
5 (Sch)	–	–	–	8

MPL, Methylprednisolone; CyA, Cyclosporin A; ATG, Antithymocyte globulin

Table 5. Complications (rejections not included)

Complications	Episodes	Patients
Herpes simplex infections with aphtous stomatitis and esophagitis	3	2
Legionellosis	1	1
Exacerbated pulmonary tuberculosis with exudative pleuritis	1	1
Pneumatosis cystoides intestinalis	1	1
Oliguria with azotemia	4	4
Severe psychosis	1	1
Mononeuritis	1	1

All patients have survived. At present the survival times are: 25 months for patient 1, 13 months for patient 2, 10 months for patient 3, 6 months for patient 4, and 3 months for patient 5.

Comment

The main indications for cardiac transplantation are end-stage coronary heart disease and end-stage congestive cardiomyopathy [5]. Among those from our experience, young patients with end-stage coronary heart disease seem to be especially suitable candidates. As compared to other patients of ours, this group offered fewer complications [9]. Accordingly, their survival rate was better.

Possible causes for the better results are: (1) the history of these patients is relatively short and (2) the impairment of cardiac function affects mainly the left ventricle. Therefore there is only a slight degree of renal and hepatic congestion, or none. This makes the postoperative immunosuppressive treatment with CyA easier and more reliable.

References

1. Britton S, Palacios R (1982) Cyclosporin A – usefulness, risks and mechanism of action. Immunol Rev 63: 5, 1982
2. Calne RY, Rolles K, White D, Thiru S, Evans D, McMasters P, Dunn D, Craddock G, Henderson R, Aziz S, Lewis P (1979) Cyclosporin A initially as the only immunosuppressant in 34 recipients of cadaveric organs. Lancet 2: 1033
3. Caves P, Stinson E, Billingham M, Rider A, Shumway N (1973) Diagnosis of human cardiac allograft rejection by serial cardiac biopsy. J Thorac Cardiovasc Surg 66: 461
4. Caves P, Schultz W, Dong E et al. (1974) A new instrument for transvenous cardiac biopsy. Am J Cardiol 33: 264
5. Jamieson S, Stinson B, Shumway N (1979) Cardiac transplantation 1979 – is it justified? Int Med 1: 18
6. Kahan B, Van Buren C, Lin S, Ono Y, Agostino G, Payne W, Boileau M, Kerman R (1982) Immunopharmacologic monitoring of CyA-treated recipients of cadaver kidneys. Transplantation 32: 36
7. Lower R, Shumway N (1960) Studies on orthotopic homotransplantation of the canine heart. S Forum 11: 18
8. Oyer P, Stinson E, Jamieson S, Hunt S, Billingham M, Scott W, Bieber C, Reitz B, Shumway N (1983) Cyclosporin A in cardiac allografting: a preliminary experience. Transplant Proc 15: 1247
9. Überfuhr P, Welz A, Reichart B, Reble B, Funccius W, Hemmer W, Kreuzer E, Gokel M (1983) Herztransplantation – 2 Jahre Erfahrung im Klinikum Großhadern der Universität München. Fortschr Med (in press)

Coronary Endarterectomy Associated with Aortocoronary Bypass

A. Thevenet and E. Baudet

Although it was the initial method of direct myocardial revascularization, coronary endarterectomy (CEA) has been abandoned in favor of aortocoronary bypass (ACBP). However in diffuse coronary artery disease a number of arteries cannot be grafted. In these conditions complementary endarterectomy makes possible a revascularization procedure in otherwise inoperable arteries.

The combined technique (CEA + ACBP) is still a controversial subject among surgeons.

This report evaluates a joint experience at two institutions (Hôpital Aiguelongue Montpellier and Hôpital Cardiologique Bordeaux).

Materials and Methods

Between 1974 and 1980, 809 patients underwent 1375 ACBPs. Among them 187 (23%) had in combination 238 endarterectomies and 393 bypass grafts.

Patients

This group of 187 patients comprises 167 males and 20 females, ranging in age from 30 to 73 years (mean 55.7). Most of them had at least two risk factors; 56.7% a stable angina and 43.3% an unstable angina. According to the NYHA classification 20 patients were in class II, 80 in class III, and 87 in class IV; that is, 89.3% in functional class III or IV.

Triple-vessel disease was observed in 75.9% of the patients and left main coronary obstruction in 11.2%. Complete occlusion of one, two, or three arteries was seen in 39% (93 of 238 endarterectomized arteries), 49.7% had one or several infarctions and two-thirds showed marked impairment of left ventricular ejection function and hypokinesia or akinesia of one or several segments.

Procedure

Operations were performed using temporary cardiopulmonary bypass (aortic and right atrial cannulations), moderate hypothermia (26 °C), cold saline pericardial irrigation, and autogenous saphenous vein.

Since September 1977, myocardial protection was achieved by injection of a cardioplegic solution at 4 °C (500 ml Ringer lactate + 10 mmol KCl in the aortic root. Distal anastomoses (and eventual endarterectomies) were performed first under continuous aortic cross clamping. Proximal anastomoses were made under tangential aortic clamping during rewarming and restoration of cardiac contractions. Additional procedures were performed and included cerebral revascularization in eight patients, mitral valve replacement in four patients, aortic valve replacement in

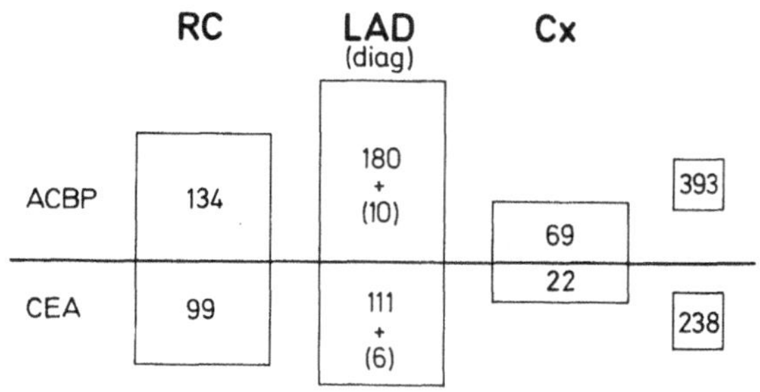

Table 1. ACBP + CEA: mean flow (%)

	RC	LAD	Cx
>50 ml/min	86.3	90.3	85.7
≤50 ml/min	13.7	9.7	14.3

four patients, excision of left ventricular aneurysm in two patients, and VSD (ventricular septal defect) closure in one patient.

There were 238 vessels endarterectomized (1.3 per patient); 99 to the right coronary artery (RC), 111 to the left anterior descending artery (LAD), 6 diagonal, and 22 to the circumflex artery (Cx), marginal or posterolateral. At the same time 393 grafts were performed (2.3 per patient), 134 RC, 180 LAD, 10 diagonal, and 69 Cx (Fig. 1). Endarterectomy was performed manually in every case. In 140 patients single vessel was endarterectomized, in 46 patients two vessels, and in 2 patients three vessels. Coronary artery bypass was single in 29 patients, double in 118 patients, triple in 40 patients, and quadruple in 2 patients.

Arteriotomy on the RC is made close to the bifurcation in posterior descending and diaphragmatic branches. A cleavage plane is established, isolating the atheromatous core from the vessel wall. Under a combination of steady traction on the core and countertraction on the outer layer, dissection progresses with a blunt dissector or spatula. After mobilization of a few centimeters of core proximally the specimen is transected. The distal part is dissected in each branch and each limb removed separately. Distal ends with the appearance of fine translucent tongues indicate separation at a site of normal intima and confirm complete removal of the core, which is also checked by means of explorers.

The LAD is approached at its middle segment and cleavage with gentle traction is used to free the specimen from the trunk and its branches (diagonal and septal), and to obtain distal patency. At the level of the marginal and posterolateral branches, endarterectomy is rarely a planned procedure but a necessary one to construct a vein bypass in an artery with a diseased wall or a short obstruction.

Flow was measured with an electromagnetic flowmeter intraoperatively in 101 patients. Mean flow was 35–130 ml/min and did not show any significant difference between bypasses with or without endarterectomy (Table 1).

Results

Hospital Mortality and Morbidity

The overall hospital mortality (within 1 month) was 3.2% (6/187). Three perioperative deaths were observed before the use of cardioplegia became routine. Those three patients had diffuse lesions and global hypokinesia. Despite prolonged circulatory assistance and intraaortic balloon pumping they could not be weaned off bypass. Two noncardiac causes of death were a massive pulmonary embolism (day 12) and a cerebrovascular accident (day 32). One patient died of unexpected ventricular fibrillation. Reversible postoperative complications were the following: four tamponades, three low-output syndromes, nine rhythm disturbances (atrial fibrillation, flutter).

Perioperative Infarction

Perioperative infarction was observed in 16 patients (8.5%), 8 anterior and 8 posteroinferior. Of these, 12 occurred in the endarterectomized territory and 4 in nonendarterectomized territory. Fifteen were diagnosed by electrocardiographic changes (new Q waves) or enzymatic elevation (CPK MB); one patient required 24 hours of balloon pumping.

Late Results

There have been 7 patients lost to follow-up. The 174 surviving patients have been followed up for 1 to 7 years (mean 40 months). Ten patients died, giving a late mortality of 5.7%: eight sudden deaths between 2 and 60 months (mean 26.3) and two cardiac failures with rhythm disturbances at 18 and 24 months. Of the patients, 82%

Table 2. NYHA functional class

	Preop.	Postop.
I	1	135+①
II	19	24+①
III	70	1
IV	74	2+②
	164	164

②, patients reoperated at 14 and 44 months

Table 3. CEA+ACBP: potency. Angiographic control of 32 patients at 1–60 months (mean 19 months)

	Total grafts	Patient	Occluded
RC	19	15	4
LAD	21	18	3
Cx	2	1	1
	42	34 (81.5%)	8

21 ACBP without CEA = 16 patent (76%)

(136/164) were asymptomatic and 15% (25/164) improved. Two patients (1.2%) became symptomatic (severe angina) at 14 and 44 months and underwent reoperation with good results.

Functional results compared to preoperative status are shown in Table 2.

Graft Patency

Control coronarography was performed in 32 patients between 1 and 60 months (mean 19) (Table 3). The overall patency rate of grafts to endarterectomized vessels was 81.5% (34 of 42 grafts), and only 76% (16 of 21 grafts) to nonendarterectomized vessels, showing the diffusion of coronary atherosclerosis in this series.

Comment

The present experience, as well as the published series [1–8] support the contention that CEA is useful and effective complementary procedure to ACBP. In diffuse coronary atherosclerosis it expands the scope of surgery, allowing bypass grafts to be performed on otherwise inoperable arteries. Enlarging the distal bed and opening collaterals, CEA gives more complete revascularization by wider distribution of the graft flow. Myocardial protection and careful attention to the technical aspects of CEA are essential. Survival, functional results, and patency rate obtained with this combined procedure indicate an expanding role for it in myocardial revascularization.

References

1. Cheanvechai C, Groves LK, Reyes EA, Shirey EK, Sones FM (1975) Manual coronary endarterectomy. J Thorac Cardiovasc Surg 70: 524
2. Hochberg MS, Merrill WH, Michaelis LL, McIntosh CL (1978) Results of combined coronary endarterectomy and coronary bypass for diffuse coronary artery disease. J Thorac Cardiovasc Surg 75: 38–46
3. Keon WJ, Akyurekli Y, Bedard P, Brais MP, Goldstein W, Beanlands DS (1979) Coronary endarterectomy: an adjunct to coronary artery bypass grafting. Surgery 86: 859–867
4. Eschenbruch EM, Schmuziger M, Tolle Naere P, Gornandt L, Hahn C (1980) Endarterectomy of the left coronary artery as a supplement surgical means of myocardial revascularization with aortocoronary bypass procedure. Thorac Cardiovasc Surg 28: 280–284
5. Miller DC, Stinson EB, Oyer PE, Reitz BA, Jamieson SW, Moreno-Cabral RJ, Shumway NE (1981) Long-term clinical assessment of the efficacy of adjunctive coronary endarterectomy. J Thorac Cardiovasc Surg 81: 21–29
6. Kamath ML, Schmidt DA, Pedraza PM, Blau FM, Sampathkumar A, Grzelak LL, Dudley Johnson W (1981) Patency and flow response in endarterectomized coronary arteries. Ann Thorac Surg 31: 28–35
7. Yacoub MH, Halim MA, Oureshi SA, Towers MK (1982) Late results of combined endarterectomy and bypass grafting for diffuse coronary artery disease. Coronary artery disease today. Proceedings of International Symposium Utrecht 1981. Excepta Medical, Amsterdam, pp 199–204
8. Thevenet A, Baudet E, Du Cailar C, Roques X, Laborde MN (1982) L'endarteriectomie coronaire associée aux pontages aorto coronariens. Ann Chir Thorac Cardiovasc 36: 587–592

Selective Treatment of Diffuse Coronary Artery Disease by a Combination of Coronary Artery Bypass Grafting and Transluminal Balloon-Catheter Dilatation

A. J. Roberts, D. G. Knauf, J. A. Alexander, R. S. Faro, R. L. Feldman, C. R. Conti, and C. J. Pepine

In 1974, Dotter and Judkins [1] introduced percutaneous transluminal balloon-catheter dilatation of lower extremity arteries. This ingenious concept stimulated Grüntzig [2] and others [3, 4] to expand its application to the coronary arteries. The term percutaneous transluminal coronary angioplasty (PTCA) was introduced and several thousand patients have subsequently undergone dilatation in the catheterization laboratory [4]. Turina [5] and Wallsh [6] were the first cardiac surgeons to report on the intraoperative use of transluminal balloon-catheter dilatation, and their pioneering efforts were followed by other surgical teams including ourselves [7–14]. The purpose of this report is to summarize the total experience at the University of Florida with balloon-catheter dilatation in conjunction with coronary artery bypass grafting (CABG) for symptomatic diffuse coronary artery disease.

Materials and Methods

Between April 1980 and October 1983, 40 patients with angina pectoris underwent intraoperative transluminal balloon-catheter dilatation and CABG. These 40 patients represented 9% of all patients having isolated CABG during that time period. A detailed description of patient selection and operative technique has been previously reported [8]. Briefly, patients were required to be symptomatic with physiologically important coronary artery stenosis (50% or greater reduction of lumen diameter) involving the proximal segment of at least one major coronary artery, along with another stenosis involving the mid-to-distal portion of the proximally narrowed artery. In these patients a USCI balloon-tipped catheter system, with a CO_2-fired pump regulating the pressure transmitted to the catheter, was utilized for dilatations. The balloon-tipped catheters varied between 1.5 to 3.0 mm in diameter in their inflated state. The catheter was positioned in the diseased artery through the arteriotomy chosen for subsequent bypass grafting. Dilatations were performed during hypothermic potassium-rich cardioplegic arrest. The arteriotomy and subsequent site for saphenous vein coronary anastomosis was made distal to the primary arterial narrowing in the proximal position of the obstructed coronary artery. Secondary or other distant arterial narrowings were the sites of balloon-catheter dilatation attempts. These secondary sites were either proximal or distal to the arteriotomy. If the balloon-tipped catheter was passed proximally (toward the aorta), this dilatation was termed retrograde. Conversely, a distal catheter passage was called an antegrade passage.

Early in our experience the concept of long-segment dilatation was employed [8]. This method was later changed to one of selective dilatation involving only the diseased arterial narrowing, provided that it could be localized intraoperatively. The reason for this change was the finding that balloon-related arterial damage could be caused by fracturing relatively normal portions of coronary arteries [15, 16]. There were 42 coronary arteries dilated in this series; the left anterior descending coronary artery in 37 cases (90%), the right coronary artery in 2, and the circumflex coronary artery in 3. Only two patients had more than one coronary artery dilated. Antegrade dilatation involving the left anterior descending coronary artery was the most frequently performed procedure, but 15 patients had combined antegrade and retrograde dilatations of this same coronary artery. A total of 57 separate dilatation procedures were performed on these 40 patients. Twenty-five patients underwent early angiography (mean 10 days postoperatively), while 13 patients underwent late catheterization (mean 12 months postoperatively). Coronary angiography, saphenous vein graft angiography, and left ventriculography were routinely performed in all patients undergoing catheterization. A description of the patient population prior to balloon-dilatation and CABG is shown in Table 1.

Results

Patient data related to events in the perioperative period are shown in Table 2. Twenty-five patients underwent early angiography. In this group, dilatations involving 25 distal arterial narrowings were studied. Fifteen (60%) were unchanged in lumen diameter with two of these patients showing evidence of intimal damage compared to the preoperative studies. Two sites (8%) were worse or narrower (none were occluded), while 8 sites (32%) were better or larger. An example of an improved dilated arterial segment in shown in Fig. 1. Four patients had retrograde dilatations that were studied early postoperatively; three were unchanged, while one improved from the preoperative status. Early vein graft patency was 97% to dilated vessels and 93% to nondilated coronary arteries. Analysis of left ventriculograms showed that regional [8] and global wall motion was unchanged compared to the preoperative condition, and no postoperative differences could be detected be-

Table 1. Preoperative patient data (April 1980–October 1983)

Follow-up: 20 ± 2 months	
Patients: 40	
Sex: 38 male, 2 female	
Age: 57 ± 1	
Functional class (NYHA): 3.4	
Prior myocardial infarction	60% (24/40)
Prior coronary bypass surgery	5% (2/40)
Associated risk factors:	
smoking	92% (36/40)
positive family history	50% (20/40)
Hypertension	50% (20/40)
diabetes	20% (8/40)
Hemodynamic data:	
ejection fraction	54.6% ± 2.6%
cardiac output	5.3 ± 0.3 liters/min
left ventricular end-diastolic pressure	15.1 ± 2.0 mmHg
Number of diseased vessels/patient	3.30 ± 0.24

Table 2. Perioperative data

Aortic cross-clamp time	67 ±4 min
Added length of cross-clamp time for coronary dilatation	4.4±0.3 min
Number of distal anastomoses/patient	3.28
Number of vessels dilated (LAD=37, R=2, C=3)	42
Sites of coronary dilatation	57 Proximal LAD=19 Distal LAD=33 R=2 C=3
Perioperative MI	2.5% (1/40)
Need for inotropic agents	10% (4/40)
Need for IABP	5% (2/40)
Mortality (early) <30 days	2.5% (1/40)
Postoperative angina <30 days	0%
Perforation	0%
False passage	0%
Inability to pass obstruction	5% (2/40)

* LAD, left anterior descending coronary artery; R, right coronary artery; C, circumflex coronary artery; IABP, intra-aortic balloon pump; MI, myocardial infarction

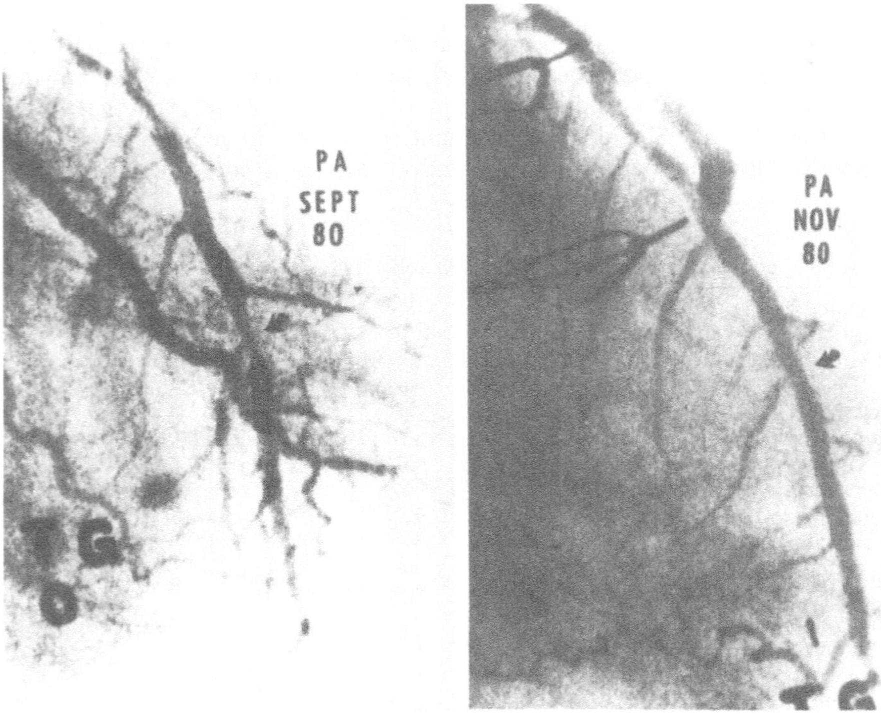

Fig. 1. Improved luminal diameter after successful intraoperative coronary dilatation.

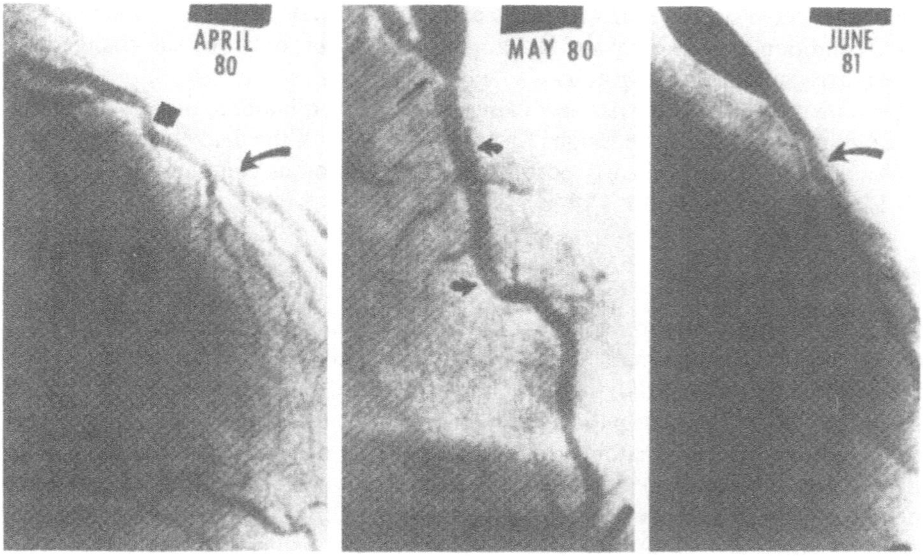

Fig. 2. Change in angiographic appearance of perioperative coronary intimal dissection during 14 month follow-up. The late angiogram shows evidence of healing and only mild stenosis.

tween those regions supplied by arteries not bypassed, bypassed without dilatation, and bypassed with dilated segments.

Late clinical follow-up (mean 30 months) revealed that three patients developed recurrent angina pectoris, three patients were known to have suffered a myocardial infarction, and one patient died with congestive heart failure. Late angiographic studies were performed in 13 patients (mean 12 months postoperatively). Thirteen vessels were analyzed after preoperative antegrade coronary artery dilatation. In comparison to the preoperative angiograms, the late arteriograms revealed that six arterial narrowings (46%) were unchanged, three (23%) were worse (one of which was totally occluded), while four (31%) were improved. Of the two segments which revealed early angiographic evidence consistent with intimal damage, both showed late evidence indicating healing. In one of these the lumen was decreased in size compared to its preoperative status by approximately 10%, while the other was unchanged compared to the preoperative luminal diameter (Fig. 2). In three patients, retrograde dilatations were observed late postoperatively; two were unchanged, while one was improved from the preoperative state. Late vein graft patency was 80% in dilated vessels and 79% in nondilated arteries. Late regional and global left ventricular wall motion remained unchanged in comparison to either of the two previous catheterization studies.

Ten patients had both early and late postoperative angiographic studies. In relation to the preoperative status, four dilated sites showed improvement in the early postoperative study. Three of these four sites remained improved, but one reverted back to an unchanged dimension at the late angiographic study. One site was narrowed but not occluded at early study and remained the same at late postoperative evaluation. Five arterial narrowings remained unchanged compared to the preoperative condition at both early and late angiography. Thus, only one site changed between early and late angiography.

Among the 25 distal arterial narrowings undergoing dilatation, there were 13 discrete lesions and 12 diffuse lesions (>2 cm in length). Of the discrete lesions, seven (53%) were improved on early postoperative evaluation as compared to only 17% (2/12) of the diffuse lesions (Table 3).

Discussion

Coronary artery bypass graft surgery has become established as a reasonable form of palliation for symptomatic coronary atherosclerosis. Although symptomatic relief is frequent after CABG, there are limitations to the effectiveness of this palliative procedure [17]. Some patients are denied surgical treatment because of inoperable coronary artery anatomy. In addition, diffuse or segmental coronary occlusive disease lends itself to incomplete revascularization, which influences long-term survival and graft patency [18]. Where segmental or diffuse coronary artery stenoses are present, the use of multiple individual vein grafts, sequential vein grafts, splitting of the distal obstruction, or endarterectomy have not been totally satisfactory. Each of these surgical techniques has its inherent technical problems at the time of surgery and an uncertain influence on long-term graft and native vessel patency.

Although the present angiographic findings after balloon-catheter dilatation appear to be relatively unimpressive compared to results with PTCA, it is probable that the surgeon is dealing with a more advanced type of atherosclerosis [19]. However, the fates of double or tandem bypass grafting and of splitting of distal obstructions in similarly diffusely diseased coronary arteries are unknown at the present time, so objective comparison of the relative efficacy of these alternative surgical techniques is not possible. Our frequency of improvement in dilated segments may appear inferior to results obtained from other studies [7, 9, 14]. The reasons for this variation are uncertain, but probably involve differences in surgical technique, patient selection, catheter design, or definition of "improvement". We have considered changes in coronary luminal diameter, while others have been concerned with coronary artery patency at the site of dilatation. Alternatively, the more extensive use of early and late angiography in our follow-up experience may more accurately define objective results. Despite the lack of a high rate of improved luminal diameter postoperatively in dilated coronary artery narrowings, the relief of chest pain in patients with such diffuse disease is frequent and graft patency as well as changes in left ventricular wall motion are comparable to results in patients with less disease undergoing coronary bypass grafting alone [18].

Table 3. Distal narrowings undergoing dilatation

	Diffuse ($n=12$)	Discrete ($n=13$)
Same	7	5
Worse	3	1
Improved	2	7

The incidence of major perioperative disruption of a dilated major coronary artery appears to be low. At least the clinical manifestations of such an event are not severe. There was only one (4%) perioperative myocardial infarction and one (2.5%) operative mortality in this series. However, the chances of a successful dilatation appears to relate in part to patient selection. Those patients with discrete distal vessel narrowing have a greater likelihood of successful dilatation compared to patients with diffusely diseased distal narrowing. We found a 53% chance of improvement in the former, and 17% in the latter. Consequently, in the presence of diffuse distal disease of the left anterior descending coronary artery, we presently favor proximal and distal CABG when possible. If this cannot be done, a long-segment endarterectomy is an alternative procedure for this problem.

We observed that the angiographic incidence of intimal dissection related to balloon-catheter dilatation may be greater than clinically appreciated. This finding has also been observed in percutaneous angioplasty methods [3]. Fortunately, when a patient is asymptomatic and intimal injury is observed angiographically soon after the dilatation procedure no specific treatment appears indicated. Based on the two patients in this series who demonstrated angiographic evidence of intimal damage, a reasonable chance for healing without important narrowing can be expected.

The serial angiographic sudies in our patients show that the early changes noted after coronary artery dilatation tend to be maintained one year later. Nine of ten dilated vessels were unchanged from early to late study. Nevertheless, the single change in classification was a downward one, with a resultant decrease in the native coronary artery lumen. Although we are encouraged to believe that late obstruction is not a prohibitive problem, further study is needed before solid conclusions can be drawn.

During a 43-month period beginning in April 1980, 9% (40/428) of our isolated CABG patients underwent intraoperative coronary artery dilatation in an attempt to improve the extent of myocardial revascularization. The added length of aortic cross-clamp time for this procedure was small (4.4 min) and it was done with relative safety. Clinical results were satisfactory, but angiographic evidence of improvement less impressive. Continued usage of intraoperative coronary artery balloon-catheter dilatation is justified and may even be encouraged. This procedure offers a satisfactory alternative to more established surgical procedures and it may improve revascularization results and extend the limits of patient selection for surgery. Furthermore, better-designed balloon-dilatation catheters [12] an the availability of intraoperative angiography [20] may enable this balloon-catheter dilatation procedure to become the procedure of choice in selected patients with discrete secondary arterial narrowings.

References

1. Dotter CT, Judkins MP (1964) Transluminal treatment of arteriosclerotic obstruction: description of a new technique and a preliminary report of its application. Circulation 30: 654–659
2. Grüntzig AR, Senning A, Siegenthaler WE (1979) Nonoperative dilatation of coronary artery stenosis. N Engl J Med 301: 61–64
3. Levy RI, Mock MB, Willman VL, Passamani ER, Frommer PL (1981) Percutaneous transluminal coronary angioplasty – a status report. N Engl J Med 305: 399–403

4. Kent K, Bentivoglio L, Block P, Cowley MJ, Dorros G, Gosselin AJ, Grüntzig A, Myler RK, Simpson J, Stertzer SM, Williams DO, Fisher L, Gillespie MJ, Detre K, Kelsey S, Mullin SM, Mock MB (1982) Percutaneous transluminal coronary angioplasty: report from the NHLBI registry. Am J Cardiol 49: 2011–2018
5. Turina M, Grüntzig A, Krayenbuhl C, Senning A (1979) The role of the surgeon in percutaneous transluminal dilation of coronary stenosis. Ann Thorac Surg 28: 103–108
6. Wallsh E, Franzone AJ, Clauss RH et al. (1980) Transluminal coronary angioplasty during saphenous coronary bypass surgery. Ann Surg 191: 234–240
7. Roberts AJ, Feldman RL, Conti CR, Selby JH, LaBrosse C, Knauf DG, Alexander JA, Watson WD, Pepine CJ (1982) Preliminary experience with intraoperative transluminal balloon-catheter dilation and coronary artery bypass grafting for the treatment of symptomatic diffuse coronary artery disease. Ann Thorac Surg 34: 504–509
8. Roberts AJ, Feldman RL, Conti CR, Knauf DG, Alexander JA, Pepine CJ (1983) Comparison of early and long-term results with intraoperative transluminal balloon-catheter dilatation and coronary artery bypass graft surgery. J Thorac Cardiovasc Surg 86: 435–440
9. Fogarty TJ, Chin A, Shoor PM et al. (1981) Adjunctive intraoperative arterial dilation. Arch Surg 116: 1391–1397
10. Mills NL, Doyle D (1982) Does operative transluminal angioplasty (OTA) extend the limits of coronary artery bypass procedure? Circulation 66 (Suppl I): 26–30
11. Katz R, Leiboff R, Aaron B et al. (1982) Intraoperative retrograde left anterior descending balloon angioplasty for reperfusion of jeopardized proximal branches. Circulation 66 (Suppl 1): 30–34
12. Wallsh E, Franzone AJ, Weinstein GS, Akan K, Clavel A, Stertzer SH (1982) Use of operative transluminal coronary angioplasty as an adjunct to coronary artery bypass. J Thorac Cardiovasc Surg 84: 843–848
13. Jones EL, King SB (1983) Intraoperative angioplasty in the treatment of coronary artery disease. J Am Coll Cardiol 1: 970–971
14. Roberts AJ, Alexander JA, Knauf DG, Faro RS, Feldman RL, Conti CR, Pepine CJ (in press) Clinical and angiographic experience with intraoperative transluminal balloon-catheter dilatation and coronary artery bypass graft surgery. J Cardiothorac Surg
15. Block PC, Baughman K, Pasternak RC, Fallon JT ((1980) Transluminal angioplasty: correlation of morphologic and angiographic findings in an experimental model. Circulation 61: 778
16. Pasternak RC, Baughman KL, Fallon JT, Block PC (1980) Scanning electron microscopy after coronary transluminal angioplasty of normal canine coronary arteries. Am J Cardiol 45: 591
17. Loop FD, Cosgrove DM, Lytle BW et al. (1979) An 11-year evolution of coronary arterial surgery (1967–1978). Ann Surg 190: 444
18. Miller DW, Ivey TD, Bailey WW, Hassel EA (1980) The practice of coronary artery bypass surgery in 1980. Circulation 62 (Suppl 3): 95
19. Turina MI: Discussion of reference [8].
20. Rainer WG: Discussion of reference [8]

The Technique of Subcutaneous Vein Harvest

A. Rashid, B. Fabri, M. R. Sastry, N. Arunachalam, and J. B. Meade

Myocardial revascularisation using reversed saphenous vein as a conduit is an established method in the surgical treatment of angina pectoris. Dissection of a leg vein using a continuous or multiple incisions [1] along the length of the vein is the most commonly used technique for vein harvest.

Patients and Results

A subcutaneous technique for saphenous vein removal was used to prepare 273 grafts for 100 consecutive patients. Their ages ranged from 36 to 68 years (mean 57) and 86 were male. Details of operative procedures are shown in Table 1. The complications following surgery are shown in Table 2. The ankle oedema was minimal and the haematomata small. Specific treatment was not required and no patient's discharge from hospital was deferred because of these complications.

Table 1. Operative procedures

Procedure	No. of patients
Quadruple bypass	13
Triple bypass	45
+ AVR	1
+ MVR	1
Double bypass	34
+ AVR	3
+ MVR	2
+ AVR + MVR + TVR	1
Total: 273 grafts	100

AVR, aortic valve replacement; MVR, mitral valve replacement; TVR, tricuspid valve replacement

Table 2. Complications of surgery

Hospital mortality	1% (double bypass + MVR)
Venospasm	0%
Ankle oedema	4%
Haematoma	2%

Operative Technique

The technique involves use of an instrument known as a "vein trap" (Fig. 1) which consists of a guide and a trimmer. The guide is a straight aortic catheter which has been specifically modified for this purpose. The trimmer consists of a handle and tip assembly (Fig. 2). The tip is blunt with an internal diameter of 9 mm. Two blades are set diametrically opposite each other 16 mm apart, the right side of the blade is the cutting edge so that it cuts when rotated in a clockwise direction. The leg is prepared for surgery in the usual fashion, externally rotated and abducted to 30°. A 3 cm longitudinal incision is made 10 cm below the knee to expose the saphenous vein, which is isolated and ligatured, and a transverse venotomy is made proximal to the ligature. The vein guide is inserted into the lumen and passed to the vicinity of the fossa ovalis. The vein and guide are identified by palpation 6–10 cm below the inguinal ligament and a 3 cm transverse incision is made to expose the vein at this site. It is mobilised and clamped, and the guide is brought through a venotomy distal to the clamp. Two ligatures are tied around the vein and guide in proximal and distal incisions and the vein is secured and divided. An assistant holds the tip of the

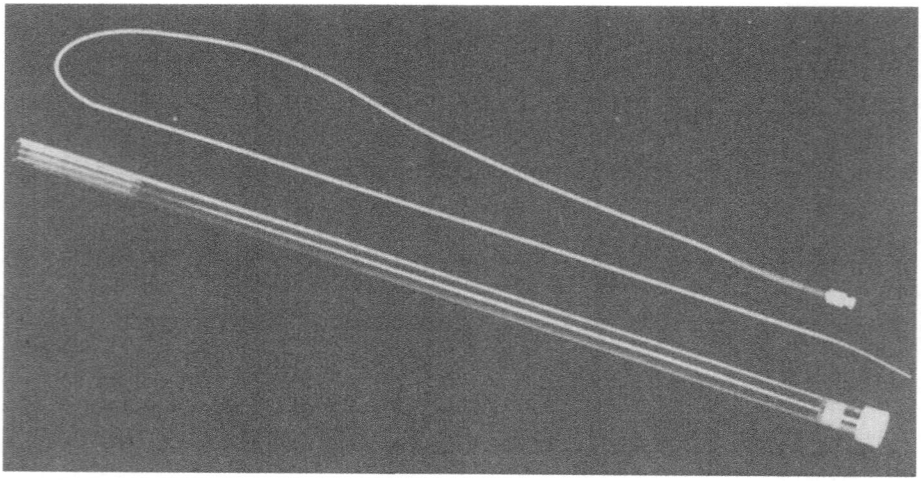

Fig. 1. The vein trap used in the subcutaneous technique of saphenous vein removal

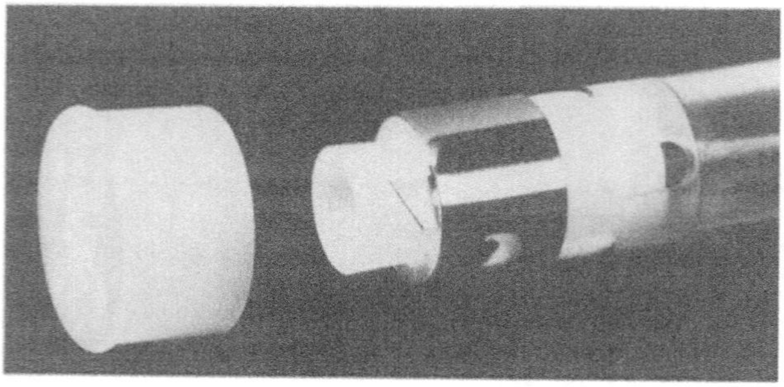

Fig. 2. Handle and tip assembly of the vein trap

guide in one hand and elevates the leg to 30° with the other. The trimmer is passed over the vein and guide into the distal incision, and the guide is held taut to prevent stretching or tearing of the vein. The trimmer is pushed in a cephalad direction, making a full 360° clockwise rotation for each 1 cm advancement over the vein. When it appears in the proximal incision the entire assembly (vein, guide and trimmer) is removed through the distal incision.

The vein is removed from the guide and excess adipose tissue is excised by sharp dissection, and the side branches are secured in the conventional manner. It is preserved in heparinised blood containing 30 mg papaverine.

The vein bed is drained using a Redivac drainage system and the incisions are closed. A crêpe bandage is applied from the base of the toes to the groin. This must extend above the proximal incision. The drain is normally removed at 24 h.

The length of vein removed is sufficient for two bypasses. Vein for four grafts is obtained by using the same technique on the other leg. When three grafts are required, the lower incision may be extended downwards and sufficient vein is dissected in the usual fashion.

Comment

The conventional method of saphenous vein harvest for myocardial revascularisation has two disadvantages; post-operative leg pain, and endothelial damage associated with venous smooth muscle spasm.

Painful leg wound complications, including ankle swelling, have been reported in 30% of patients [2]. Wound infection is not uncommon, and skin necrosis has occasionally necessitated skin grafting procedures [3]. The subcutaneous technique, by eliminating the need for long or multiple incisions, has in our experience reduced the incidence of these complications.

A healthy venous endothelium is essential to early graft patency. Experimental studies have shown that venous smooth muscle contraction subsequent to vein removal causes intraluminal endothelial protrusions, and smooth muscle cytoplasmic extensions into the subendothelial spaces which lift, separate and desquamate the endothelial cells [4]. Endothelial damage decreases the fibrinolytic activity of the intima, causing deposition of platelets and fibrin, thus resulting in thrombosis and early graft occlusion [5]. Study of vein graft specimens obtained at surgery and autopsy suggest that 70% of occlusions during the first year are secondary to thrombus formation overlying areas of endothelial desquamation [6]. Recent studies relate graft patency rates to the methods of vein harvest and preparation [7].

Our initial experience with this subcutaneous technique suggests that by minimising manipulation and dissection venous smooth muscle spasm is abolished. This should reduce endothelial damage and thus improve graft patency.

Acknowledgement. We wish to acknowledge the help of Mrs. S. F. Rudge in preparing this manuscript.

References

1. Ochsner JL, Mills NL (1978) Coronary artery surgery. Lea and Febiger, Philadelphia, p 154
2. Ochsner JL, Mills NL (1978) Coronary artery surgery. Lea and Febiger, Philadelphia, p 161
3. DeLaria GA, Hunter JA, Goldin MD, Serry C, Javid H, Najafi H (1981) Leg wound complications associated with coronary artery surgery. J Thorac Cardiovasc Surg 81: 403–407
4. Baumann FG, Catinella FP, Cunningham JN, Spencer FC (1981) Vein contraction and smooth muscle cell extensions as causes of endothelial damage during graft preparation. Ann Surg 194 (2): 199–211
5. Acinapura AJ, Porter JM, Futrell W, Silver D (1966) The effect of local vascular trauma on fibrinolysis. Am Surg 32: 762–766
6. Unni KK, Kottke BA, Titus JL, Frye RL, Wallace RB, Brown AL (1974) Pathologic changes in aorto-coronary saphenous vein grafts. Am J Cardiol 34: 526–532
7. Catinella FP, Cunningham JN Jr, Srangaram RK, Baumann FG, Nathan IM, Glassman FA, Knopp EA, Spencer FG (1982). The factors influencing early patency of coronary artery bypass vein grafts (correlation of angiographic and ultrastructural findings) J Thorac Cardiovasc Surg 83: 686–700

Flow in Saphenous Vein Bypass Grafts

W. H. Prioleau, Jr., R. A. Horney, L. D. Voegele, and P. Hairston

Flow in saphenous vein bypass grafts was determined using a electromagnetic flowmeter from Carolina Medical Electronics. Following cardiopulmonary bypass, peak flow in grafts during diastole was recorded once the systolic pressure was over 90.

Vascular Bed

Important determinants of the size of a vascular bed served by a graft include the distribution of the coronary artery grafted, its size, degree of distal vascular disease, degree of proximal coronary occlusion, and myocardial function.

Another factor found to be of importance in determining the size of a vascular bed was the presence of total occlusion of the coronary artery as opposed to high grade partial occlusion. Median flow was 40 ml/min in 61 patients with partial occlusion of the left anterior descending (LAD) artery and 14.5 ml/min in 20 patients with total occlusion of the LAD artery ($p < 0.001$; Fig. 1). In an analysis of flows where the LAD was totally occluded, low flows correlated with severe myocardial dysfunction ($p < 0.02$), and flows over 25 ml/min were present only in vessels which were 1.5 mm or greater in size [1].

Flow and Types of Coronary Anastomosis

The end-to-side anastomosis (ESA) was used in all single grafts and for the terminal anastomosis in sequential grafts. The flow in single grafts was: LAD, 42.01 ± 4.86 ml/min (mean $\pm$ 2 SE); right coronary artery (RCA), 41.98 ± 6.37 ml/min; and circumflex (CX), 37.21 ± 6.61 ml/min.

In sequential grafts where the vein graft lay parallel to the RCA for the side-to-side anastomosis (SSA) and the ESA was a termination of the graft to the CX (Fig. 2), the mean flow was 62 ml/min, insignificantly less than the 70 ml/min found by adding the flows of single RCA and CX grafts in a similar group of patients ($p = 0.15$).

In sequential grafts where the vein graft crossed the distal branches of RCA and CX at right angles, diamond-type anastomoses were constructed. Longitudinal incisions were made in both artery and vein and a continuous suture of 7-0 prolene was used. In this group of patients all grafts originated from the left side of the aorta. The vessel most distant from the aorta received the ESA regardless of whether it was bigger or smaller than the vessel or vessels between the aorta and the ESA which received an SSA (diamond). The mean flow in two-vessel sequential grafts with a diamond anastomosis was 51 ml/min as opposed to 74 ml/min for single grafts to comparable vessels in another group of patients ($p < 0.01$).

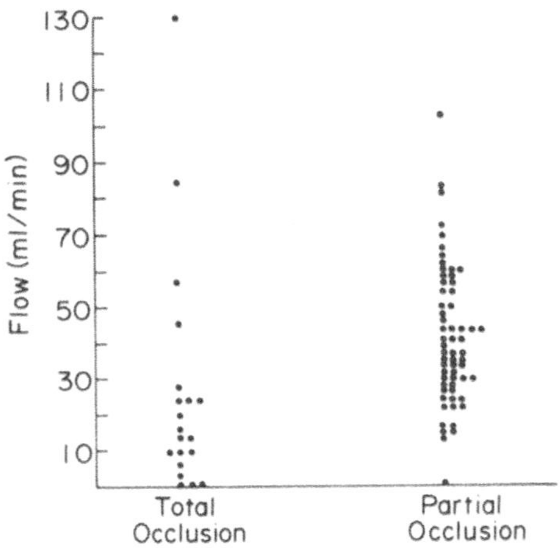

Fig. 1. Flows in LAD grafts in the presence of total and partial occlusion of the LAD (Prioleau et al. [1])

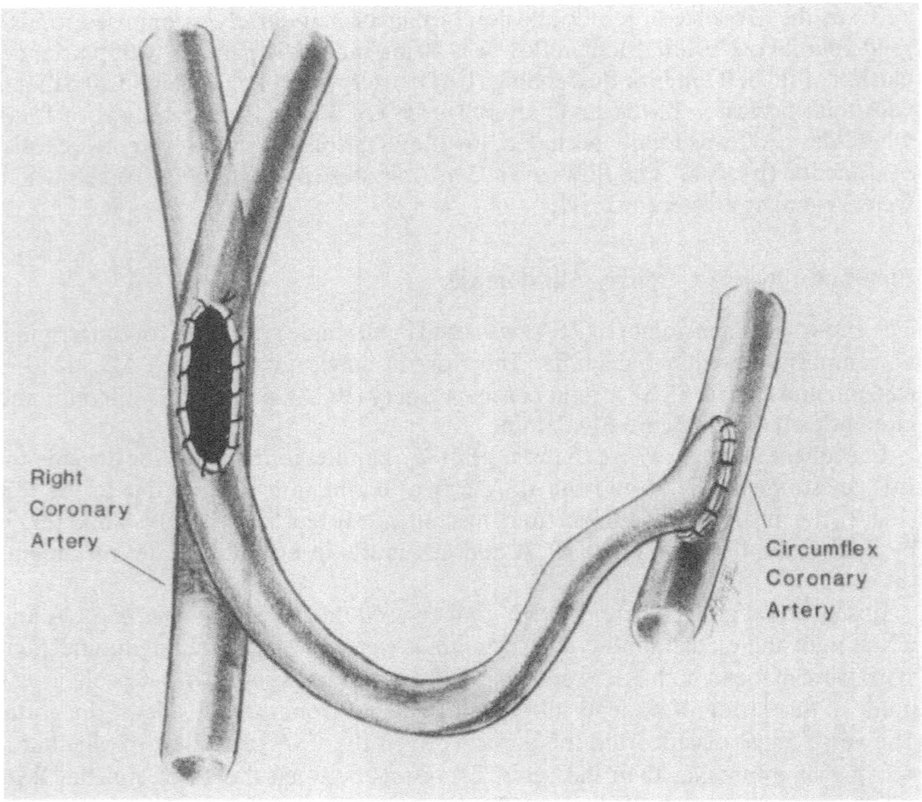

Fig. 2. A sequential graft with a side-to-side anastomosis to the RCA and an end-to-side anastomosis to the CX

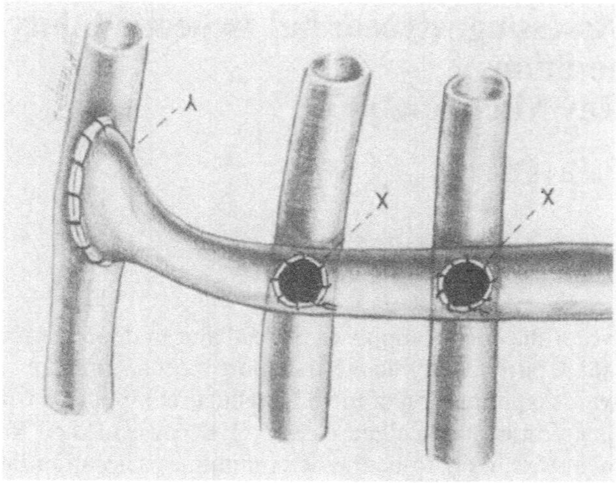

Fig. 3. A sequential graft with two diamond anastomoses (flows indicated by x) and an end-to-side anastomosis (flow indicated by y).

To determine whether the lower flow per anastomosis in the sequential group was related to a population bias (more severe disease or smaller vessels in those patients with sequential grafts) or whether the decrease in flow was related to impaired flow through the SSA diamond anastomosis, the sequential grafts were expressed as simultaneous equations. Letting x equal the flow through the SSA and y equal the flow through the ESA, the mean flow of 31 grafts with two distal anastomoses $(x+y)$ was 51 ml/min and the mean flow in 19 grafts with three distal anastomoses $(2x+y)$ was 69 ml/min (Fig. 3). The mean flow in the diamond SSA was then 18 ml/min and the mean flow in the ESA was 33 ml/min. Although not a statistical analysis, the results of the simultaneous equations suggested that the decreased flow in sequential grafts with diamond anastomoses may not be equally shared by SSA and ESA. Furthermore, the mean ESA flow of 33 ml/min suggested by the simultaneous equations was close to the mean ESA flow of 37 ml/min found in another group of patients who received a single graft to the posterior circulation.

To determine if continuous suture technique was causing the low flow in sequential grafts, a group of 12 operations were done with interrupted suture for the diamond anastomosis. The mean flow with continuous suture was 51.2 ml/min and with interrupted suture 52.5 ml/min, an insignificant difference.

In conclusion, the data suggest that there may be some streaming effect in the vein graft, permitting better flow in the ESA than the SSA where the vein graft is anastomosed to a coronary artery at right angles. Where the vein graft and coronary artery lie parallel to one another as in the case of an SSA to the RCA, the flow in the sequential grafts is approximately the same as the flow through a single graft. In no situation was the mean flow in sequential grafts superior to the mean flow expected from multiple single grafts.

Acknowledgement. The authors wish to thank Karen Y. Tempel for illustrations.

Reference

1. Prioleau WH, Jr., Clark S, Gross A, Voegele LD, Hairston P (1982) Flow in coronary artery bypass grafts to totally and partially occluded left anterior descending coronary arteries. Ann Thorac Surg 34 (5): 490–492

A New Method of Assessing Myocardial Ischemic Injury During Cardiac Operations: Electron Probe X-Ray Microanalysis*

E. Anyanwu, E. R. Krefting, and H. Dittrich

Introduction

Ischemia leads to breakdown of the energy supply in the cell and to depression of the Na-K-ATPase activity [6]. Consequently active transport mechanisms are inhibited, with a tendency towards equilibration of the intracellular components with the constituents of the volume-limited extracellular space [5]. Because of their low molecular weights, the elements are likely to be the determining equilibration factors. Intracellular element assay can therefore be used to provide information about the changes in the composition and concentration of the intracellular elements. If it is combined with extracellular element assay, the intracellular element profile should furnish information about the integrity of the cells and their membranes. Electron probe X-ray microanalysis is a one-stage analytical method avoiding the errors inherent in a multistage procedure. The following elements can be assayed: calcium (Ca), sodium (Na), phosphorus (P), sulfur (S), chlorine (C1), potassium (K), and magnesium (Mg).

The Principle of Electron Probe X-ray Microanalysis in Biological Tissues

Energy is released when electrons travel through matter. If the inner shell (eg., K shell) of an atom is ionized, the hole in this shell is filled up by an electron from one of the outer shells (eg., L or M shell). During this transition, a definite amount of energy characteristic for each atom is set free. This energy can be released as X-rays. The energy of these X-rays is characteristic for each element. To identify the X-rays an energy dispersive (ED) or wavelength dispersive (WD) system can be used. In the ED system, each X-ray quantum produces an electronic signal proportional to its energy. This energy is counted in the corresponding channel of a multichannel analyzer. Thus the whole X-ray spectrum is obtained. In the WD system, the X-rays are diffracted by a suitable crystal. Because of the geometrical conditions (interference of the X-rays), only the quanta of one wavelength are counted at any one setting. By rotating the crystal different wavelengths (energies) can be counted consecutively with the WD system, while the ED system allows the simultaneous recording of the whole X-ray spectrum. On the other hand, the WD system has a much better spectral resolution (about 4 eV) than the ED system (about 150 eV) and a much better signal-to-background ratio. Thus adjacent lines can be separated and the elements with small concentrations detected. The intensity Px of the characteristic X-rays is proportional to the concentration of an element in thin specimens. Be-

* Supported with funds from the Sonderforschungsbereich SFB 104 Teilprojekt B2 (Dittrich)

cause the thickness of the sections of the tissues may be uneven, the intensity *Px* of the characteristic X-rays is divided by the intensity *W* of a suitable range of the X-ray continuum. *W* is proportional to the thickness of the specimen, therefore the ratio *Px/W* is independent of the section thickness [4]. Thus a quantitative assessment of the element in question is feasible. Other authors [2, 3] have employed electron probe X-ray microanalysis to study element concentration shifts in normal and injured myocardium.

Analytical Procedure

Transmural biopsies are obtained from the myocardium and immediately shock-frozen in propane cooled with liquid nitrogen at about −190 °C. The shock-frozen specimens are cut to a thickness of about 4 μm with a cryostat at a temperature of −30 °C (temperature of specimen holder and knife: −45 °C). Each section is subsequently transferred onto a thin plastic foil (pioloform, supplied by Hert. Munich, Germany) stretched over a special tissue holder (aluminium tube, 9 mm in diameter). The preparation is covered by a second thin foil and gently pressed for good alignment between the section and the supporting foil. The specimens are transferred to the specimen stage of an evaporator (Edwards 306) cooled by liquid nitrogen. Here the frozen sections are dried at a pressure of about 10^{-6}mb, following which they are coated with carbon. Suitable flat sections are examined. For the element analysis, the WD system (CAMECA MS 46) and ED System (EDAX 707) are employed. Using the scanning mode, microcompartments for the analysis are selected. A suitable area for the analysis ranges from 2×2 to $10 \times 10\ \mu m^2$, at a probe current of about 7 nA and 15 to 35 keV electron energy. During a typical investiga-

Table 1a. Intracellular calcium assay during myocardial ischemia: temperature 37 °C

	Control	0 min	2.5 min	5 min	10 min	15 min
n	68	24	26	22	40	18
MV	22	33	27	23	41	39
SD	20	19	37	28	28	8

	20 min	30 min	60 min	120 min	180 min
n	24	14	22	24	20
MV	24	53	39	72	31
SD	28	47	8	36	11

Table 1b. Intracellular calcium assay: temperature 10 °C

	Control	5 min	20 min	60 min	90 min	180 min
n	38	18	18	16	20	20
MV	32	34	39	31	46	56
SD	15	8	7	14	19	18

MV, mean value; SD, standard deviation
Results expressed as *Px/W* values (ratio of the intensity of the characteristic X-rays and the intensity of a suitable range of the X-ray continuum) and multiplied by 10^4 for clarity.

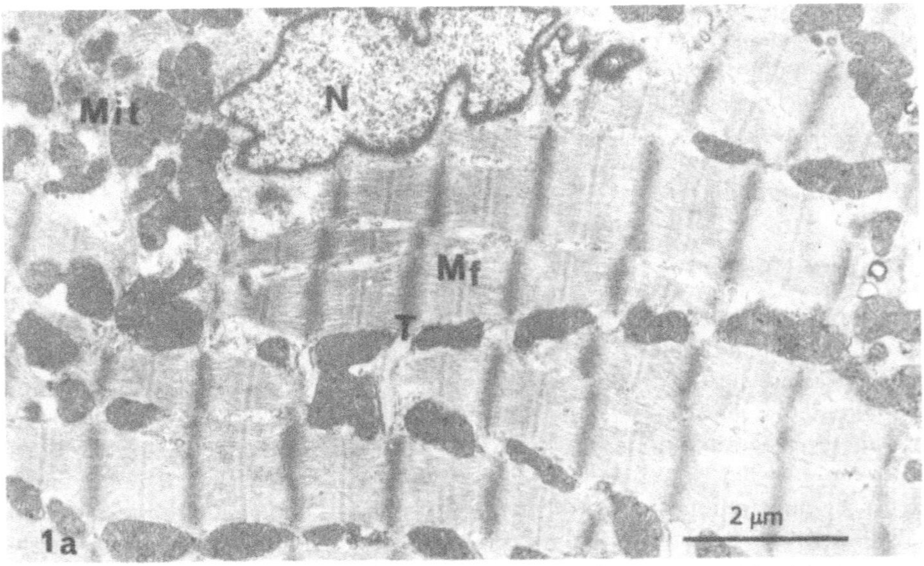

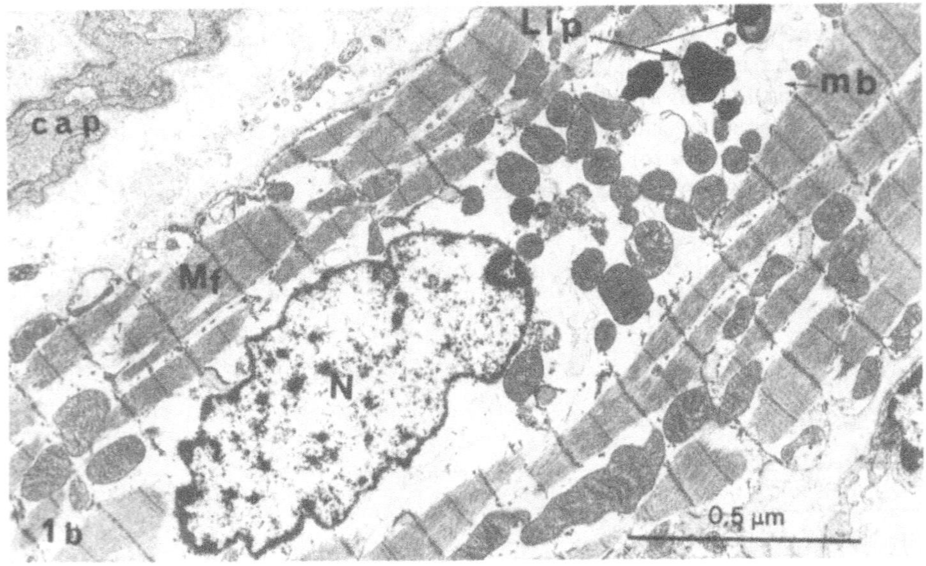

Fig. 1a. Ultrastructure of the canine myocardium before ischemic arrest. The myofilaments *(Mf)* are in a state of contraction. The mitochondria *(Mit)* present with numerous matrix granules. The crests are sharply defined. Temperature: 37 °C; **b** Ultrastructure of the same myocardium following 5 min ischemia. The myofilaments *(Mf)* already display focal areas of lysis leaving the Z lines virtually isolated. The nucleus *(N)* is slightly electrolucent and has accumulations of ribosome-sized granules. The mitochondrial crests are blurred in appearance. The mitochondria lack normal granules. Myelin bodies *(mb)* have already formed within the myocyte. *cap*, capillary; *Lip*, lipofuscin. Temperature: 37 °C

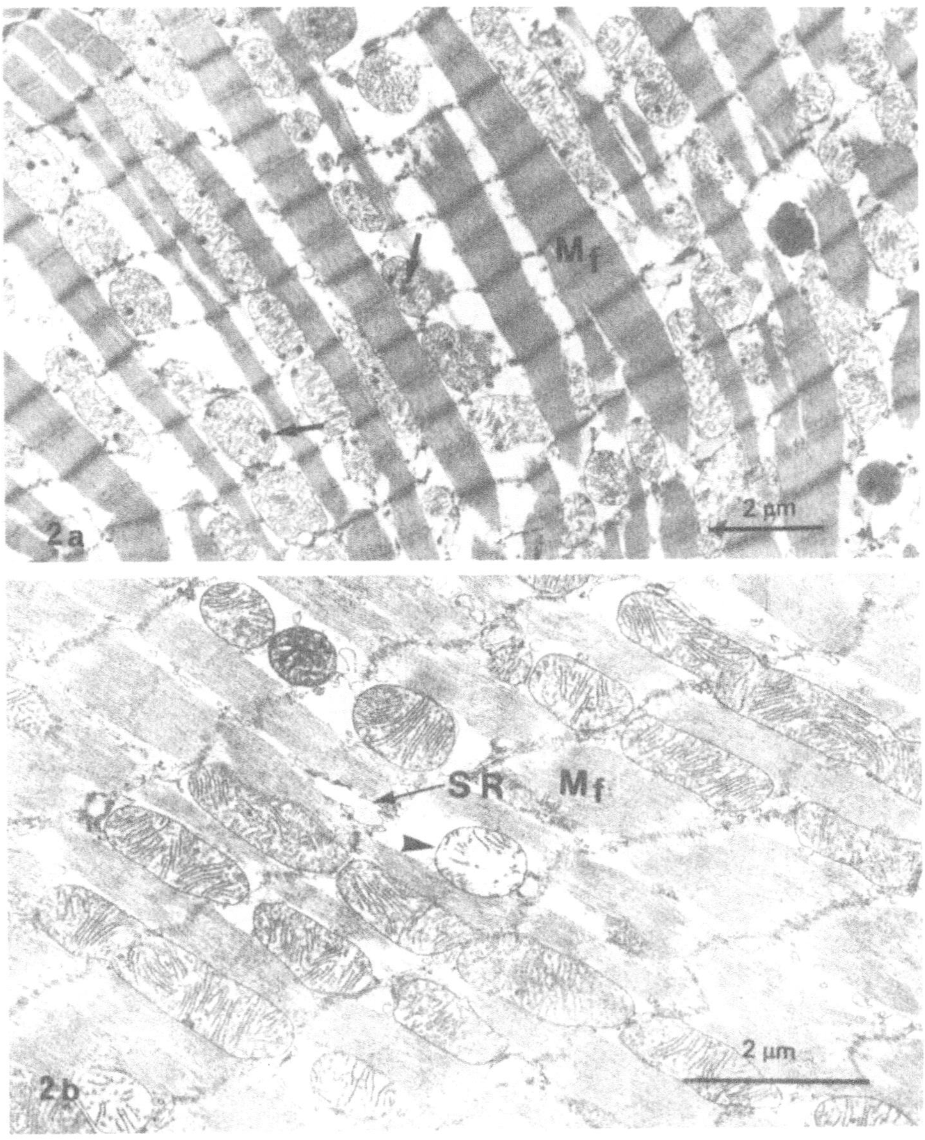

Fig. 2 a. Ultrastructure of the myocardium following 15 min of ischemia. Note the increased distance between the bundles of myofilaments *(Mf)*, and more extensive areas of microfilamentolysis. The mitochondria demonstrate multiple crest fragmentation, cristolysis, light matrix, lack of normal granules, and an abundance of flocculent dense bodies *(arrow)*. Temperature: 37 °C; **b** After 30 min, the cells generally display rarefaction of the myofilaments *(Mf)*. The sarcoplasmic reticulum *(SR)* is slightly widened. The mitochondrial matrix is electrolucent, shows crest fragmentation and complete cristolysis *(arrow)*. Of particular importance is the conspicuous absence of the flocculent densities described in Fig. 2 a. Temperature: 37 °C.

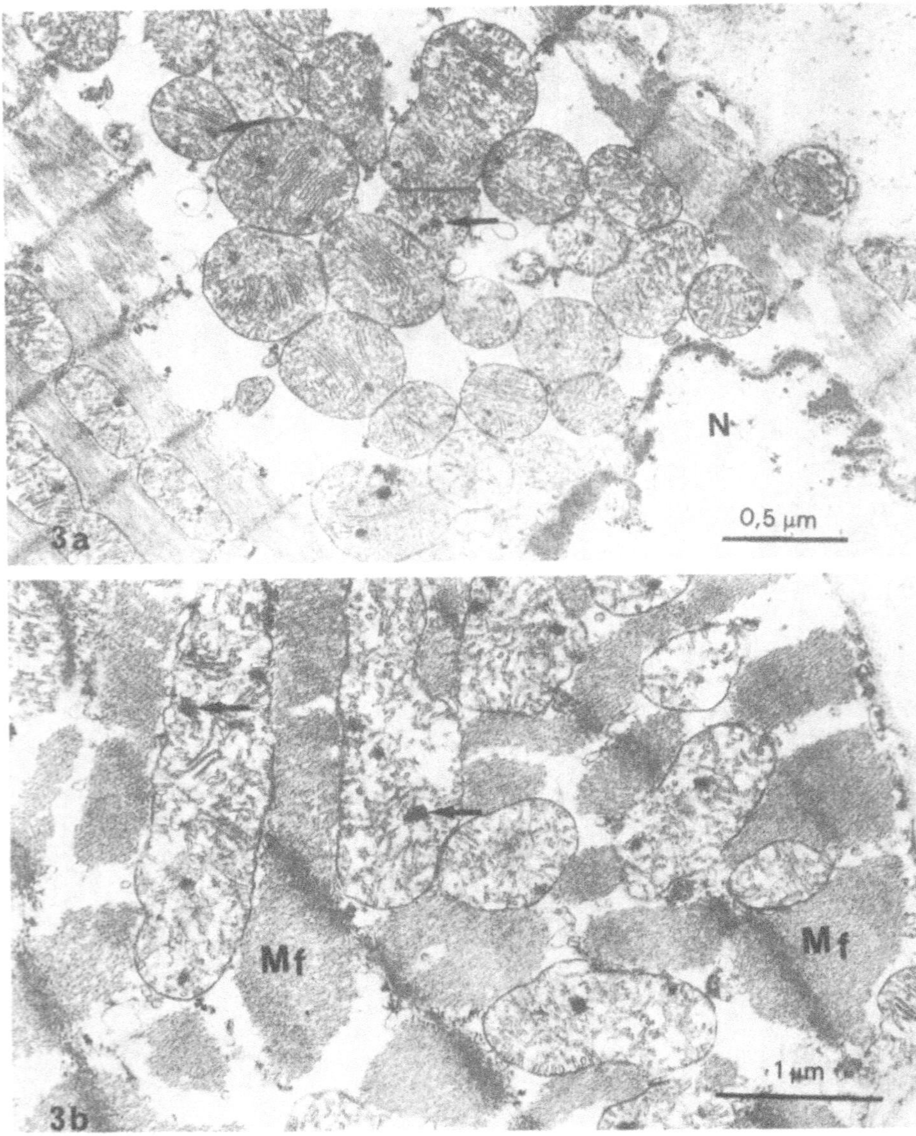

Fig. 3a. After 60 min of ischemia, one observes complete nuclear clearing and margination of the chromatin material *(N)*. Within the mitochondria fine granular calcium precipitation – calcium spicules – are present *(arrow)* Temperature: 37 °C. **b** At 120 min, these densities still persist and appear coarser *(arrow)*. Cristolysis and myofilamentolysis are prominent features. *Mf*, myofilaments. Temperature: 37 °C

tion biopsies were taken from the left ventricles of normally beating canine hearts and from the same ventricle immediately following ischemic cardiac arrest. Subsequent biopsies were taken at defined ischemic intervals (2.5, 5, 10, 15, 20, 30, 40, 60, 90, 120, and 180 min) and at selected myocardial temperatures (37 °C and 10 °C). Eight dogs were used for the experiments. Similarly, biopsies were obtained from the left ventricles of human hearts before cardiopulmonary bypass (control), during ischemia, and after reperfusion, and analyzed as described above. The hearts were arrested by a calcium-free cardioplegic solution as previously described [2]. Biopsies were obtained at the same time for ultrastructural studies. The assessment of myocardial ischemic injury was in accordance with known cirteria [1].

Results and Discussion

During the first 10 min of normothermic ischemia, the intracellular Ca content was practically unchanged. Thereafter, the Ca concentration within the cells fluctuated (Table 1). Peak contents were recorded at 10, 30 and 120 min intervals, whereas the mean values at 15, 60, and 180 min were comparatively low – though higher than the intracellular Ca content of the normal beating nonischemic heart (control). A comparison of the mean values using Student's t-test showed that the difference between the peak and the control values was statistically significant ($p < 0.001$). The ultrastructural studies, aside from demonstrating the concurrent emergence of flocculent densities and calcium spicules (Figs. 1–3) in the mitochondria at the time of the Ca peaks, also showed scarcity of the flocculent densities and disappearance of the Ca spicules during periods of low intracellular Ca concentration. These densities were lacking in other parts of the myocardial cell. Up to 120 min, the degree of ischemic mitochondrial damage correlated positively with the accumulation of amorphous densities and Ca spicules.

Table 2. Intracellular element analysis: ischemia Temperature 37 °C

	n	Na		Mg		P		S		Cl		K	
		MV	SD	MV	SD	MV	SD	MV	SD	MV	SD	MV	SD
Control	19	124*	79	121	81	1896	315	381	94	800	136	3104	371
0.0 min	11	44	57	173	53	2089	90	569	59	521	50	3220	109
2.5 min	14	157	77	186	86	2210	142	513	70	696	142	3410	144
5 min	15	123	64	123	87	2075	223	519	63	793	203	3170	296
10 min	12	117	83	170	92	2253	162	577	49	550	70	3390	127
20 min	12	248	86	134	116	1958	261	728	72	1089	162	2224	492
40 min	12	149	57	101	110	2172	199	567	138	654	58	3229	305
60 min	11	152	73	65	82	2121	113	495	31	658	142	3410	194
120 min	15	163	51	105	95	2124	137	454	88	729	60	3030	210
Temperature 10 °C													
Control	12	219	16	97	112	2075	203	669	111	869	204	3100	442
5 min	12	108	74	124	72	1931	69	693	86	545	58	3080	127
60 min	12	251	145	189	130	2168	107	730	66	758	85	3290	130
90 min	12	156	61	209	127	1914	134	692	160	846	107	3100	140
180 min	14	215	68	130	107	2049	206	776	123	1002	178	2885	866

Refer to table 1 for further explanation.

Table 3a. Intracellular element assay

		Calcium					
		Sp 1			Sp 3		
		n	MV	SD	*n*	MV	SD
RS	BI	10	0.042	0.011	10	0.045	0.009
	FI	8	0.014	0.006	8	0.0062	0.005
	AR	8	0.020	0.005	8	0.022	0.005
SH	BI	8	0.044	0.025	8	0.053	0.022
	FI	8	0.012	0.006	8	0.010	0.004
	AR	8	0.016	0.007	8	0.018	0.008
TH	BI	16	0.041	0.030	16	0.048	0.036
	FI	16	0.020	0.007	16	0.025	0.010
	AR	14	0.024	0.006	14	0.027	0.009
LNJ	BI	58	0.021	0.014	58	0.027	0.018
	FI	57	0.012	0.005	57	0.015	0.007
	AR	53	0.014	0.007	53	0.015	0.009
		Sodium					
		Sp 4			ED		
RS	BI	10	0.459	0.120	5	0.156	0.048
	FI	8	0.150	0.032	4	0.119	0.017
	AR	8	0.517	0.057	4	0.181	0.027
SH	BI	8	0.550	0.088	6	0.181	0.023
	FI	8	0.342	0.138	6	0.141	0.046
	AR	8	0.282	0.143	6	0.127	0.029
TH	BI	16	0.541	0.102	8	0.197	0.051
	FI	16	0.278	0.035	8	0.160	0.014
	AR	14	0.576	0.064	7	0.204	0.026
LNJ	BI	58	0.471	0.150	29	0.205	0.040
	FI	57	0.297	0.089	30	0.164	0.029
	AR	53	0.332	0.150	30	0.159	0.037

BI, before ischemia; FI, following ischemia; AR, after reperfusion; RS, SH, TH, LNJ, patients whose myocardium was analyzed; Sp 1, Sp 3, Sp 4, wavelength dispersive systems; ED, energy dispersive system

The ischemic myocardium at 10 °C (hypothermia) showed no significant intracellular Ca accumulation up to 60 min of ischemia. After 90 and 180 min, the Ca content was significantly higher than the control value ($p < 0.01$ and $p < 0.001$, respectively). Flocculent densities and Ca spicules were still lacking in the mitochondria after 180 min.

At 37 °C the other elements, Na, S, P, Mg, and K, showed equivocal changes throughout the experiment (Table 2). Chlorine dropped initially, rose again and remained practically unchanged. The results obtained at 10 °C were similar to those at 37 °C. The results stated here were consistent in all dog hearts studied, but the time during which the element shifts (primarily Ca shifts) occurred varied slightly, reflecting the individual resistance of the myocardium to ischemia.

Table 3b. Intracellular element assay

Chlorine (ED)

	n	MV	SD	n	MV	SD	n	MV	SD	n	MV	SD
BI	5	0.291	0.036	6	0.285	0.040	8	0.310	0.099	29	0.229	0.048
FI	4	0.128	0.018	6	0.270	0.085	8	0.123	0.016	30	0.153	0.058
AR	4	0.290	0.038	6	0.276	0.056	7	0.299	0.060	30	0.188	0.058
Patient	RS			SH			TH			LNJ		

Potassium (ED)

	n	MV	SD	n	MV	SD	n	MV	SD	n	MV	SD
BI	5	0.632	0.022	6	0.426	0.171	8	0.533	0.068	29	0.769	0.164
FI	4	0.958	0.065	6	0.436	0.233	8	0.563	0.094	30	1.034	0.200
AR	4	0.787	0.174	6	1.00	0.161	7	0.606	0.127	30	0.938	0.164
Patient	RS			SH			TH			LNJ		

Phosphorus (ED)

	n	MV	SD	n	MV	SD	n	MV	SD	n	MV	SD
BI	5	0.669	0.100	6	0.609	0.070	8	0.619	0.124	29	0.768	0.081
FI	5	0.733	0.051	6	0.681	0.086	8	0.642	0.065	30	0.766	0.103
AR	8	0.751	0.081	6	0.655	0.045	7	0.700	0.122	30	0.679	0.108
Patient	RS			SH			TH			LNJ		

Sulfur (ED)

	n	MV	SD	n	MV	SD	n	MV	SD	n	MV	SD
BI	5	0.306	0.272	6	0.155	0.040	8	0.148	0.052	29	0.120	0.026
FI	4	0.133	0.031	6	0.205	0.049	8	0.112	0.027	30	0.097	0.027
AR	4	0.105	0.017	8	0.159	0.038	7	0.104	0.043	30	0.107	0.028
Patient	RS			SH			TH			LNJ		

Refer to Table 3 for abbreviations

Table 3c. Extracellular element assay: representative results

Patient:	INJ	n	MV	SD	n	MV	SD	
Calcium	(Sp 1)							*Calcium* (Sp 3)
	BI	35	0.028	0.013	35	0.037	0.018	
	FI	39	0.130	0.079	39	0.144	0.103	
	AR	13	0.086	0.045	13	0.104	0.056	
Sodium	(Sp 4)							*Sodium* (ED)
	BI	35	0.560	0.162	29	0.190	0.043	
	FI	39	1.201	0.634	51	0.376	0.153	
	AR	13	1.855	0.983	8	0.516	0.271	
Phosphorus	(ED							*Sulfur* (ED)
	BI	29	0.730	0.112	29	0.123	0.027	
	FI	51	0.500	0.307	51	0.155	0.135	
	AR	8	0.557	0.368	8	0.137	0.054	
Chlorine	(ED)							*Potassium* (ED)
	BI	29	0.324	0.127	29	0.810	0.154	
	FI	51	0.523	0.338	51	0.756	0.322	
	AR	8	0.815	0.753	8	0.638	0.255	

Refer to Table 3 for abbreviations

Table 3d. Comparison of any two mean values (Student's t-test)
Intracellular element assay

Patient	Ca (Sp 1)			Ca (Sp 3)			Na (Sp 4)		
	BI/FI	BI/AR	FI/AR	BI/FI	BI/AR	FI/AR	BI/FI	BI/AR	FI/AR
RS	+3	+3	−1	+3	+3	−3	+3	−	−3
SH	+2	+1	−	+1	+2	−1	+2	+3	+
TH	+1	+1	−	+1	+1	−	+3	−	−3
LNJ	+3	+2	−	+3	+3	−	+3	+3	−
	Na (ED)			Cl (ED)			K (ED)		
	BI/FI	BI/AR	FI/AR	BI/FI	BI/AR	FI/AR	BI/FI	BI/AR	FI/AR
RS	+	−	−1	+3	+	−2	−2	−	+
SH	+	+2	+	+	+	−	−	−2	−3
TH	+	−	−2	+2	+	−3	−	−	−
LNJ	+3	+3	+	+3	+2	−1	−3	−3	+1

Extracellular element assay

Ca (Sp 1)			Ca (Sp 3)			Na (Sp 4)		
BI/FI	BI/AR	FI/AR	BI/FI	BI/AR	FI/AR	BI/FI	BI/AR	FI/AR
−3	−3	+	−3	−2	+	−3	−3	−
Na (ED)			Cl (ED)			K (ED)		
BF/FI	BI/AR	FI/AR	BI/FI	BI/AR	FI/AR	BI/FI	BI/AR	FI/AR
−3	−1	−	−3	−	−	+	+	+
+3	+	−	P (ED)					
−	−	+	S (ED)					

Range of significance: 1, 1%–5%; 2, 0.1%–1%; 3, less than 0.1% sign before digit: mean value before virgule significantly higher (lower) than that after it
+1, +, −, −1: differences not significant

Table 3 illustrates the results which can be expected from individual patients following cardioplegic arrest. The intracellular Ca content during ischemia was always lower than the control values (before cardiopulmonary bypass). Na and Cl behaved similarly, while the mean intracellular K concentration rose. During reperfusion, the behavior of these elements was the reverse of the behavior during ischemia. These elemental shifts were mostly significant (Table 3). The concentrations of S and P were practically unchanged. A comparison of the two analytical systems used, as illustrated by Na assay, shows that the WD system is much more sensitive than the ED system (Table 3a). From the results of the extracellular element assay (Table 3c), the Ca concentration during ischemia was higher than the control value. Na and Cl behaved similarly, but the K content dropped. P and S showed only insignificant shifts, whereas those of Ca, Na, and Cl were highly significant ($p < 0.001$). The shift in K was not significant ($p > 0.05$).

The extracellular compartment is small compared with the intracellular compartment. Consequently extracellular element assay is not routinely carried out because of yet unsolved technical barriers.

Summary and Conclusions

During normothermic myocardial ischemia, Ca accumulated within the cells in stages corresponding to peaks, between which the intracellular Ca content did not significantly rise above the control level.

Ultrastructural studies showed that the Ca peaks corresponded in time with the appearance of amorphous densities and Ca spicules within the mitochondria.

The degree of ischemic mitochondrial injury correlated with the accumulation of flocculent densities and calcium peaks. The intracellular concentrations of the elements Na, Cl, Mg, S, P and K did not show significant shifts either during normothermic or hypothermic ischemia.

Hypothermia drastically slowed down the rate of intracellular Ca accumulation and preserved myocardial ultrastructure. Cardioplegic cardiac arrest allowed a selective movement of the elements Ca, Na, Cl, and K across the myocardial cellular membrane. The restoration of the element concentrations to their control values proves that the cells suffered reversible or little ischemic injury.

Finally, because of its positive correlation with the degree of ischemic myocardial injury – as assessed ultrastructurally – the electron probe X-ray microanalysis is a reliable method of studying myocardial ischemic injury.

References

1. Anyanwu E, Konermann Ch, Klinke F, Dittrich H (1983) The influence of non-coronary collateral blood supply on the electively arrested heart during ischemia and reperfusion. Res Exp Med (Berl) 182: 111–126
2. Anyanwu E, Kreftiŋg ER, Dittrich H (1983) Myocardial intra- and extracellular calcium changes following cardioplegic cardiac arrest. Res Exp Med (Berl) (In press)
3. Hagler H, Burton K, Buja L (1981) Electron probe X-ray microanalysis of normal and injured myocardium: methods and results. In: Hutchinson TE, Somlyo AP (eds) Microprobe analysis of biological systems. Academic, New York p 127
4. Hall TA (1971) Microprobe assay of chemical elements. In: Oster G (ed) Physical techniques in biochemical research, 1 A, 2nd edn. Academic, New York, p 157
5. Trump BF, Mergner WJ, Kahng MW, Saladino AJ (1976) Studies of the subcellular pathophysiology of ischemia. Circulation 53 (Suppl 1): 17–25
6. Willerson JT, Scales F, Mukherjee A, Platt M, Templeton GH, Fink GS, Buja LM (1977) Abnormal myocardial fluid retention as an early manifestation of ischemic injury. Am J Pathol 87: 159–188

Direct Revascularization of the Septal Arteries: Preliminary Report on 112 Patients

S. Caparrotti, O. Alfieri, W. Brands, J. Defauw, R. De Geest, P. Knaepen, F. Vermeulen, M. Zembala

Recent studies have shown that a policy of complete revascularization improves long-term results of surgery for coronary artery disease [1, 2, 5, 7]. However, when obstruction involves septal arteries, most cardiac surgeons do not perform direct grafting of these arteries. In the majority of patients the ischemic interventricular septum can be revascularized indirectly with grafts to the left anterior descending coronary artery (LAD) or the posterior descending artery, but there are situations, like those depicted in Fig. 1, in which direct revascularization of the septal arteries is either advisable or mandatory to achieve complete revascularization. In our institution septal arteries have been revascularized directly when indicated.

Clinical Material

From May 1, 1976 to December 31, 1982, 4820 patients underwent myocardial revascularization procedures at St. Antonius Hospital. One hundred and twelve (2.3%) received direct septal artery revascularization. Selection of the patients for this procedure was based on angiographic criteria:

- Appropriate caliber of the septal artery (Fig. 2 shows the most usual variation in our patients)
- Poor communication between LAD and septal artery due either to a stenosis (>60%) of the septal artery itself or to obstructive LAD lesions in the proximity of the origin of the septal artery (Fig. 1)

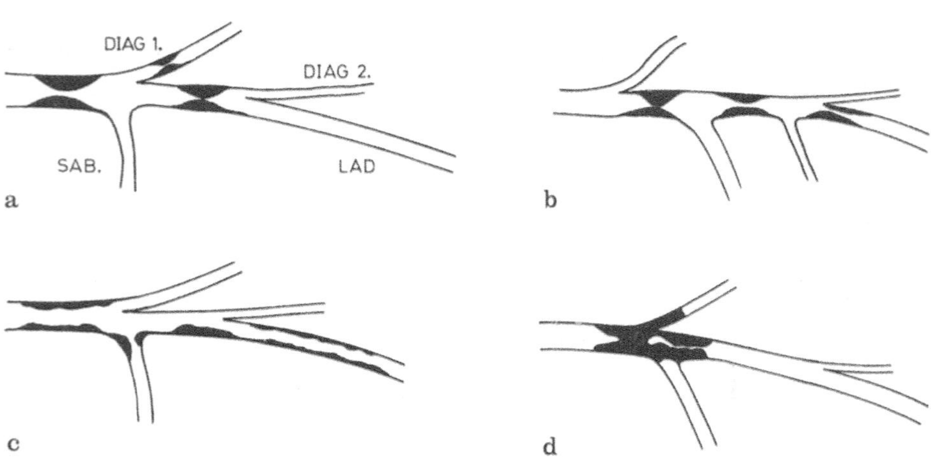

Fig. 1. Some examples of common septal artery branch lesions

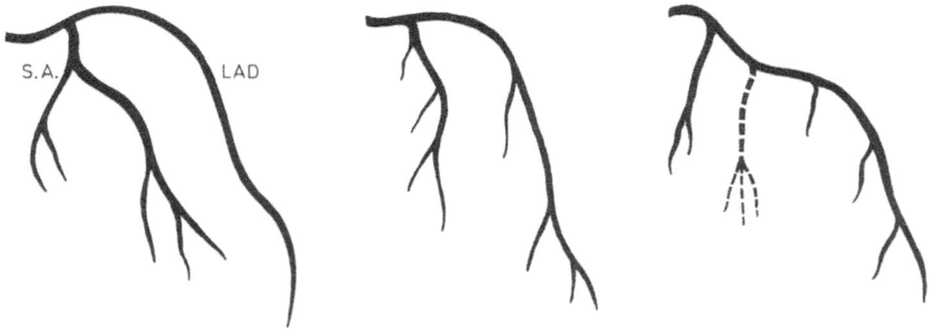

Fig. 2. Some of the most common septal artery configurations

Table 1. Septal artery revascularization, patient variables

	Group I Intermit. Aort. occl.	Group II Cardioplegia
Age (years)	55.0 ± 8.05	60.3 ± 7.45
Sex ratio (F/M)	9/59	6/38
No. D. A. per patient	5.0 ± 1.43	5.4 ± 1.26
XCL time	77 ± 23.5 min.	91 ± 28.8 $p = <0.01$
ETOB	195 ± 61.1 min.	164 ± 53 $p = <0.01$

D. A., distal anastomoses; XCL time, aortic cross-clamp time; ETOB, elapsed time of bypass

- Descending posterior artery diffusely diseased or not graftable because of small diameter (< 1.25 mm)

All operations were done with cardiopulmonary bypass. In regard to the method of myocardial preservation, intermittent aortic occlusion with systemic hypothermia (25°–28 °C) was used before July 1979, and cold cardioplegia since then.

The patients operated on with intermittent aortic occlusion numbered 68 (group I), while those who had cold cardioplegia for myocardial protection numbered 44 (group II). Data concerning the age, sex, number of distal anastomoses per patient, cross-clamp time, and elapsed time of cardiopulmonary bypass are presented for the two groups in Table 1.

The Operation

Dissection of the septal artery is currently done after aortic cross clamping during cardioplegic arrest (this accounts for the significantly longer aortic occlusion in group II).

Identification of the proximal LAD in the fatty tissue is usually facilitated by the presence of calcifications in this tract of the artery. The exact point of origin of the septal artery from LAD is localized from its angiographic relationship with the origin of the diagonal arteries, which are visible at the surface of the heart. The dissection is carried out at the right side of the LAD.

Table 2. Septal artery revascularization, graft construction (no. of patients = 112)

Single graft to septal	106	95%	"pure" single graft	88
			Y-graft	18
Sequential side to side graft to septal	6	5%		
In total: 582 distal anastomoses				
Average distal anastomoses per patient: 5.2				

Since septal arteries usually closer to the right than to the left ventricular endocardium, care must be taken not to enter the right ventricle. Once the septal artery has been identified, adequate exposure is obtained, retracting the fatty tissue with pledgetted sutures and taping the LAD proximally and distally to the septal artery.

All patients who had direct revascularization of a septal artery had diffuse coronary artery disease and received multiple distal anastomoses (average: 5.2 per patient).

In 106 patients the septal artery was revascularized by means of a single graft (88 "pure" single grafts and 18 "Y" grafts), while in 6 patients the septal artery received a laterolateral anastomosis from a graft ending on the distal LAD (Table 2).

Associated procedures were performed in seven patients of group I (two had mitral valve replacement, four had left ventricular aneurysmectomy, and one had carotid endarterectomy) and in three patients of group II (each had a left ventricular aneurysmectomy).

Results

The overall hospital mortality was 6.2% (7 out of 112). All patients who died were in group I. The cause of death was low cardiac output in three patients and multiple organ failure in four patients. Hospital complications in surviving patients included postoperative low cardiac output (four in group I and one in group II), perioperative myocardial infarction (four patients), supraventricular rhythm disturbances (26 patients), and requirement of prolonged ventilatory support (seven patients).

All patients who survived the operation have been followed up for a period ranging from 10 months to 7 years (average 3.8 years). Three late deaths have occurred, two due to acute myocardial infarction and one to pulmonary embolism.

Twelve patients had recurrent angina, and one of them underwent reoperation 3 years after the initial procedure. In this patient the graft to the septal artery was the only patent graft. The remaining 11 patients can be managed satisfactorily with medical treatment, although 7 of them have a positive exercise test.

Eighteen unselected patients were angiographically studied early postoperatively, and in 16 the septal artery graft was patent (89%). In the 11 symptomatic patients restudied 25 ± 7 months postoperatively, 7 septal artery grafts were patent (64%).

Discussion

Selection of patients for direct septal artery revascularization is based on the anatomical pattern of the blood supply to the ventricular septum. The blood supply to the human interventricular septum was described in 1958 by James and Burch, who showed that the blood flow to the septum is assured by septal branches of LAD and descending posterior artery. The septal branches of the LAD vascularize 80% of the septal muscle, while the branches of the descending posterior artery supply blood to the proximal septum, where the AV node and the His bundle are located, and represent a source of important potential collateral circulation toward the LAD area. Stoney et al., reviewing 100 coronary angiograms, found that a rather large septal artery supplying most of the interventricular septum is present in 30% of the cases [6].

However, direct septal artery revascularization was performed in less than 2% of the patients operated on for coronary artery disease by Stoney et al. [6] and by Bedard et al. [3]. Direct septal artery revascularization was done in 2.3% of the coronary operations in our institution.

Restrictive criteria of patient selection are justified by the fact that the surgical technique is demanding and requires experience. The hospital mortality was not negligible in this series, but the deaths occurred exclusively in patients operated on years ago with suboptimal myocardial protection.

The hospital mortality in patients who had septal artery revascularization was not significantly different from the hospital mortality in patients who required extensive myocardial revascularization (more than five distal anastomoses) before the introduction of cold cardioplegia as method of myocardial preservation [1]. The fact that no patient died out of the 44 in group II is very encouraging. Certainly when the myocardium is adequately protected during the aortic occlusion, direct septal artery revascularization can be performed safely without an increased hospital mortality and morbidity. Therefore a policy of complete revascularization should include direct grafting of septal arteries where indicated.

References

1. Alfieri O, Vermeulen F, Knaepen P, De Geest R, Huysmans H, Schaepkens van Riempst A (1980) Extensive myocardial revascularization – influence of cardioplegia. Thorac. Cardiovasc. Surg 28: 343–347
2. Alfieri O, Van Swieten H, Ascoop C, De Geest R, Knaepen P, Schaepkens van Riempst A, Vermeulen F (1982) Technique and operative results of extensive myocardial revascularization. In: Bruschke et al. (eds) Coronary artery disease today: diagnosis, surgery and prognosis. Excerpta Medica, Amsterdam, pp 279–284
3. Bedard P, Keon W, Brais M, Goldstein W (1980) First septal artery: direct or indirect grafting. Circulation 62 [Suppl 1]: 116–118
4. James T, Burch G (1958) Blood supply of the human interventricular septum. Circulation 17: 391–395
5. Liddle V (1981) Perspectives in coronary artery surgery. J Thorac Cardiovasc Surg 81: 1–10
6. Stoney WS, Vernon RP, Aflord SC Jr, Burrus GR, Thomas CS (1976) Revascularization of the septal artery. Ann Thorac Surg 21: 2–6
7. Vermeulen F, Alfieri O, Van Brussel B, Frey R, De Geest R, Pieké R, Knaepen P, Schaepkens van Riempst A (1982) Late results of complete versus incomplete revascularization. In: Bruschke et al. (eds) Coronary artery disease today: diagnosis, surgery and prognosis. Excerpta Medica, Amsterdam, pp 285–291

The Use of Timolol in Reducing the Incidence of Supraventricular Arrhythmias After Coronary Artery Bypass Surgery*

R. J. Vecht, J. Ikwueke, E. P. Nicolaides, C. Liassides, and J. Cleary

Introduction

A review of 13 publications dealing with the development of supraventricular arrhythmias after coronary artery bypass graft yielded a mean overall incidence of 27.5% (Table 1) [1–12]. In the U.S.A. some 100000 such operations are performed yearly [13] and something on the order of 30000 patients develop this postoperative complication. These arrhythmias often require cardioversion and invariably drug therapy. They can cause a drop in arterial pressure which could have deleterious effects on graft haemodynamics and subsequent long-term patency.

We conducted a retrospective analysis of 102 patients operated on at St. Mary's Hospital in 1981. The incidence of postoperative supraventricular arrhythmia was 18.2%, two-thirds of arrhythmias occurring in the first 24 h (Table 2).

The role of digoxin given prophylactically before surgery or postoperatively is still controversial [2, 3, 7, 10, 14, 15]. There is evidence that continued administration of beta-blocking agents after surgery reduces the incidence of postoperative supraventricular arrhythmias [4, 6, 12, 14]. The purpose of the present study was to establish whether timolol given 24 h after coronary artery bypass grafting had a suppressive anti-arrhythmic effect.

Materials and Methods

Patients undergoing exclusive coronary artery bypass grafting (132) were randomised postoperatively (when able to take oral medication) to receive double-blind timolol 10 mg b.d. or matched placebo. Exclusion criteria included hypotension (systolic < 90 mmHg), bradycardia (< 48 beats/min) and the standard contra-indications for receiving beta blockers.

Results

During the period of this trial, 225 patients underwent coronary artery bypass grafting of these 132 patients were randomised: 66 receiving timolol and 66 placebo. Excluded from the trial were 93 patients, 77 of these were closely followed up.

In the placebo group 13 patients developed supraventricular arrhythmias (19.7%) compared to 5 patients given timolol (7.5%; $p < 0.05$). In the group of 77 excluded from the trial, 14 patients exhibited supraventricular arrhythmias (18.2%; 71.4% of

* This work was supported by a grant made available by Merck, Sharpe & Dohme Ltd.

Table 1. Incidence of arrhythmias after CABG: review of 13 publications, 1974–1982

Year	Author	No. of pts	%SVT	%VT/VF
1974	Angelini [1]	75	13.3	13.3
1975	Rose [2]	15	40.0	6.6
1976	Johnson[a] [3]	66	25.7	5.0
1979	Boudoulas[a] [4]	50	30.0	–
1979	Michelson [5]	50	28.0	4.0
1979	Salazar[a] [6]	22	50.0	–
1979	Tyras[a] [7]	79	11.4	–
1980	Stephenson[a] [8]	136	18.0	5.0
1980	Oka[a] [9]	52	38.4	–
1981	Csicsko[a] [10]	270	15.2	1.8
1981	Buxton [11]	99	29.0	–
1981	Mohr[a] [12]	48	40.0	–
1981	St. Mary's	102	18.2	6.8
	Total	1064	Mean 27.5	Mean 6.0

SVT, supraventricular tachychardia; VT, ventricular tachychardia; VF, ventricular fibrillation; pts, patients

[a] Randomised studies, control groups only considered

Table 2. Incidence of arrhythmias in 102 patients undergoing coronary artery bypass graft (St. Mary's 1981)

	No. pts	A. fib	A. tachy.	A. flut	VT	VF	V. bigem.
Preoperative	102	–	–	–	–	–	–
Operative	102	–	–	–	–	6	–
Postoperative	99						
early	–	8	3 (1 DC)	1	1(DC)	–	1
late		4 (1 DC)	4 (3 DC)	3 (1 DC)	–	–	–

Incidence of SVA = 18.2%
Incidence of early SVA = 66.6%

Abbreviations: pts, patients; A. fib, atrial fibrillation; A. tachy, atrial tachycardia; A. flut, atrial flutter; VT, ventricular tachycardia; VF, ventricular fibrillation; V. bigem, ventricular bigeminy; DC, direct current cardioversion

these occurring within 48 h). In the trial groups, there were no significant differences with regard to age, sex, pre-operative blood pressure, cardiothoracic ratio or operative details such as duration of cardiopulmonary bypass or aortic cross-clamping.

The mean time of administration of trial medication was 21.7 h in the placebo group and 23.4 h in the timolol group (*P*: N.S.) Of the 18 patients who developed supraventricular arrhythmias, only one was not on beta blockers prior to surgery.

Discussion

There is a universal incidence of supraventricular arrhythmia after coronary artery bypass graft of approximately 30%, giving rise to an established morbidity without, as yet, an accepted mode of prevention. The use of digoxin either prophylactically or postoperatively has been advocated by some and shown to have adverse effects by others [2, 3, 7, 10, 14, 15]. In 102 patients given digoxin routinely at St. Mary's Hospital in 1981, the incidence of postoperative supraventricular arrhythmia was similar to that seen in the 66 patients receiving placebo, who were not digitalised.

Several studies have now shown the benefit of postoperative beta blocker administration. Combining digoxin and propranolol also appears effective [14]. We have shown conclusively in a randomised double-blind study that postoperative administration of timolol significantly reduced the incidence of supraventricular arrhythmia, particularly in patients who were on beta blockers before surgery. We encountered no serious side effects other than hypotension in five patients, who reverted spontaneously after withdrawal of timolol. We believe that earlier administration of timolol after surgery would have resulted in a still lower incidence of supraventricular arrhythmia since, in the majority, this complication occurred in the first 48 h postoperatively.

Acknowledgements. We wish to thank the physicians and surgeons whose patients were included in the trial, in particular, Mr. S.C. Lennox, Mr. R. Sapsford, Mr. R. Stanbridge, Dr. E.M.M. Besterman, Dr. P.H. Kidner. Our thanks are also extended to Miss M. Petrie for secretarial assistance.

References

1. Angelini P, Feldman MI, Lufschanowski R, Leachman RD (1974) Cardiac arrhythmias during and after heart surgery: diagnosis and management. Prog Cardiovasc Dis 16 (5): 469–495
2. Rose MR, Glassman E, Spencer FC (1975) Arrhythmias following cardiac surgery: relation to serum digoxin levels. Am Heart J 89 (3): 288–294
3. Johnson LW, Dickstein RA, Fruehan CT, Kane P, Poots JL, Smulyan H, Webb WR, Eich RH (1976) Prophylactic digitalisation for coronary artery bypass surgery. Circulation 53 (5): 819–822
4. Boudoulas H, Lewis RP, Snyser GL, Karayannocos P, Vasko JS (1979) Beneficial effects of continuation of propranolol through coronary bypass surgery. Clin Cardiol 2: 87–91
5. Michelson EL, Morganroth J, Mac Vaugh H (1979) Postoperative arrhythmias after coronary artery and cardiac valvular surgery detected by long-term electrocardiographic monitoring. Am Heart J 97 (4): 442–448
6. Salazar G, Frishman W, Friedman S, Patel J, You Tse Lin, Oka Y, Frater RWM, Becker RM (1979) β-Blockade therapy for supraventricular tachyarrhythmias after coronary surgery: a propranolol withdrawal syndrome? Angiology 30: 816–819
7. Tyras DH, Stothert JC, Kaiser GC, Barnes HB, Codd JE, Willman VL (1979) Supraventricular tachyarrhythmias after myocardial revascularisation: a randomised trial of prophylactic digitalisation. J Thorac Cardiovasc Surg 77 (2): 310–314
8. Stephenson LW, MacVaugh H, Tomasello DN, Josephson ME (1980) Propranolol for prevention of post-operative cardiac arrhythmias: a randomised study. Ann Thorac Surg 29: 113–116
9. Oka Y, Frishman W, Becker RM, Kadish A, Strom J, Matsumoto M, Orkin L, Frater R (1980) Clinical pharmacology of the new beta adrenergic blocking drugs, part 10. Beta adrenoceptor blockade and coronary artery surgery. Am Heart J 99 (2): 255–269
10. Csicsko JF, Schatzlein MH, King RD (1981) Immediate postoperative digitalisation in the prophylaxis of supraventricular arrhythmias following coronary artery bypass. Thorac Cardiovas Surg 81: 419–422

11. Buxton AE, Josephson ME (1981) The role of P Wave Duration as a predictor of postoperative atrial arrhythmias. Chest 80: 68–73
12. Mohr R, Smolinsky A, Goor DA (1981) Prevention of supraventricular tachyarrhythmias with low dose propranolol after coronary bypass. J Thorac Cardiovasc Surg 81: 840–845
13. Roberts WC, Mason DT, Engle MA, Cohn LM (1982) Cardiology 1982. Yorke Medical p 69
14. Mills SA, Poole GV, Breyer RH, Holliday RM, Lavender SW, Blanton KR, Hudspeth AS, Johnston FR, Cordell AR (1983) Digoxin and propranolol in the prophylaxis of dysrhythmias after coronary artery bypass grafting. Circulation 68 (Suppl 11): 222
15. Chee TP, Prakash NS, Desser KB, Benchimol A (1982) Post-operative supraventricular arrhythmias and the role of prophylactic digoxin in cardiac surgery. Am Heart J 104: 974

Effect of the Bypass Pump Priming Fluid on the Metabolic Response to Open-Heart Surgery

C. K. McKnight, M J. Elliot, D. T. Pearson, M. P. Holden, and K. G. M. M. Alberti

Introduction

The metabolic response to open-heart surgery has been extensively studied during the past 30 years, and yet there are wide quantitative differences in the reported hormonal and metabolite changes.

Although it has been shown that the response is modified by different anaesthetic techniques [1, 2], pulsatile flow [3] and hypothermia [4] during bypass, there is a lack of controlled studies to investigate the possibility that the nature of the cardiopul-

Table 1. Composition of the bypass pump-priming fluids used in the various groups

Priming fluids			
Group A			
Hartmann's solution	Na^+	131	mmol/l
(lactate/no glucose)	K^+	5	mmol/l
	Ca^{++}	2	mmol/l
	Cl^-	111	mmol/l
	lactate	29	mmol/l
Group B			
Hartmann's solution/5% dextrose	dextrose	25	g/l
(lactate/glucose)	Na^+	66	mmol/l
	K^+	2.5	mmol/l
	Ca^{++}	1	mmol/l
	Cl^-	56	mmol/l
	lactate	15	mmol/l
Group C			
Plasmalyte 148 (Travenol)	Na^{++}	140	mmol/l
(no lactate/no glucose)	K^+	5	mmol/l
	Ca^{++}	5	mmol/l
	Mg^{++}	1.5	mmol/l
	Cl^-	80	mmol/l
	Acetate	27	mmol/l
Group D			
Solution 11 (Travenol)	dextrose	25	g/l
(no lactate/glucose)	Na^{++}	102	mmol/l
	K^+	5	mmol/l
	Ca^{++}	2.5	mmol/l
	Mg^{++}	2	mmol/l
	Cl^-	107	mmol/l
	gluconate	5	mmol/l
	phos-phate	1	mmol/l

monary bypass pump-priming fluid may also modulate this response. In order to investigate the effect of different pump primes on the metabolic response to open-heart surgery we carried out the following study

The Study

Twenty-four well-matched adult patients undergoing elective heart valve replacement were investigated. All patients were free of hepatic, metabolic and renal disease, and all had a normal pre-operative glucose tolerance test. No patient was taking β-blockers. The same surgical, anaesthetic and perfusion techniques were used in all cases, with hypothermic (28 °C), pulsatile cardiopulmonary bypass.

The patients were randomly allocated to receive one of the four crystalloid pump primes described in Table 1, which includes all the commonly used primes in the United Kingdom. Blood samples were drawn at frequent intervals from 1 day pre-operatively to 7 days postoperatively for the assay of cortisol, glucagon, growth hormone, insulin and intermediary metabolites.

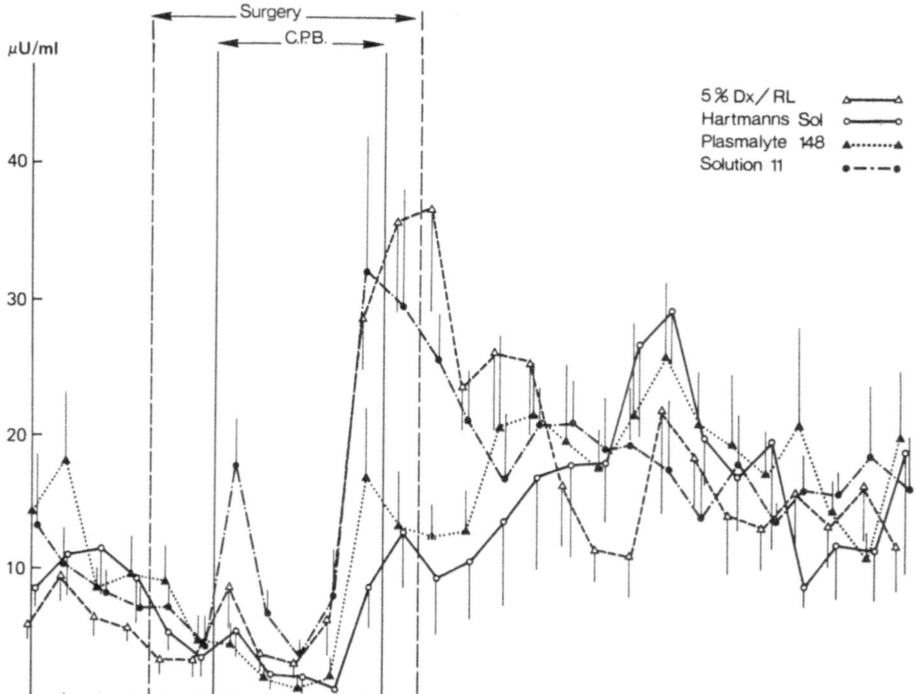

Fig. 1. Insulin levels for the four patient groups. *P. O. D.* postoperative day; *C. P. B.*, cardiopulmonary bypass; *5%DX/RL*, Hartmann's solution/5% dextrose

Results

There were no significant differences between groups in cortisol, glucagon or growth hormone levels at any stage during the study. Cortisol started to rise with the skin incision and reached a peak on the first postoperative day. Glucagon levels only started to increase 4 h after the end of surgery but also peaked on the first postoperative day. Growth hormone values increased steadily during surgery reaching a maximum 5 min before the end of cardiopulmonary bypass, and returning to normal over the first 8 h postoperatively.

The serum insulin response of the four groups is depicted graphically in Fig. 1. Serum insulin levels fell in all groups during the hypothermic phase of bypass. With rewarming there was a marked increase in insulin, with significantly higher values in the two groups allocated glucose-containing primes. This difference had disappeared by 4 h after the end of surgery. Insulin levels remained significantly elevated for the week following surgery when compared with pre-operative values.

The blood glucose levels for the four groups are shown in Fig. 2. Those groups allocated to receive glucose-containing primes had markedly elevated blood glucose levels for the duration of bypass (of the order of 25–30 mmol/l), but there was no significant difference between groups from 4 h postoperatively.

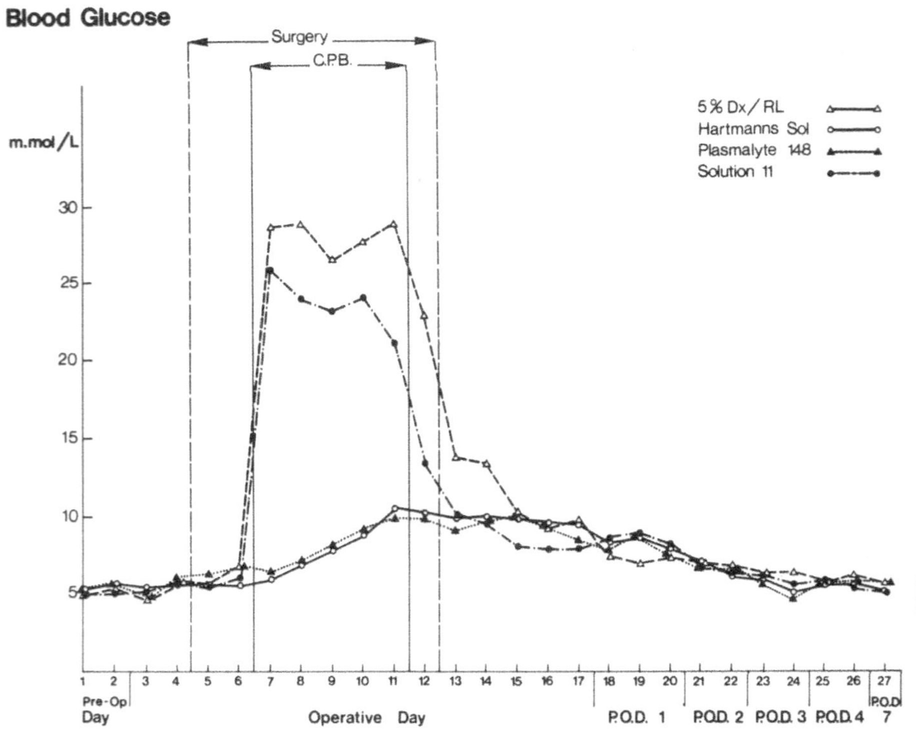

Fig. 2. Blood glucose levels for the four patient groups. *P. O. D.*, postoperative day; *C. P. B.*, cardiopulmonary bypass; *5% DX/RL*, Hartmann's solution/5% dextrose

Blood glucose levels in all groups were significantly elevated until the 3rd day after the operation, and this, along with the elevated insulin levels, demonstrates prolonged postoperative insulin resistance. Similarly, the presence of lactate in the priming fluid resulted in lactate levels during bypass that were significantly higher than in patients with non-lactate-containing primes, but all differences between the groups had disappeared by 2 h after the end of surgery. Serum levels of alanine (the major gluconeogenic precursor to arise from muscle) and glycerol (the major gluconeogenic precursor to arise from fat) showed no significant differences between groups at any stage.

Conclusion

Our study has shown that the nature of the crystalloid cardiopulmonary bypass pump-priming fluid had little effect on the hormonal response to open-heart surgery, except for transiently elevated insulin levels at the end of the prodedure when glucose-containing primes were used. In addition, the differences in intermediary metabolites that occurred during bypass were related merely to their inclusion in the prime, and in no case did any difference between groups extend for more than 4 h postoperatively.

References

1. Walsh ES, Paterson JL, O'Riodan JBA, Hall GM (1981) Effect of high dose fentanyl anaesthesia on the metabolic and endocrine response to cardiac surgery. Br J Anaesth 53: 1155–1164
2. Brandt MR, Korshin J, Prange-Hansen A, Hummer L, Nistrup-Modsen S, Rygg I, Kehlet H (1978) Influence of morphine anaesthesia on the endocrine-metabolic response to open heart surgery. Acta Anaesthesiol Scand 22: 400–412
3. Taylor KM, Wright GS, Reid JM, Bain WH, Caves PK, Walker MS, Grant JK (1978) Comparative studies of pulsatile and non-pulsatile flow during cardio-pulmonary bypass: II. The effects on adrenal secretion of cortisol. J Thorac Cardiovasc Surg 75 (4): 574–578
4. Moffitt EA, Sessler AD, Molnar GD, McGoon DC (1971) Normothermia versus hypothermia for whole body perfusion: effects on myocardial and body metabolism. Anesth Analg (Cleve) 50 (4): 505–516

Hemodynamic Results with Hemofiltration in Postoperative Cardiac Surgical Patients

F. Coraim, H. Kassal, G. Pauser, F. Stellwag, and E. Wolner

Introduction

Cardiogenic shock in the postoperative period of cardiac surgery still seems to be a life-threatening complication despite counterpulsation and potent pharmacological treatment [17, 22, 27, 30, 31, 33]. Effective catecholamine medication usually increases myocardial oxygen consumption [4, 15, 17, 18, 22, 27, 30, 33]. Focal necroses within the myocardial structure can sometimes be detected after treatment [24, 25, 27, 28] and tachycardia may also increase oxygen consumption [4, 17, 18, 22, 29–31, 33]. Hypoxia, acidosis, and ischemia as a result of hemodynamic deterioration will be seen in almost all organs [10, 11, 13, 14]. These unfavorable conditions are most deleterious to organs in the splanchnic region [9, 12, 19–21, 29]. They produce as a result toxic peptides like myocardial depressant factor (MDF) and lysosomal enzymes [1, 2, 6–9, 12, 19–21, 26, 29, 32]. These peptides seem to be the humoral component of the shock state, whose effect is usually considered only with regard to hemodynamics. Counterpulsation lowers myocardial oxygen consumption by reducing afterload and increases coronary blood flow, especially in the diastole [2, 27, 31, 33, 34]. Nevertheless toxic peptides remain in the circulation [4, 6, 7], and paralyze the peripheral vascular compartment [4, 6, 7, 27]. Counterpulsation at this point produces almost no effect [2, 4–7]. The resulting circulus vitiosus will lead to further deterioration [11].

Hemofiltration (HF) seems to be a good method to eliminate these peptides from the circulation [4, 8, 23]. A mechanism which is not yet well understood helps to restore the membrane potential and metabolism of the cell [11].

Method

The femoral vessels are connected via an arteriovenous cannulation to a hemofiltration cartridge (Amicon D20) mounted bedside. Continuous heparinization is used to the arterial line (10 units/kg body weight. The volume of hemofiltrate containing the toxic peptides [5–8] (MDF) and shock mediators is immediately replaced by crystalloid solutions administered intravenously. Toxic peptides and substances with molecular weights lower than 10000 daltons can pass through the filter [32, 33]. A quantitative analysis of these peptides using a modified Biuret method [9, 16] shows a distinct increase in shock patients (Figs. 1, 2). The MDF-containing fraction shown in our curve as peak B was isolated from plasma by gel filtration and ion exchange chromatography [9, 12, 20, 26]. The same method was used to determine MDF concentrations in the hemofiltrate. A bioassay using the papillary muscle of a guinea pig shows the decreased contractility after application of hemofiltrate from a shock patient (Fig. 3) compared to hemofiltrate from a control subject (Fig. 4).

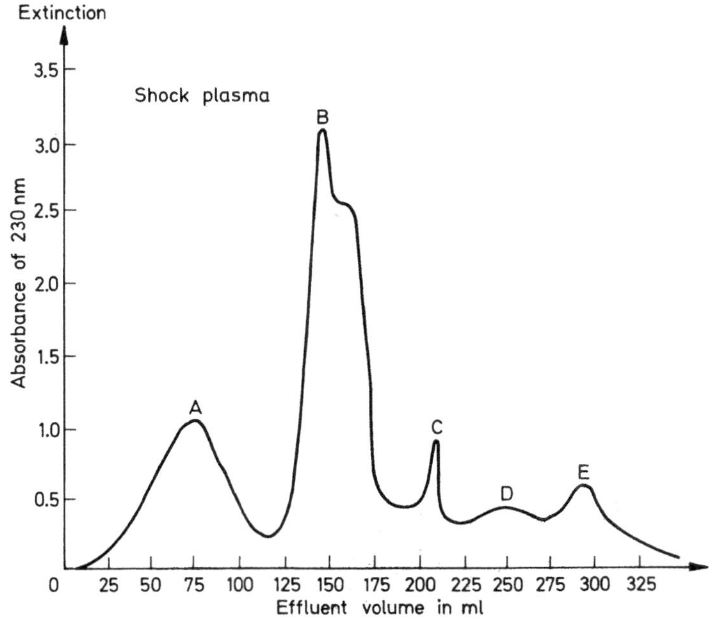

Fig. 1. Chromatographic pattern of low molecular weight peptides in a patient with postoperative cardiogenic shock. Peak *B* represents the extinction activity of toxic peptides (MDF).

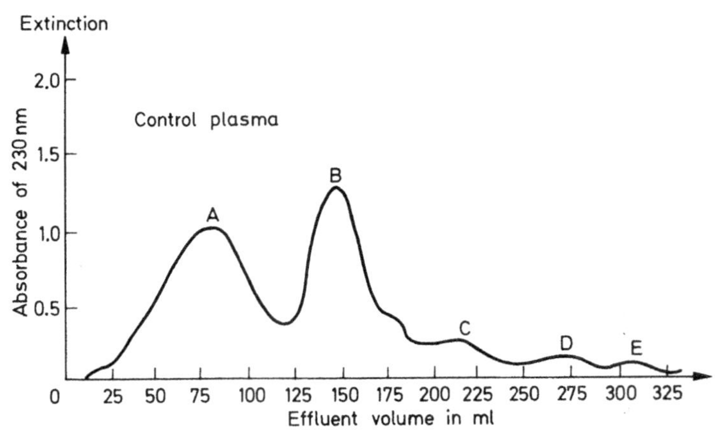

Fig. 2. Chromatographic pattern of low molecular weight peptides in a control group subject without increased toxic peptide activity.

We used HF in 23 patients of 31–74 years of age (mean age 53 years). There were 3 females and 20 males. There were five patients treated after aortic valve replacement (AVR), five patients after mitral valve replacement (MVR), four patients after aortocoronary bypass procedures, and nine after combined operations. All patients had developed cardiogenic shock soon after surgery and did not respond to cate-

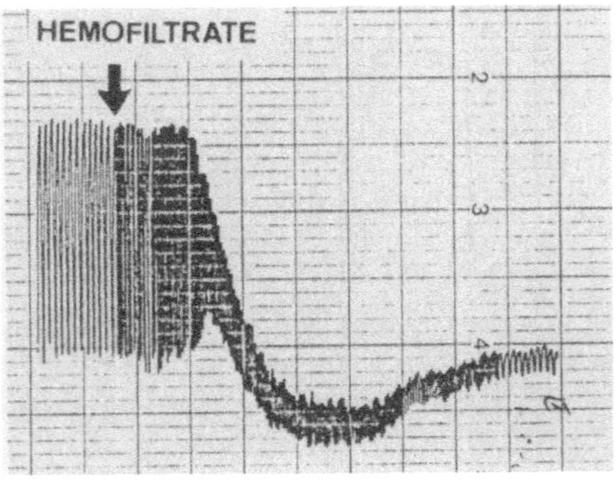

Fig. 3. Decreased contractility in an isolated guinea pig papillary muscle after treatment with hemofiltrate from a shock patient.

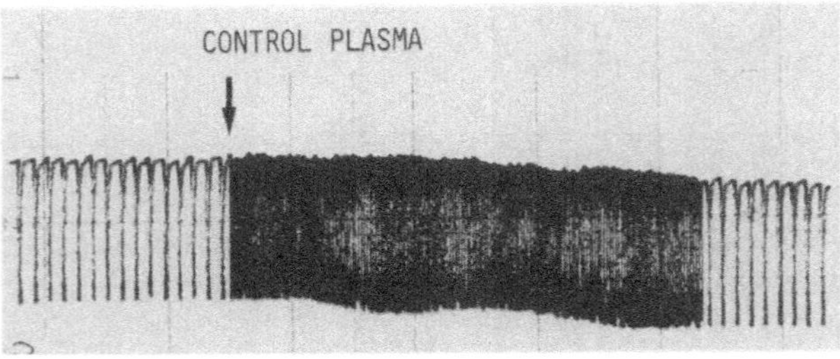

Fig. 4. Unchanged contractility of a guinea pig papillary muscle after application of a hemofiltrate sample from a control subject.

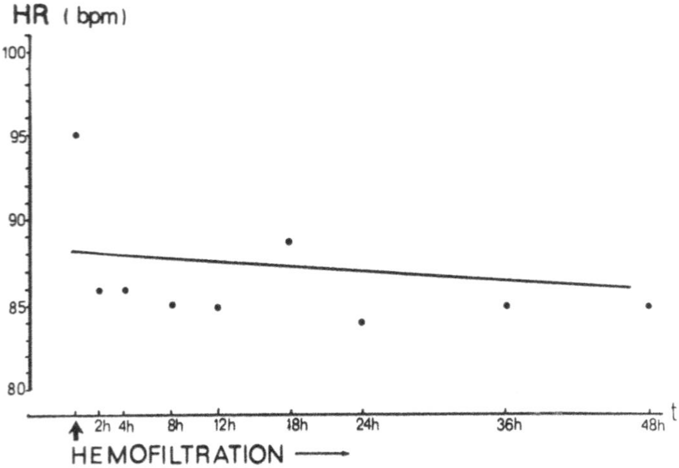

Fig. 5. Heart rate (HR) changes in 23 patients after HF

cholamine treatment. Ten patients had additional intraaortic balloon pump treatment. Swan-Ganz catheters were inserted in nine patients. Hemodynamics were evaluated using the standard procedures of a postoperative care unit. The following hemodynamic parameters were registered on line, stored, and calculated in a computer: mean arterial pressure ($\bar{p}$Art), left atrial mean pressure (LAP), pulmonary artery mean pressure (PAMP), central venous pressure (CVP), cardiac index CCT), stroke volume index (SVI), left ventricular stroke work index (LVSWI), total peripheral resistance (TPR), and pulmonary vascular resistance (PVR).

Hemodynamic Results

Heart Rate

The heart rate showed a significant decrease from 95 ± 3.9 (SD) bpm before HF to 86 ± 3.3 bpm after 2 h. After 24 h the rate was 84 ± 3 bpm (11.2% slower) (Fig. 5).

Left atrial Mean Pressure, Pulmonary Artery Mean Pressure, and Central Venous Pressure

The decreases in LAP, PAMP, and CVP were highly significant (Fig. 6; $p < 0.01$). LAP, which was 26 ± 1.5 (SD) mmHg before HF, decreased to 20 ± 4 mmHg (minus 24%) after 2 h. After 24 h a value of 19 ± 3 mmHg was reached (minus 27%). The

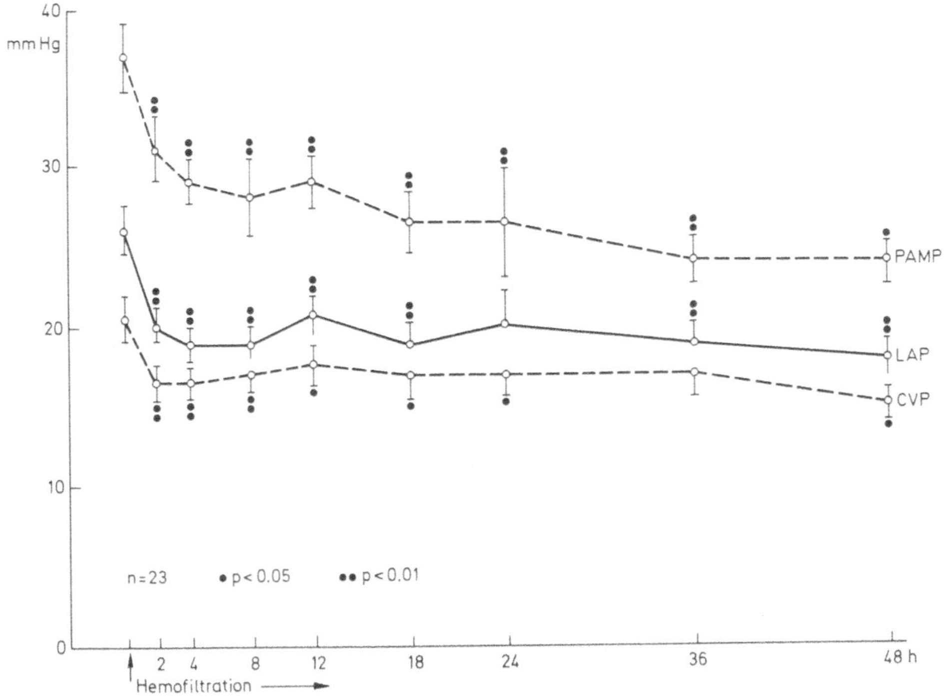

Fig. 6. Pulmonary artery mean pressure *(PAMP)*, left atrial pressure *(LAP)*, central venous pressure *(CVP)* in our series ($n = 23$) before and during HF

PAMP decreased from 37±2.5 mmHg before HF to 30±2.1 mmHg after 2 h (minus 19%). The tendency to decrease continued, and the PAMP reached 26±3.5 mmHg (minus 30%) after 24 h.

Mean Arterial Pressure

The p̄Art (Fig. 7) increased from 52±1.5 (SD) mmHg before HF up to 66±5.3 mmHg (plus 20%) after 2 h and to 77±4.2 mmHg (plus 45%) after 24 h and remained constant thereafter ($p<0.01$).

Left Ventricular Stroke Work Index

The LVSWJ (Fig. 8) increased from 23.5±3.4 (SD) g/min/m² to 33±1.3 g/min/m² after 2 h (plus 68%) and reached 45.4±2.3 g/min/m² (plus 93%) after 24 h ($p<0.01$)

Total Peripheral Resistance and Pulmonary Vascular Resistance

The TPR (Fig. 9) was 433±256 (SD) dyne s cm^{-5}. After 2 h of HF the TPR increased to 582±263 dyne s cm^{-5} and to 628±238 dyne s cm^{-5} (plus 45%) after 24 h. These data suggest a severe peripheral paralysis before HF. A continuous increase of TPR is seen during HF treatment. A 99% significant decrease of the PVR was seen in our patients, indicating a good oxygen diffusion improvement in the

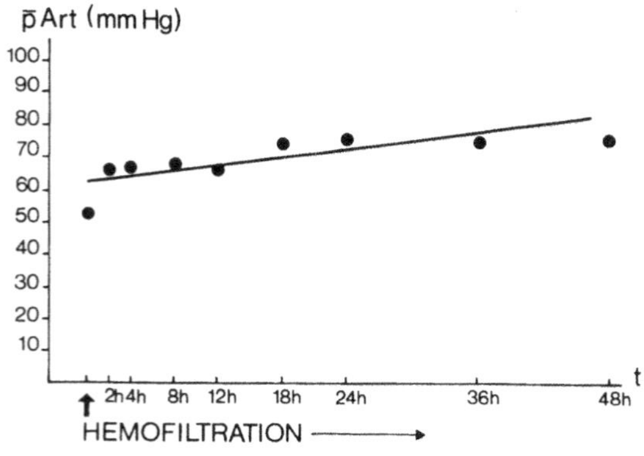

Fig. 7. Mean arterial pressure *(p̄Art)* in 23 patients before and during HF

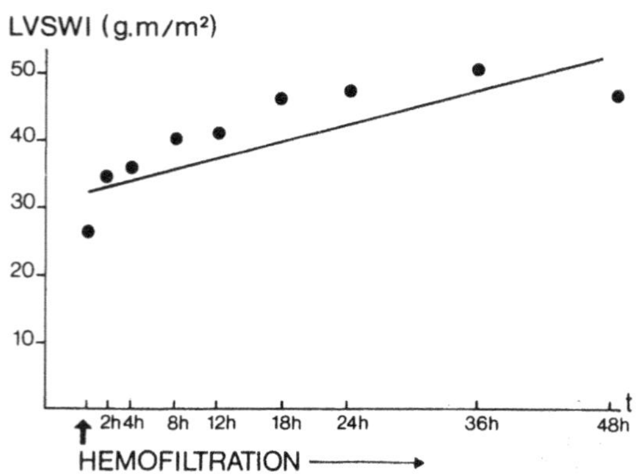

Fig. 8. Left ventricular stroke work index *(LVSWI)* in nine patients during HF

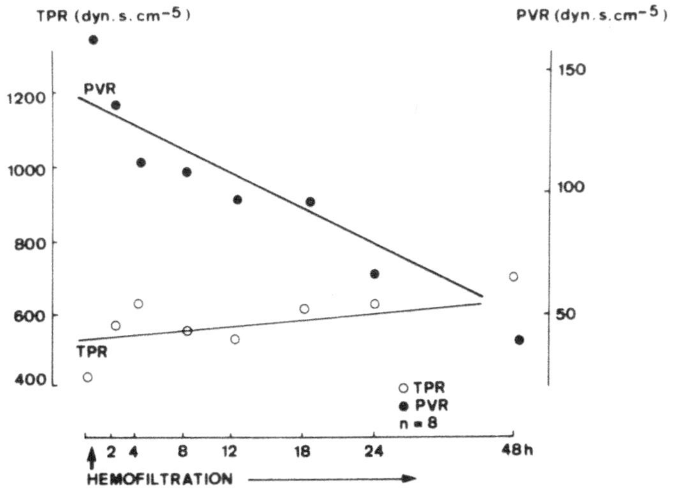

Fig. 9. Total peripheral vascular resistance *(TPR)* compared to pulmonary vascular resistance *(PVR)* in our patients ($n=9$).

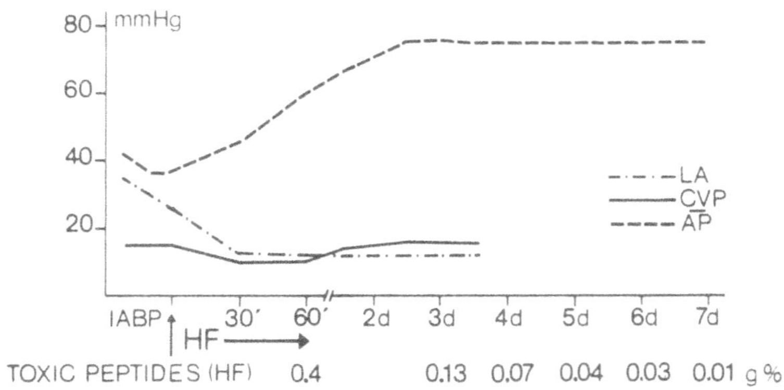

EPINEPHRINE	0.48	0.64	0.48	0.24	0.24	0.048	0.012	0	0	0	mcg/kg/min
DOBUTAMINE	54	44	40	27	23	23	6.7	4.5	0	0	mcg/kg/min
DOPAMINE	16	16	12	10	5	2.4	2.4	0	0	0	mcg/kg/min

Fig. 10. Hemodynamics in a postoperative patient undergoing HF, with concomitant reduction of catecholamines. *LA*, left atrial pressure; *CVP*, Central venous pressure; $\overline{AP}$, mean arterial pressure; *IABP*, intraaortic balloon pumping.

lung. Figure 10 shows some hemodynamic data of a 48-year-old male after AVR. HF was started 24 h after surgery. The primary postoperative treatment with high doses of catecholamine and intraaortic balloon pumping did not produce any result. The catecholamine dosage could be decreased immediately after HF was started. At the same time the amount of toxic peptides eliminated in the hemofiltrate decreased gradually. The patient's overall situation became better. Of the patients

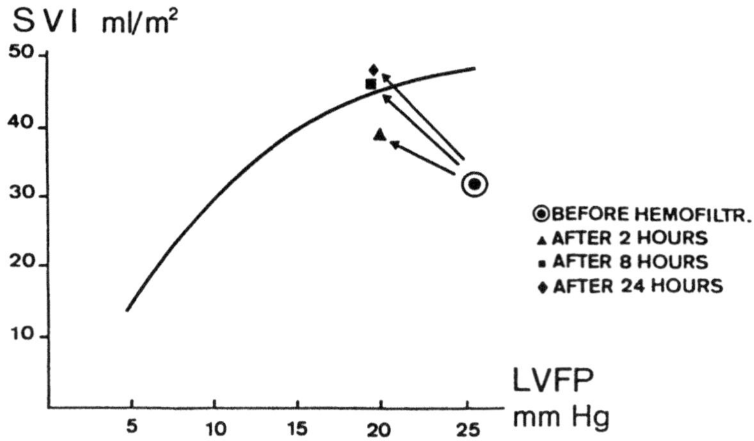

Fig. 11. Left atrial pressure *(LAP)* changes (ΔLAP in HF group patients compared to a control group).

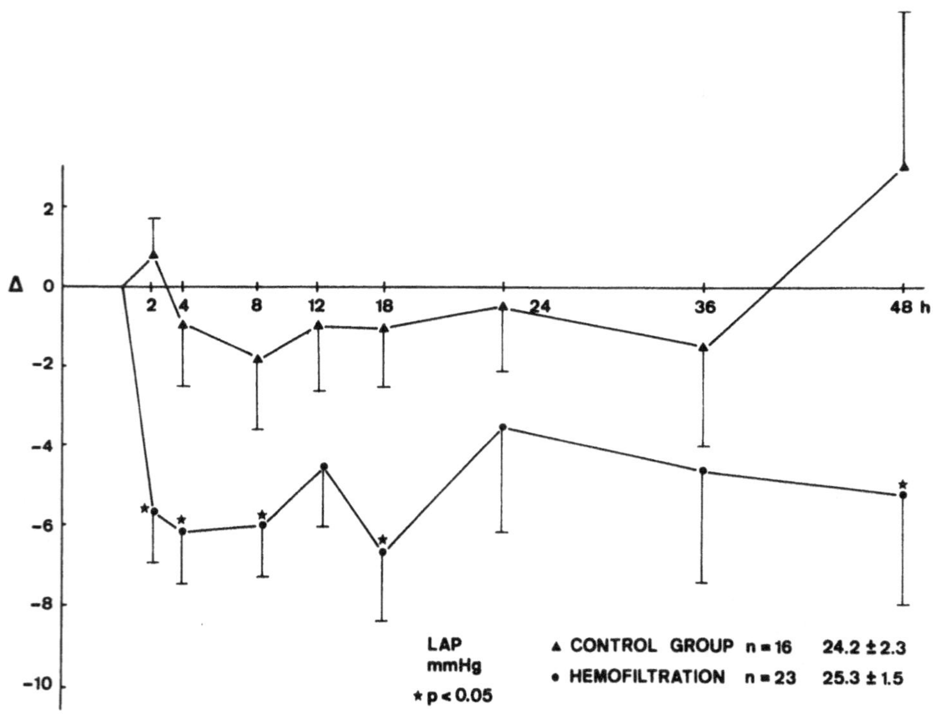

Fig. 12. Stroke volume index *(SVI)* and left ventricular filling pressure *(LVFP)* before and after HF (Starling's law).

treated with HF, two died within 12 h from cardiogenic shock. The shock state was successful treated in 21 patients. Eight of this group died in the hospital within 2 to 4 weeks, from causes other than cardiogenic shock. Thirteen patients recovered successfully and left the hospital. We compared this group with a control group having similar basic conditions after heart surgery. HF was not available for them at that time. Out of this control group of 16 patients, 10 died and only 6 recovered.

Discussion

The data presented show a significant improvement of hemodynamics with HF in patients with cardiogenic shock after various cardiac surgical procedures involving extracorporeal circulation [5–8].
The LAP, an important hemodynamic parameter indicating the functional state of the left ventricle, showed a significant decrease in our series with HF compared to a control group (Fig. 11). Considering the SVI and the left ventricular filling pressure (LVFP) according to Starling's law before and after HF, a distinct shift to the left side is noticed (Fig. 12). Improved subendocardial perfusion [15, 18] and improved contractility follow. As shown above, HF is able to eliminate toxic peptides like MDF and lysosomal enzymes [1, 3, 5–10, 12–14, 18, 20, 26, 29, 32] which are proven to have a negative inotropic effect as well as to be deleterious to oxygen exchange in the lung [13, 14, 18]. After elimination of toxic peptides the arterial pressure increases. At the same time coronary perfusion is much better and organ perfusion guaranteed. The peripheral paralysis may gradually decrease.

All these preliminary data indicate an obvious improvement in all our patients treated with HF for postoperative cardiogenic shock. Therefore we conclude that the concept of elimination of toxic humoral products from the circulation in cardiogenic shock seems to be at least as important as counterpulsation and catecholamine treatment.

References

1. Addonizio VP, Strauss JF, Chang LF, Fischer CA, Colman RW, Edmunds LH (1982) Release of lysosomal Hydrolases during simulated extracorporeal circulation. J Thorac Cardiovasc Surg 84: 28
2. Blanke H, Rentop P, Karsch KR, Hellberg T, Kirchhoff PD, Kreuzer H (1980) Invasive Diagnostik und Therapie im kardiogenen Schock: Kreislaufschock. Anesth Intensivmed 125: 127
3. Brand ED, Lefer AM (1966) Myocardial depressant factor in plasma from cats in irreversible post-oligemic shock. Proc Soc Exp Biol Med 122: 200
4. Bruckner JB, Hess W, Oser G, Schmidt D, Schneider E, Schweichel E (1976) Kreislaufveränderungen und Sauerstoffversorgung des Herzens unter Dopamin. Dopamin-Symposium, Mainz, 1976, Supp p 73
5. Coraim F, Duma St, Fina U, Krisch I (1983) Die Wirkung von Katecholaminen vor und nach Haemofiltration beim kardiogenen Lungenoedem. Wien Klin Wochenschr 133 (Suppl): 74
6. Coraim F, Haider W, Krisch I, Wolner E (1983) Haemofiltration während der extrakorporalen Zirkulation. 1. Herzchirurgie Symposium Zürs

7. Coraim F, Haider W, Stellwag F, Wolner E (1983) Die Wirkung der Haemofiltration auf den postoperativen pulmonalen Gasaustausch nach Herzoperationen. 1. Herzchirurgie Symposium Zürs
8. Coraim F, Stellwag F, Deutsch M, Wolner E (1983) Die Haemofiltration nach herzchirurgischen Eingriffen – Haemodynamische Ergebnisse. 1. Herzchirurgie Symposium Zürs
9. Curtis MT, Lefer AM (1983) Actions of opiate atnagonists with selctive receptor interactions in hemorrhagic shock. Circ Shock 10: 131–145
10. Eisenbach J (1974) Die Problematik des postischaemischen Organschadens am Beispiel der temporären Lungenischaemie. 7. Neue Aspekte der Trasylol Therapie. Schattauer, Stuttgart, p 127
11. Erdmann N (1972) Pathophysiologie der zellulären Sauerstoffversorgung im Schock. In: Frey R, Stossek K, (eds) Der Schock und seine Behandlung. Fischer, Stuttgart, p 91
12. Glenn TM, Lefer AM, Martin JM, Lovett WL, Morris JN, Wangensteen SL (1971) Production of myocardial depressant factor in cardiogenic shock. Am Heart J 82: 78
13. Heine H (1980) Allgemeine Grundlagen des intestinal induzierten Schocks. I. Medizinische Gespräche, 29. November 1980, Bamberg
14. Heine H, Trenkel K, Arbogast R, Eisenbach J (1980) Funktionelle Morphologie von Endstrombahn und Transitstrecke. Probleme beim Schock. Med Welt 15: 558
15. Hess W, Brückner JB, Faber du Fauz JV, Schmidt D, Tarnow J (1979) Hämodynamische Wirkung von Dobutamin und Dopamin bei Patienten mit koronarer Herzkrankheit. Anaesthesist 28: 316
16. Hirs CHW (1967) Detection of peptides by chemical methods. Methods Enzymol 11: 325
17. Halloway E, Stinson EA, Derby CC, Harrison DC (1975) Action of drugs in patients early after cardiac surgery. I. Comparison of isoproterenol and dopamine. Am J Cardiol 35: 656
18. Horpacsy G, Schnells G (1982) Die Bedeutung der lysosomalen Enzyme in der experimentellen und klinischen Schockforschung. Intensive Care Med 1: 12
19. Lefer AM (1973) Blood-borne humoral factor in the pathophysiology of circulatory shock. Circ Res 32: 87
20. Lefer AM, Glenn TM (1972) Interaction of lysosomal hydrolases and a myocardial depressant factor in pathogenesis of circulatory shock. In: Forscher BK, Lillehei RC, Stubbs SS (eds) Shock in low and high flow states. Excerpta Medica, Amsterdam, p 88
21. Lefer AM, Martin J (1970) Relationship of plasma peptides to the myocardial depressant factor in hemorrhagic shock in cats. Circ Res 26: 59
22. Litwak RS, Kuhn LA, Gadboys KL, Lukban SB, Sakurai H (1968) Support of myocardial performance after open cardiac operations by rate augmentation. J Thorac Cardiovasc Surg 56: 484
23. Mann H, Schultes R, Homburg A, Raguse T, Rantenbach R (1978) Haemofiltration in Intensivmedizin. Intensivtherapie 2: 15
24. Morales AR, Fine G, Taber RE (1967) Cardiac surgery and myocardial necrosis. Arch Pathol 83: 71
25. Najafi H, Henson D, Dye WS, Javid H, Hunter JA, Callghan R, Eisenstein JOC (1969) Left ventricular hemorrhagic necrosis. Ann Thorac Surg 7: 550
26. Okuda M, Yamada T, Hosono K (1975) activity of myocardial depressant factor and associated lysosomal abnormalities in experimental cardiogenic shock. 8. New aspects of trasylol therapy. Schattauer, Stuttgart, pp 183–199
27. Reichart B, Türk R, Alt E, Kemkes B, Kreuzer E, Holtz J, Franke N, Schmucker P (1981) Treatment of acute left heart failure using dobutamine and intraaortic counterpulsation. Intensive Care Med 3: 133
28. Robert WC, Morrow AG (1967) Causes of early postoperative death following cardiac valve replacement. J Thorac Cardiovasc Surg 54: 422
29. Sicuteri F, DelBianco PL, Curradi C, Monetti G (1975) The kinin system in cardiogenic shock. 8. New aspects of trasylol therapy. Schattauer, Stuttgart, pp 357–369
30. Sonneblick EH, Downing SE (1963) Afterload as a primary determinant of ventricular performance. Am J Physiol 204: 606
31. Spiller P, Bormkoel K, Kreutzer H, Neuhaus KL, Niessen HW, Schulte HD (1975) Intra-

aortic balloon pumping in cardiogenic shock after cardiac surgery. Thoraxchirurgie 23: 364–367
32. Stephen L, Wangensteen S, De Holl JD, Stephen BS, Kriechel F, Martin J, Lefer AM (1970) Influence of hemodialysis on myocardial depressant factor in hemorrhagic shock. Investigate Surg 6: 935
33. Vivie de R, Hellberg K, Kettler D, Kirchhoff PG (1975) Diagnostic and therapy of postoperative cardiac low-output-syndrome by means of intraaortic Balloon pumping (IABP) or external counterpulsation (ECP) – a comparison. Thoraxchirurgie 23: 367–371
34. Wolner E (1972) Die mechanische Kreislaufunterstützung in Experiment und Klinik. Wien Klin Wochenschr 84 Suppl 1: 26

Myocardial Preservation by Preoperative Administration of High Amounts of Insulin

W. Haider, W. Schütz, A. Moritz, W. Sandtner, M. Semsroth, and J. Slany

Introduction

The ability of the myocardium to shift under conditions of reduced oxygen tension from oxidative lipolytic to anaerobic glycolytic energy sources is an important survival mechanism [12]. This is based on the fact that on the path of anaerobic glycolysis from glucose to pyruvate two molecules of ATP are consumed, but two times two molecules are produced, which amounts to a net gain of at least two molecules of ATP without oxygen.

An improvement of the myocardial survival conditions should occur if this metabolic switching is anticipated:

1. By enlarging the myocardial glycogen depots prior to ischemia, and
2. By ensuring the utilization of those depots during ischemia.

Both are accomplished by insulin, since it enhances glycogenesis (by activating glycogen synthetase) as well as facilitating glycolysis by activiating several glycolytic enzymes.

Table 1. Different trials to achieve better myocardial preservation by means of an augmented myocardial glycogen content

	Treatment	Subjects	Results	
Austen et al. [2]	20% glucose into aorta	dogs ECC	myoc, glucose uptake ↑	l. ventric. function↑ (starling curve)
Scheuer et al [11]	reserpine 24 h prior to perfusion	rats isolated perfused heart	myoc. glycogen ↑ Myoc. ATP↑	LVEDP ↓ DP/DT ↑
Weissler et al. [12]	insulin (100 mu/ml) into perfusate	rats isolated perfused heart	after 30 min anoxia: myoc. CP ↑ Myoc, ATP ↑	L. ventric. pressure ↑ DP/DT ↑
Hewitt et al. [5]	fat diet 3 days prior to ECC	dogs ECC	after 30 min ischemia: myoc. glycogen ↑	CO ↑ DP/DT ↑
Opie et al. [9]	glucose insulin (40–60 u/l) potassium 3 min after cor. ligation	baboons LAD-ligation 10% myoc. infarction	myoc. ATP 15% ↑ CP 15% ↑ glycog: 25% ↑	incidence of ventric. fibrillation ↓
Lolley et al. [6]	glucose + fat diet overnight	patients ACBP	myoc. glycogen ↑	arrhythmias vasopressorneed ↓
Pasque et al. [10]	ribose infusion preop.	rats isolated perfused heart	myoc. ATP ↑	aortic pressure ↑ CO ↑

Abbreviations: U, units; ECC, extracorporeal circulation; CP, creatine phosphate; ACBP, Aortocoronary bypass; LVEDP, left ventricular end-diastolic pressure; LAD, left anterior descending coronary artery; cor,

Several trials have been made in the last 10 years by various investigators [2, 5, 6, 9–12] using different methods in order to obtain better myocardial preservation by means of an augmented myocardial glycogen content. As summarized in Table 1, every one of these approaches has achieved more or less of an increase in the myocardial glycogen content, and increased myocardial content of energy-rich phosphates has been achieved as well as improvement in several inotropic parameters.

While we had long been familiar with the *therapeutic* administration of high doses of insulin, in this study we tried to obtain enlarged myocardial glycogen stores by the administration of high doses of insulin in a *preventive* way.

Materials and Methods

We investigated 16 patients (aged 33–67 years) undergoing mitral valve replacement, in two randomized groups. The patients' data, clinical grades according to the New York Heart Association (NYHA) classification, time of extracorporeal circulation (75–81 min), and aortic cross-clamp times (39–44 min) were nearly identical in both groups. The first group, used as control, received Ringer's lactate; whereas the second group (insulin group) received from onset of anesthesia until aortic cross clamping (an average of 80 min) a 250 ml 33% glucose infusion containing 160 units insulin (Actrapid Novo) at a rate of 40 drops/min (0.5 g glucose/kg/h, 1 unit insulin/kg per h). After an average 26 min ischemic period, a papillary muscle tip was cut out and immediately plunged into liquid nitrogen (Fig. 1). The myocardial content of ATP, ADP, and creatine phosphate (CP) was determined.

Results

The myocardial content of ATP remained significantly higher in the insulin group (7.98 ± 0.82 µmol/g wet weight vs 4.54 ± 0.79 µmol/g) as did the myocardial content of CP (6.78 ± 1.06 µmol/g vs 5.16 ± 1.72 µmol/g). The myocardial content of ADP was a little lower in the insulin group (Fig. 2).

The calculated ATP/ADP quotient was thus significantly higher in the insulin group (5.53 ± 0.83 vs 2.61 ± 0.52), as was the energy charge potential (ECP (0.919 ± 0.009 vs 0.857 ± 0.016) (Fig. 3).

The mean serum potassium level in both groups varied between 3.8 and 4.8 mEq/liter. Because of the intracellular shifting of potassium by insulin it was necessary, however, to add a much greater amount of potassium in the insulin group: the average amount of potassium substitution in the insulin group during surgery was 72 ±

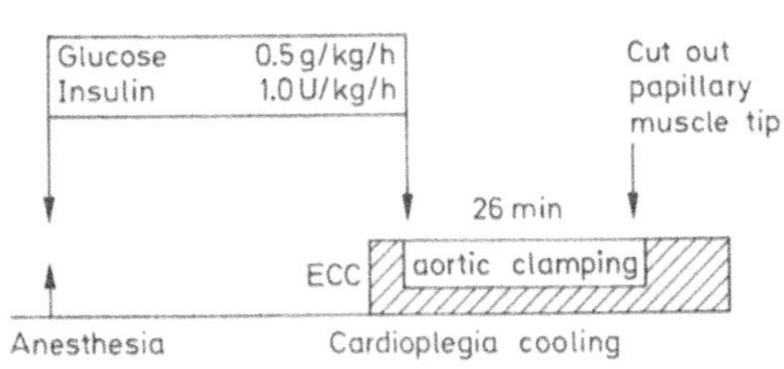

Fig. 1. Time schedule of the study. *ECC*, extracorporeal circulation.

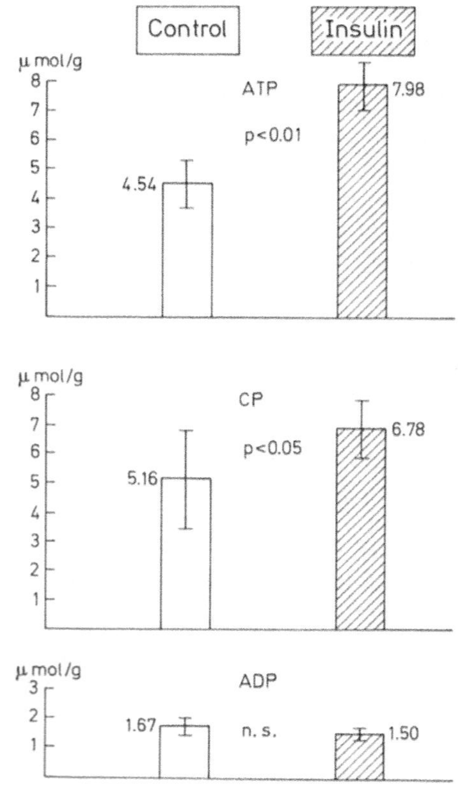

Fig. 2. Myocardial content of *ATP*, *ADP*, and *CP* (creatine phosphate) after an average 26 min ischemia in two groups of patients ($n = 16$) undergoing mitral valve replacement.

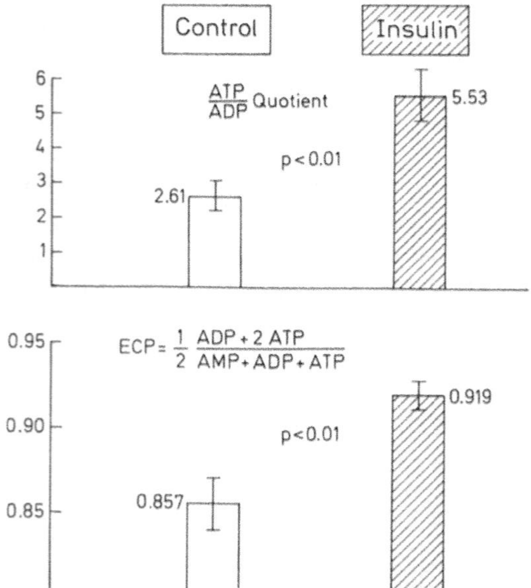

Fig. 3. *ATP/ADP* quotient and *ECP* (energy charge potential) in left ventricular myocardium after an average 26 min of ischemia in patients ($n = 16$) undergoing mitral valve replacement.

28 mEq, and 93 ± 27 mEq postoperatively until the morning of the first postoperative day (total 165 mEq), while the control group required only 52 ± 20 mEq during surgery and 50 ± 17 mEq postoperatively (total 102 mEq).

Discussion

The reasoning behind the preventive administration of insulin prior to myocardial ischemia is based on the assumption that the switching of myocardial metabolism from fat to carbohydrate utilization takes place not only through the pathophysiologic mechanism of hypoxia [8], but already at the beginning of insulin administration. In our study this was about 80 min before the ischemic event took place. Thus the metabolic shifting towards glycolysis, carried out automatically by the heart in ischemia, will be anticipated.

Since the ECP [1] is a cellular expression of the capacity for biosynthetic reactions [3], it can be assumed that the myocardial cells in the insulin group are in better energetic condition compared to those of the control group. Although there is no question about the absolute effect of cardioplegia and cooling, the increased energy provided from ATP and CP will guarantee the synthesis of vital enzymes as well as the function of cellular organelles like the mitochondria [7]. Thus myocardial cell viability is preserved and myocardial damage is prevented during ischemia by an increased anaerobic metabolism [5, 9].

A protective effect on the myocardium was also shown with the preventive administration of massive insulin doses (20 units/kg per h) in dogs prior to the onset of an experimental extracorporeal circulation, which caused a more rapid regeneration of the heart. This was proven by evaluation of Starling curves after weaning off extracorporeal circulation [4].

The increased lactate production with an augmented glycolytic flux is countered by the cardioplegia infusion during the entire aortic cross-clamp time followed by good washout during the whole period of ischemia.

Conclusion

It is concluded that high insulin administration together with glucose and potassium prior to the onset of extracorporeal circulation lead to an augmented anaerobically utilizable energy provision for the myocardium (glycogen, ATP, CP) and a maintained cellular energy charge, indicating improved myocardial preservation from hypoxic damage.

With this approach myocardial preservation can be achieved not only by decreasing the ischemic energy demand, i.e., cooling (decrease of myocardial metabolism) and cardioplegia (blockade of myocardial metabolism), but also by increasing the ischemic energy provision, i.e., an enlargement of the myocardial energy charge through preoperative insulin administration.

References

1. Atkinson DE (1968) The energy charge of the adenylate pool as a regulator parameter. Interaction with feedback modifiers. Biochemistry 7: 4030–4034
2. Austen WG, Greenberg JJ, Piccinini JC (1965) Myocardial function and contractile force affected by glucose loading of the heart during anoxia. Surgery 67: 839–845
3. Fürst P, Bergström J, Vinnars E, Schildt B, Holmström B (1978) Intracellular amino acids and energy metabolism in catabolic patients with regard to muscle tissue. In: Johnston IDA (ed) Advances in parenteral nutrition. MTP-Press, Lancaster, pp 85–106
4. Haider W, Duma S, Fina U, Eckersberger F, Spiss C, Wolner E (1982) Myocardial protection by preoperative high insulin supply. Anaesthesia, volume of summaries. 6th European Congress of anaesthesiology, 8–15 September 1982, London, p 159
5. Hewitt RL, Lolley DM, Adrouny GA, Drapanas TH (1974) Protective effect of glycogen and glucose on the anoxic arrested heart. Surgery 75: 1–19
6. Lolley DM, Ray JF III, Myers WO, Sautter RD, Tewksbury DA (1979) Importance of preoperative myocardial glycogen levels in human cardiac preservation. J Thor Cardiovasc Surg 78: 678–687
7. Maroko PR, Libby P, Sobel BE, Bloor CM, Sybers HD, Shell WE, Covell JW, Braunwald E (1972) Effect of glucose-insulin-potassium infusion on myocardial infarction following experimental coronary artery occlusion. Circulation 45: 1160–1175
8. Morgan HE, Henderson MJ, Regen DM, Park CR (1961) Regulation of glucose uptake in muscle. J biol Chem 236: 253–261
9. Opie LH, Brynell K, Owen P (1975) Effects of glucose, insulin and potassium infusion on tissue metabolic changes within first hour of myocardial infarction in the baboon. Circulation 52: 49–57
10. Pasque MK, Spray TL, Pellom GL, Van Trigt P, Peyton RB, Currie WD, Wechsler AS (1982) Ribose enhanced myocardial recovery following ischemia in the isolated working rat heart. J Thorac Cardiovasc Surg 83: 390–398
11. Scheuer J (1975) Some metabolic approaches to improving myocardial performance during cardiac hypoxia. In: Roy PE, Rona G (eds) The metabolic contractions. University Park Press, Baltimore, pp 195–207
12. Weissler AM, Altschuld RA, Gibb LE, Pollack ME, Kruger FA (1973) Effect of insulin on the performance and metabolism of the anoxic isolated perfused rat heart. Circ Res 32: 108–116

Myocardial Preservation in Emergency Coronary Surgery

N. Bleese, V. Döring, P. Kalmar, H.-J. Krebber, D. Mathey, and G. Rodewald

Patients who have had acute myocardial infarction or are suffering from unstable angina are candidates for emergency coronary artery surgery. These patients run a high risk of postoperative myocardial insufficiency due to an extremely reduced ischemic tolerance of the myocardium, which is critically impaired even before the revascularization. The perioperative management and especially the intraoperative myocardial preservation of these patients should therefore prevent any additional loss of myocardial function or structure. Our method of myocardial preservation combines hypothermic cardioplegic arrest with maintenance of an oxidative myocardial metabolism. This is done by either intermittent or – if technically feasible – continous cardioplegic coronary perfusions and allows all distal and central vein anastomoses to be performed during a single period of cardiac arrest [1, 2].

In contrast to electively performed coronary artery surgery – at which the myocardium has at least a compensated blood supply and therefore central vein anastomosis can safely be performed on the beating or fibrillating heart during the reperfusion period – the energy-depleted heart in emergency coronary patients should be arrested as soon as possible under the conditions mentioned above and kept arrested for the whole time of revascularization, in order to minimize the oxygen requirements of the impaired myocardium. Thus resuscitation of these hearts should not be done before completion of both distal and central vein anastomoses.

Table 1. Composition of the Hamburg cardioplegic solution for continuous coronary perfusion[a]

Hydroxyethyl starch	6%
Magnesium aspartate	2 mmol/liter
Procaine-HCL	4 mmol/liter
$CaCl_2$	0.5 mmol/liter
KCL	4 mmol/liter
$NaHCO_3$	25 mmol/liter
Glucose	10 mmol/liter
Mannitol	200 mmol/liter
6-methylprednisolone[b]	250 mg/liter
Total Na^+ content	50 mmol/liter
Osmolarity	320 mosmol/liter
Oncotic pressure	35 mmHg
pH at 37 °C	7.40
pO_2 (2 vol% at 20 °C)	> 600 mmHg

[a] Dr. E. Fresenius, D-6380 Bad Homburg v. d. H.;
[b] Urbason, Hoechst AG, D-6000 Frankfurt/Main 71

Method

The composition of the "Hamburg" cardioplegic solution is shown in Table 1.

Preparation of the Cardioplegic Solution

Immediately before use, 25 mmol/liter sodium bicarbonate and 250 mg/liter 6-methylprednisolone are added to the solution, which is bubbled with 95% oxygen plus 5% carbon dioxide at room temperature through a long multiperforated metal cannula. It will take about 30 min to oxygenate the perfusate and equilibrate the pH value. After that the perfusate is cooled down to 4 °C in an ice box. The perfusate is not equilibrated with 0_2 at 4 °C, in order to prevent cytotoxic effects of hyperbaric oxygen and the formation of bubbles in the case of too-rapid rewarming of the perfusate in tubes or in the coronary arteries. The perfusion system consists of the bottles with cardioplegic perfusates in the ice box, and one or two pressure-controlled roller pumps, depending on whether the perfusion is performed via aortic root or via the coronary ostia after aortotomy [1, 2].

Surgical Procedure

After total bypass is achieved, the tube system for the cardioplegic coronary perfusion is precooled prior to the beginning of the actual perfusion, so that the temperature of the cooled perfusate at the end of the pipe system does not exceed 10 °C.

Before the aorta is cross clamped, both venae cavae are snared and the body temperature is reduced to 32 °C. Right and left ventricles are drained, and the pulmonary artery is closed using a tape tourniquet. Cardioplegic perfusion is performed via the aortic root and the perfusion pressure is measured directly in the aorta. In order to avoid edema of the myocardium the pressure in the aortic root should not exceed 30 mmHg. The perfusion is performed using a fixed Sarns aortic vent cannula. In addition, surface cooling is performed either with 5% mannitol or ice-sludge made of 0.9% NaCl. The heart is insulated. The temperature of the myocardium is checked with a thermistor probe, and when the temperature is down to 20 °C or lower, initial cardioplegic coronary perfusion is stopped. At least every 15–20 min we perform regular cardioplegic reperfusion for about 3 min in order to reestablish cardioplegia, wash out metabolic waste products, and keep the myocardial temperature at a constand level.

Table 2. Intraoperative protocol for myocardial protection – the "Hamburg Approach"

Initial hypothermic cardioplegic coronary perfusion (6–8 min)
myocardial temperature: 15° –20 °C

← Surface cooling

↓

- either: regular intermittent cardioplegic reperfusions (every 20 min)
- or: continuous cardioplegic perfusion (if technically possible and medically necessary)

In patients suffering preoperatively from severe low cardiac output or cardiogenic shock, the cardioplegic arrest should be induced as soon as possible if ECG abnormalities persist under the supportive conditions of the extracorporeal circulation, and the cardioplegic coronary perfusion should be performed either continuously or as long as possible during the period of cardiac arrest, in order to maintain an oxidative metabolism (Table 2).

Intracoronary Thrombolysis

Since February 1980 more than 200 patients with signs and symptoms of acute myocardial infarction were submitted to our protocol of intracoronary lysis with streptokinase. Indications for thrombolysis were: (a) acute, transmural infarction (b) symptoms of less than 3 h duration and (c) absence of Q waves in ECG. The patients were taken to the catheterization lab, heparin was started as a bolus of 10000 units subcutaneously and coronary angiography was started at the vessel most likely to be occluded. Before lysis, intracoronary 201-thallium scintigraphy was performed in most cases. Intracoronary lysis was started at an infusion rate of 4000 units per min and continued for about 30–45 min. A guide wire was used to perforate the thrombus, and second intracoronary 201-thallium scintigraphy was performed after reestablishing coronary blood flow, and the procedure was concluded by biplane left ventricular angiography. In almost 75% of the patients the intracoronary thrombolysis has proved to be effective but leaves the initial stenosis unchanged; reocclusions are therefore quite likely. Despite successful lysis within 3–4 h after onset of the myocardial infarction, an irreversible necrosis in the center of the impaired myocardial region could be demonstrated in every case.

Aortocoronary vein grafts cannot resuscitate these necrotic cells, but can improve the function of impaired myocardium which is still viable, and can, above all, prevent reinfarction after reocclusion.

Table 3. Isolated coronary surgery (1981–1983) hospital mortality

	n	Causes of death					
		Myocardial infarction[a] *n*	Low output *n*	Others		Total *n*	(%)
Elective procedure	706	8	3	Techn. problems Pulm. embolism Cerebral insult	3 1 1	16	(2.3)
Emergency procedure (without thrombolysis)	77		4	Postop. arrhythmia	1	5	(6.5)
Emergency procedure[b] (following thrombolysis)	56		1	Bronchopneumonia	1	2	(3.6)
Total	839	8	8		7	23	(2.7)

[a] New intra- or postoperative myocardial infarction;
[b] In all cases preoperative myocardial infarction was demonstrated

The indications for early coronary artery surgery following intracoronary lysis are:

1. Imminent reocclusion
   Secondary to subtotal stenosis
   Residual thrombus
   Intermittent spasm
2. Lysis for complication of percutaneous transluminal coronary angioplasty
3. Unstable angina
4. Multiple vessel disease

However, at least a 50% reduction of the initial filling defect in the intracoronary 201-Thallium scintigram was found to be an essential condition for early surgery. Out of 200 patients who had undergone lysis therapy, 56 were selected for early operative revascularization. Out of this group 33 patients (59%) were operated upon within 24h after myocardial infarction, 14 patients (25%) within 2 days, and 9 patients (16%) between 3 and 12 days.

Results

Since January 1981, 839 patients have undergone isolated coronary artery surgery with the Hamburg approach of cardioplegic coronary perfusion. The overall hospital mortality (including 30 days postoperatively) was 2.7% (Table 3). Out of the whole group 706 patients were electively operated – hospital mortality: 2.3% (16), 77 patients were operated on an emergency basis without preceding intracoronary thrombolysis, the hospital mortality rate was 6.5% (5), and 56 patients with intracoronary thrombolysis had a hospital mortality of 3.6% (2).

In patients who had undergone intracoronary thrombolysis the average cardioplegic coronary perfusion time was extended to about 50% of the aortic cross-clamp time (Table 3) and in 50% of the patients both distal and central vein anastomoses were completed during cardiac arrest.

Causes of Death

In the elective group there were eight fatal perioperative myocardial infarctions – but only three deaths due to severe myocardial insufficiency (Table 3). In the emergency group without thrombolysis the main cause of death was low cardiac output, while in the emergency group operated following lysis therapy there were two deaths, one from low cardiac output and one from bronchopneumonia.

Table 4. Myocardial protection following intracoronary thrombolysis

Ischemic time[a] (min)	Cardioplegic perfusion time (min)	Mortality *n* (%)
Mean 35 ± 22	19 ± 14	
Range 5–92	3–73	2 (3.6)

[a] In 50% of the patients, all (distal and central) vein anastomoses were made during cardiac arrest

Discussion

The effectiveness of a method of myocardial protection can be measured best by the incidence of postoperative myocardial insufficiency in patients who already have critically impaired myocardial performance before the operation. In these patients a prolonged or – if possible – continuous aerobic cardioplegic perfusion becomes more and more the method of choice [1, 2, 4].

The maintenance of a basal metabolism results in a preservation of myocardial fine structure, which is of considerable importance in these patients who have only borderline myocardial tolerance of ischemia.

Our data show that prolonging the duration and increasing the rate of cardioplegic reperfusions during the cardiac arrest reduces the time of ischemia and permits operations not only in patients with severe myocardial insufficiency, but also following myocardial infarction [3]. This is demonstrated by the relatively low mortality rate and the absence of new intra- and postoperative infarctions in the emergency groups.

References

1. Bleese N, Döring V, Kalmar P, Pokar H, Polonius M-J, Steiner D, Rodewald G (1978) Intraoperative myocardial protection by cardioplegia in hypothermia. J Thorac Cardiovasc Surg 75: 405
2. Bleese N, Döring V, Rodewald G (1982) Crystalloid cardioplegia experience with the Hamburg approach. In: Engelmann M, Levitzky S (eds) A textbook of clinical cardioplegia. Futura, New York
3. Krebber HJ, Mathey DG, Schofer J, Rodewald G (1983) Indication for early aorto-coronary bypass surgery after successful intracoronary lysis. Thorac Cardiovasc Surg 31: 53
4. Rosenkranz ER, Vinten-Johansen J, Buckberg GD, Okamoto F, Edwards H, Bugyi H (1982) Benefits of normothermic induction of blood cardioplegia in energy-depleted hearts, with maintenance of arrest by multidose cold blood cardioplegic infusions. J Thorac Cardiovasc Surg 84: 667

Thermographic Evaluation of Cardioplegia Diffusion in Coronary Patients

C. Gagliardi, D. Pantaleo, C. Del Naja, P. Rocco, and N. Spampinato

Thermographic studies of exposed hearts have been published in which variations in regional blood flow and uneven myocardial cooling are described in patients with coronary artery disease undergoing coronary revascularization [1, 2].

Cold potassium cardioplegia has been proven to enhance myocardial protection during the ischemic period in cardiac surgery [3]. In coronary obstructive disease, however, distribution of cardioplegic solution is affected by the coronary disease. Severe stenosis or total occlusion of coronary branches obviously reduces the perfusion of the corresponding myocardial territory. Even temperature recording by means of needle thermistors inserted into the myocardium fails to give complete information on global myocardial cooling.

Thermographic evaluation has rarely been used for this purpose, mainly because of logistics problems. The thermographic camera is bulky and fits awkwardly into an already crowded operating room.

We tried thermographic evaluation of the heart under several conditions, using a germanium-coated mirror which keeps the camera away from the operating table and does not abstruct the work of the surgical team (Fig. 1).

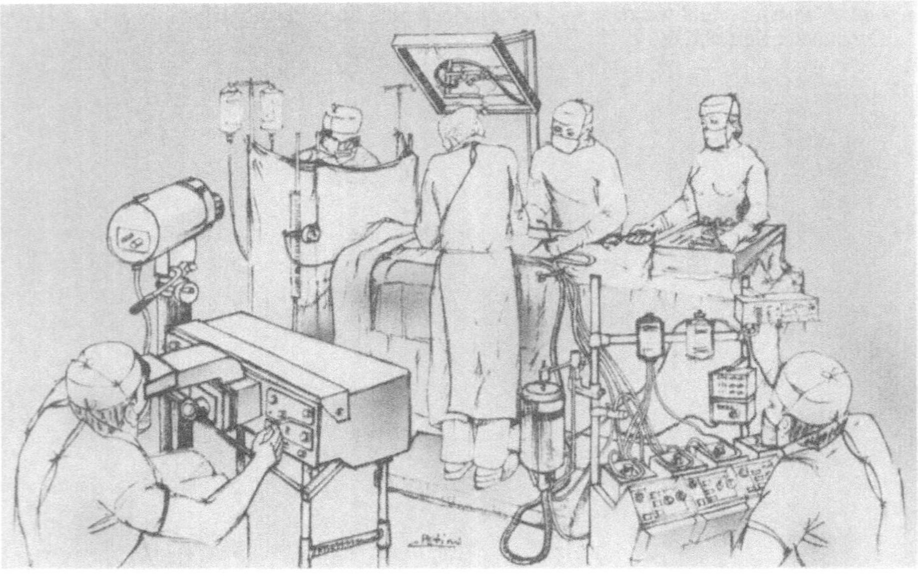

Fig. 1. Accomodation of thermographic camera and germanium-coated mirror in the operating room

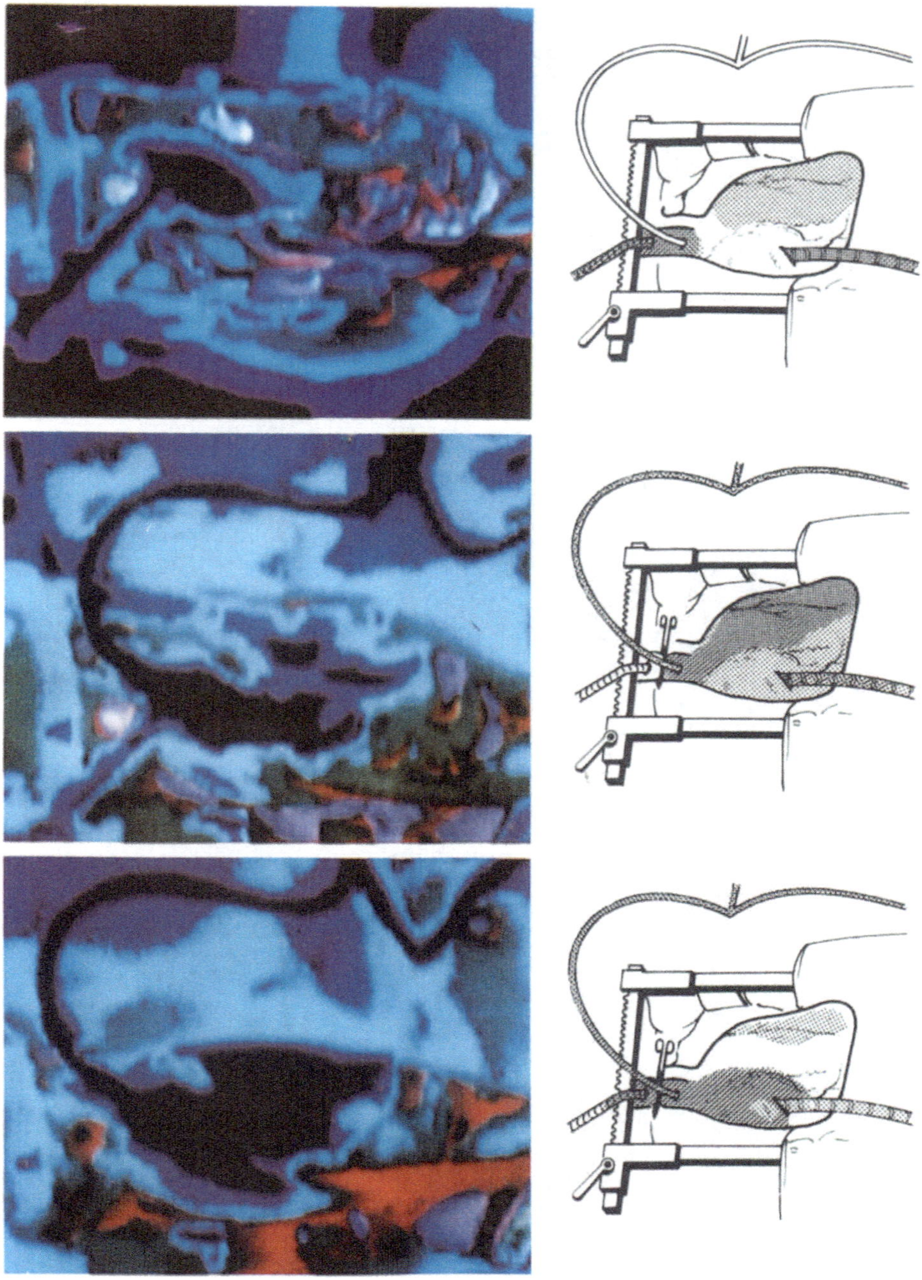

Fig. 2. Progressive cooling of the myocardium while cold cardioplegic solution is infused

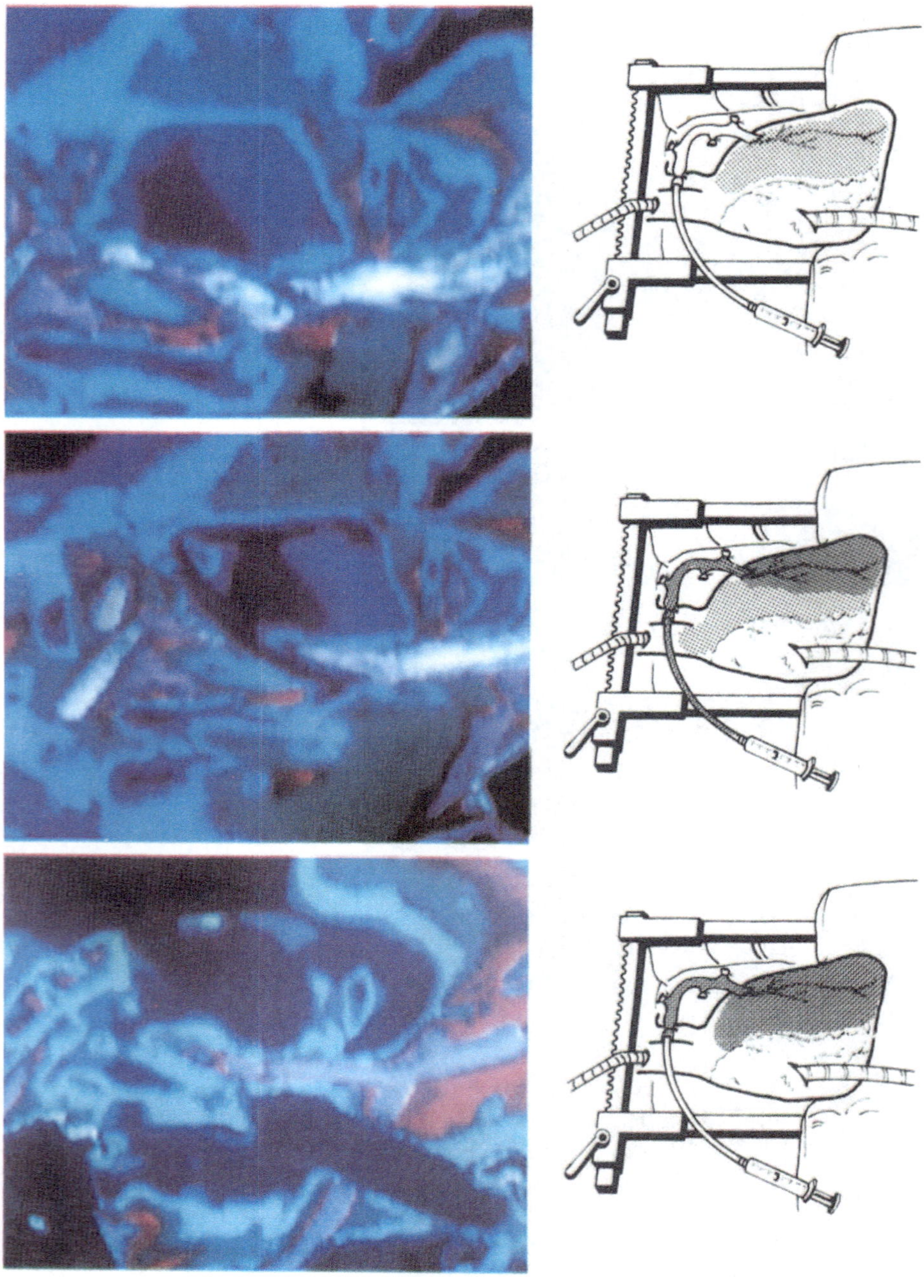

Fig. 3. After completion of the distal anastomosis, cold potassium cardioplegia is injected into the proximal end of the vein to check graft patency by means of progressive cooling of perfused area

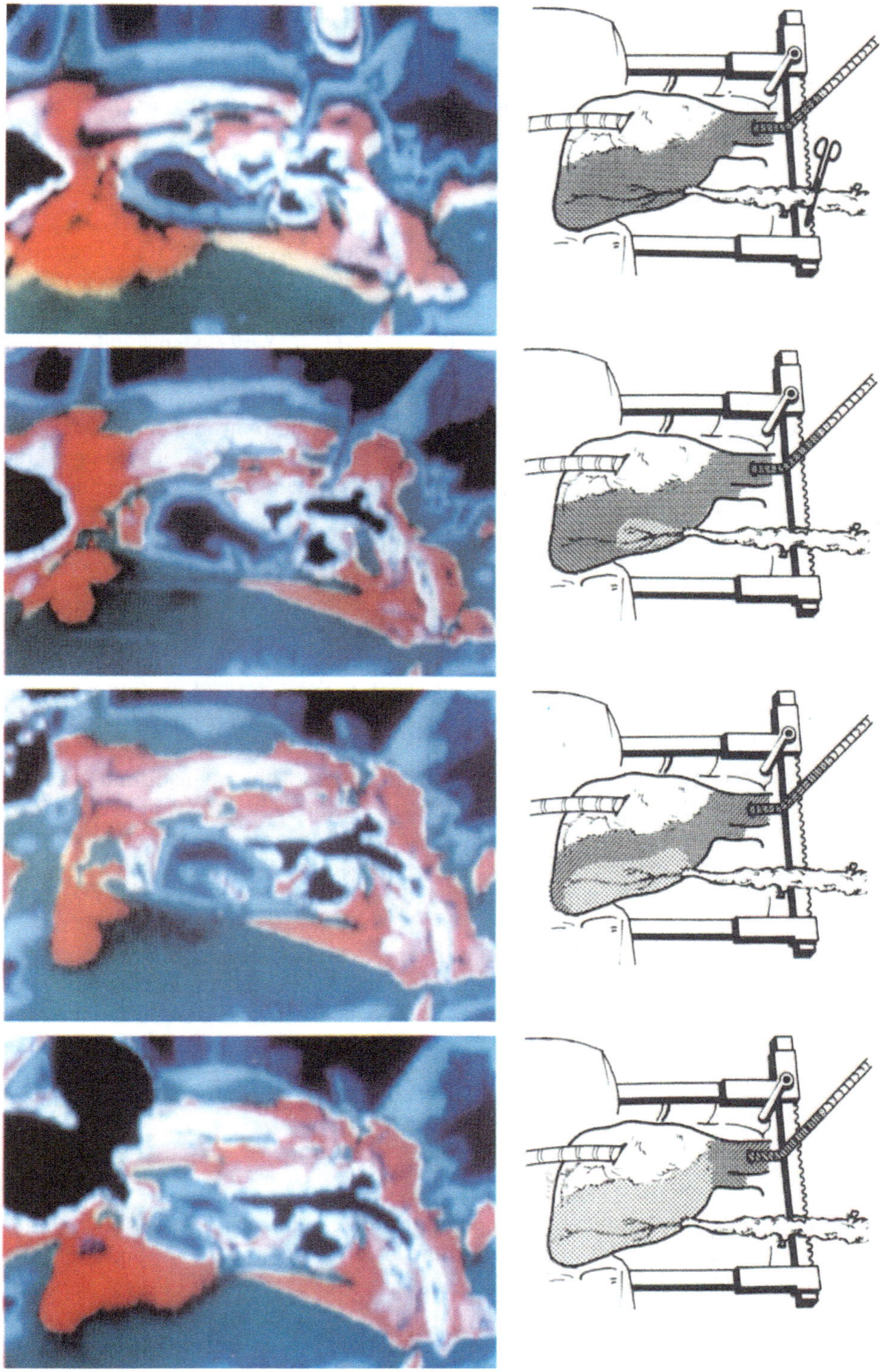

Fig. 4. With an IMA graft, release of the clamp from the mammary artery allows rewarming of revascularized area, so proving graft patency

Thermographic evaluation of the heart, besides providing useful data on cardioplegic diffusion in the myocardium, can be very useful in assessing patency of saphenous vein grafts and internal mammary artery (IMA) anastomoses without flow measurements which can sometimes be cumbersome and often are not perfectly reliable.

Materials and Methods

During aortocoronary bypass grafting, a thermographic camera (AGA Thermovision mod. 680) is placed behind the surgeon. A germanium-coated mirror is placed on the opposite side behind the first assistant, oriented in such a way as to show the heart to the camera. The discomfort for the surgical team with such accomodation is very tolerable. A cold point (the so-called black point) is placed near the heart as a baseline temperature indicator. The patient is placed on cardiopulmonary bypass and the cardioplegic solution is administered with a pump through a plastic needle (gauge 12) in the aortic root. Usually 120–160 ml/min are given according to the severity of coronary obstruction and the pressure of the infusion, which should not exceed 180 mmHg.

Seriate pictures are taken. Because development of the photographs is immediate (Polaroid-type), it can be judged from the colors (cold appears dark blue) if there are areas of the myocardium which are still not perfectly cooled. To observe the diaphragmatic or posterior aspect of the left ventricle, the heart can be rotated and elevated to expose that area to the mirror. Additional cardioplegic solution is added until the left ventricle appears completely cooled. Some topical cooling is usually added to speed up the process; this is done by pouring cold saline solution in the pericardial sac (Fig. 2).

Besides the ability to record the complete cooling of the myocardium after administration of cardioplegic solution, there are further advantages in using a thermographic camera. In case of a saphenous vein graft the injection of cold cardioplegic solution into the vein once the distal anastomosis is completed shows an immediate cooling of the territories perfused by the graft, giving proof that the graft functions (Fig. 3).

During an IMA anastomosis proof of patency can be obtained in a different way. The temperature of the heart is maintained at 10°–20 35, while the circulating blood is usually in moderate hypothermia (25°–27 °C). When the IMA anastomosis is completed, releasing the bulldog clamp on the mammary artery allows the relatively warm systemic blood to perfuse the myocardium: this appears on the thermographic image as a warm spot in the perfused territory (Fig. 4).

Comments

Thermographic evaluation in the operating room can be useful for assessing complete cardioplegic cooling of the heart and patency of saphenous vein and IMA grafts. Obviously this technique cannot be used routinely because of the time necessary to carry out the procedure, the delay in operative time, and the scarcity of available thermographic apparatuses. The advantages of this procedure can be employed in those cases in which coronary lesions are widely diffused and the long time of aortic cross clamping necessary to perform multiple grafts requires accuracy in homogeneous myocardial cooling. Furthermore, graft patency can easily be checked, to confirm the effectiveness of myocardial revascularization.

References

1. Ekroth R, Berggren H, Südow G, Wojciechowski J, Zackrisson BF, William-Olsson G (1980) Thermographic demonstration of uneven myocardial cooling in patients with coronary lesions. Ann Thorac Surg. 29: 341–345
2. Robicsek F, Masters TN, Svenson RH, Daniel WG, Daugherthy HK, Cook JW, Selle JG (1978) The application of thermography in the study of coronary blood flow. Surgery 84: 858–864
3. Engelman RM, Auvil J, O'Donoghue MJ, Levitsky S (1978) The significance of multidose cardioplegia and hypothermia in myocardial preservation during ischemic arrest. J Thorac Cardiovasc Surg 75: 555–563

Magnesium Augmentation During Reperfusion for the Reduction of Postischaemic Myocardial Damage*

AH. Brown and J. Kitchen

Introduktion

The surgical benefits of the dry immobile heart provided by ischaemia are offset by ischaemic damage. Adequate cooling and cardioplegia have minimised this damage but during reperfusion it is manifested and worsened [1, 2]. At this stage, however, the surgeon has regained his control of the extracellular environment of the heart and can either restore or destroy the partially damaged cells.

These cells have impaired membranes and calcium ingress or electrolyte imbalance further damages them. Inotropic agents [3] worsen this damage whereas the early restoration of membrane integrity by adequate normothermic perfusion [4] minimises it. Recovery is also improved by electrochemical inhibition [5, 6] or secondary cold blood cardioplegia [7]. The agent for electrochemical inhibition after cardioplegia should not be potassium, which worsens the calcium paradox, [8] or cold, which would perpetuate membrane incompetence. Magnesium, however, is negatively inotropic [9] and antagonises the effects of calcium on tension [10] at most calcium concentrations [11]. These effects of magnesium are seen in concentrations of 5–10 mmol/litre [12]. Worsening reperfusion damage is characterised by lowered intracellular magnesium and raised calcium levels [13]. Magnesium has already shown its benefit at the stage of cardioplegia in preventing the calcium paradox [14, 15] and protecting the cells against catecholamine or calcium increase [16]. Diuretics [17] and cardiopulmonary bypass [18] reduce magnesium, which increases the likelihood of benefit from the augmentation of magnesium during reperfusion.

Experimental Method

Greyhounds weighing 20–30 kg were premedicated with droperidol (2–3 mg) and fentanyl (50–75 µg) and anaesthetised with 30–40 µg/kg pentobarbitone. Endotracheal ventilation with 60/40 nitrous oxide/oxygen mixture was done while the chest was opened by a median sternotomy and, after intravenous administration of 3 µg/kg heparin, the right atrium and ascending aorta were cannulated for bypass and the low ascending aorta cannulated for pressure monitoring. Cardiopulmonary bypass was established with a Temptrol Q 100 oxygenator and a Pemco pump. The descending aorta, brachiocephalic trunk, subclavian artery and superior and inferior venae cavae were ligated and divided; the heart was fibrillated electrically and the pulmonary veins divided. The perfused but fibrillating heart was then excised

* The laboratory work was funded by the Newcastle upon Tyne Medical Research Committee, the National Heart Research Fund and the Wellington (New Zealand) Medical Research Foundation.

and placed in a funnel which returned escaped blood to the oxygenator, which was filled to capacity with the animal's blood. A purse-string suture in the mitral valve retained a balloon in the left ventricle, which was connected to a pressure transducer and graduated syringe. When enough measured saline had been put into the balloon to raise the intraventricular pressure to 10 mmHg the heart was defibrillated, an average of 5 min from the time of fibrillation. Surface electrocardiographic leads and a septal temperature probe were affixed (Fig. 1) and connected to the multichannel recorder (Devices M19) already attached to the arterial and intraventricular pressure transducers (Bell and Howell). In this recorder the intraventricular pressure was inscribed on a 0–250 mm (0–33.5 kPa) and a 0–25 mm (0–3.4 kPa) Hg range and as a differentiated +/− 2500 mm (335 kPa)/s Hg range trace. The aortic root was perfused at 13 kPa (100 mmHg) and the heart rate maintained near 100 by pacing if necessary. Blood gas and pH levels were maintained within normal limits. An isovolumetric ventricular function test was made by raising the end-diastolic pressure from 0 to 2 kPa (0–15 mmHg) with 5-ml increments of fluid into the balloon. Perfusion was then stopped and the aortic root instilled with St. Thomas' solution at 4 °C and 7 kPa (50 mmHg) pressure until the myocardial temperature was 15 °C. This temperature was maintained with plastic-wrapped ice for the next 90 min, while the pump prime was saved and the oxygenator kept filled with Hartmann's solution. The oxygenator prime was returned and rewarmed at the end of the 90 min ischaemic period and its pH and blood gas levels confirmed as satisfac-

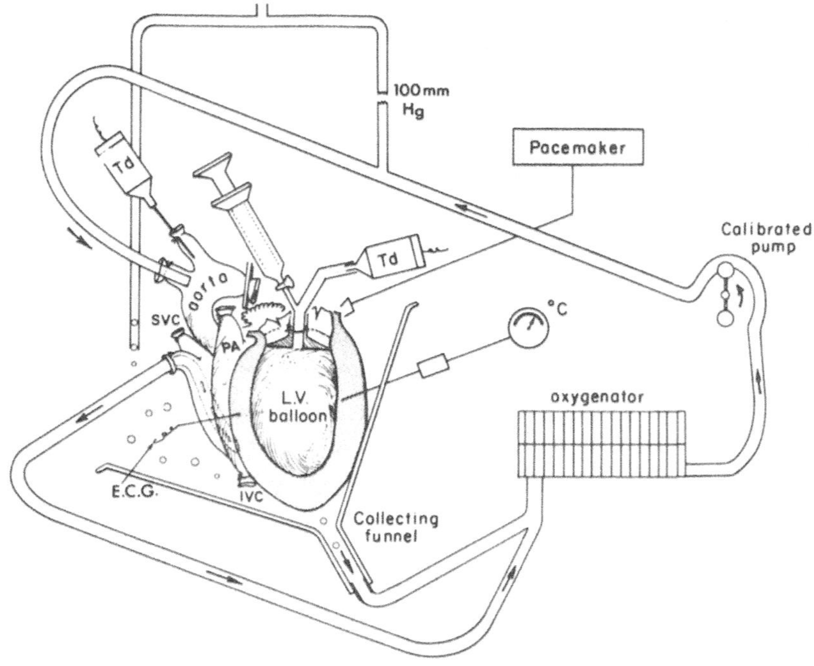

Fig. 1. Diagram of the isolated heart preparation; *100 mmHg* indicates an overflow column which limits the head of pressure which can be applied to the coronaries. *Td*, transducer; *SVC*, superior vena cava; *totC*, thermistor; *PA*, pulmonary artery; *L. V.*, left ventricle; *IVC*, inferior vena cava; *E. C. G.*, electrocardiograph.

tory. The heart was then removed from its cold situation and reperfused with the normothermic blood at 13 kPa (100 mmHg) pressure. In the hearts randomly allotted to the experimental series an infusion of 50% magnesium sulphate solution was added to the blood in the aortic root from a syringe by hand or syringe pump at a rate calculated to raise the magnesium concentration of the infusate by 4 mmol/litre. The coronary flow was known accurately from the calibrated perfusion pump; a total of 16 mmol of magnesium were added. This magnesium addition was not done in the control hearts. In all hearts the diastolic ventricular pressure was maintained between 0.66 and 1.3 kPa (5–10 mmHg) and the slow-running polygraph watched until the systolic pressure and rate of rise of pressure had established a plateau. Ventricular function was retested as before, and the perfusion was then stopped and the left ventricle dissected free for measurement of its volume and weight.

Calculations

The peak systolic tension was found for each volume/pressure combination from the formula $t = pr/2h$ (t = midwall tension, p = peak systolic pressure, r = internal radius, h = wall thickness). The wall thickness had been found by adding the ventricular volume to the intraventricular bolloon volume to obtain the outer total volume; the inner and outer radii were then derived from $v = 4/3\,\pi r^3$ and the wall thickness was the difference between these radii. Regression formulae were calculated of the end-diastolic pressure against: the peak systolic pressure, the peak rate of rise of pressure, the intraventricular volume and the peak systolic tension. The values for each of these indices of ventricular function were read at the end-diastolic pressure of 10 mmHg and the postischaemic recovery values were expressed as percentages of the initial ones. The mean and standard error of each group could then be calculated for the final percentage compliance (volume), velocity (dp/dt) and force (pressure and tension) and the significance of the differences between the groups expressed with Student's t-test.

Results

The results are shown in Table 1.

Compliance. The hearts reperfused with augmented magnesium levels had final compliance values of 111.8% of the initial values, whereas those reperfused without magnesium augmentation had a mean of 83.7% of initial values; this difference was not, however, statistically significant.

Peak Systolic Pressure. The hearts reperfused with augmented magnesium had 85.7% recovery of peak systolic pressure; the controls had 48.8% of their initial contractile force. This difference was significant at the 5% level.

Tension. The magnesium-augmented hearts recovered 96.5% of their capability to generate tension; the controls only recovered 38% of this. This difference was significant at the 2.5% level.

Table 1. Results

	Group 1: Controls	Group 2: Magnesium augmentation	p
Volume			
n	7	9	
Mean	83.7	111.8	
S.E.	21.4	11.6	0.15–0.1
Pressure			
n	7	10	
Mean	48.8	85.7	
S.E.	8.3	15.8	<0.05
Tension			
n	7	9	
Mean	38	96.5	
S.E.	4.16	23.2	<0.025
Contractile velocity (dp/dt)			
n	7	10	
Mean	45.4	69	
S.E.	4.16	23.2	0.2–0.15

Contractile Velocity (p/t). The experimental group recovered 69% of their initial contractile velocity whereas the controls recovered 45.4%. This difference was not, however, statistically significant.

Results expressed as percentages of initial indices of ventricular function after 90 min of cold cardioplegic ischaemic arrest followed by maximal recovery with normothermic, normotensive reperfusion with or without 4 mmol/litre added magnesium in the reperfusate

Discussion

Although efficient cardioplegia minimises the damage from the global ischaemia conducive to accurate intracardiac surgery, the inevitable reperfusion still unveils and exaggerates this damage. Surgical stress raises catecholamines and reduces myocardial magnesium levels [19]. Cardiopulmonary bypass raises catecholamines [20, 21] and ACD blood lowers magnesium levels, as does ischaemic heart disease [22]. The addition of magnesium stabilises the catecholamines in the heart and prevents the release of noradrenalin [23]. Arrhythmias can be reduced in open-heart surgery with additional magnesium [24]. There is thus good theoretical justification for magnesium augmentation during the vulnerable phase of reperfusion.

Our experiment confirms the benefit of additional magnesium. We also noted that contractile force was at least as profoundly depleted by the ischaemia/reperfusion sequence as compliance or contractile velocity. This global insult not only stiffens the ventricle, reducing the velocity of contraction and relaxation, but also weakens it. A relaxing agent like magnesium might have been expected to produce spurious improvement in diastolic compliance. The demonstration of benefit to contractile force in this experiment supports the claim that the protection from magnesium was real.

The clinical application of this work should interfere little with current practice. The probable myocardial blood flow can be calculated from the estimated size of the heart and magnesium then injected into the aortic root at a rate which would raise the concentration in the (normothermic, normotensive) reperfusate by 4 mmol/litre for the first 4 min of reperfusion. An alternative method, differing rather more from the experimental one and interfering rather more with the current routine, would be to use separate aortic root perfusion and add 4 mmol/litre magnesium solution to the reservoir. This method would also ensure that the reperfusion was truly normothermic and at normal perfusion pressures, which is also important [4]. If feasible, the latter technique is therefore probably preferable.

Acknowledgements. We are grateful to Betty Copley for her technical assistance in the laboratory.

References

1. Cerra FB, Lajos TZ, Montes M, Siegel JH (1975) Hemorrhagic infarction: a reperfusion injury following prolonged myocardial ischaemic anoxia. Surgery 78: 95–104
2. Schaper J, Hehrlein F, Schleper M, Theidemann KU (1977) Ultrastructural alterations during ischemia and reperfusion in human hearts during cardiac surgery. J Mol Cell Cardiol 9: 175–189
3. Lazar HL, Foglia RP, Mangonaro AJ, Buckberg GD (1978) Detrimental effects of premature use of inotropic drugs to discontinue cardiopulmonary bypass. Surg Forum 29: 276–282
4. Brown AH, Morritt GN, Hammo M (1982) Avoidance of reperfusion injury after cardioplegia. Thorax 37: 275–279
5. Danforth WH, Naegle S, Bing RJ (1960) Effects of ischemia and reoxygenation on glycolytic reactions and adenosine triphosphate in heart muscle. Circ Res 8: 965–971
6. Follette DW, Steed DL, Foglia RP, Fey KH, Buckberg GD (1977) Reduction of post-ischemic myocardial damage by maintaining arrest during initial reperfusion. Surg Forum 28: 281–283
7. Lazar HL, Buckberg GD, Manganaro AJ, Foglia RP, Becker H, Mulder GG, Maloney JV (1979) Reversal of ischemic damage with secondary blood cardioplegia. J Thorac Cardiovasc Surg 78: 688–697
8. Pernot AC, Ingwall JS, Menasche P, Grousset C, Bercot M, Mollet M, Piwnica A, Fossel ET (1981) Limitations of potassium cardioplegia during cardiac ischemic arrest: a phosphorus nuclear magnetic resonance study. Ann Thorac Surg 32: 536–545
9. Furukawa Y, Chiba S (1981) Effects of magnesium on the isolated, blood perfused atrial and ventricular preparations of the dog heart. Spn Heart J 22: 239–246
10. Shine KI (1979) Myocardial effects of magnesium. Am J Physiol 237: 413–23
11. Kerrick WGL, Donaldson SKB (1972) Effects of magnesium on submaximal calcium activated tension in skinned fibres of frog skeletal muscle. Biochem Biophys Acta 272: 117–124
12. Wacker WEC, Parisi AF (1968) Magnesium metabolism. N Engl J Med 278: 712
13. Shen AC, Jennings RB (1972) Myocardial calcium and magnesium in acute ischemic injury. Am J Pathol 67: 417
14. Hearse DJ, Stewart DA, Braimbridge MV (1978) Myocardial protection during ischemic cardiac arrest; the importance of magnesium in cardioplegic infusates. J Thorac Cardiovasc Surg 75: 877–885
15. Kalmar P, Bleese N, Doring V, Gerckrn G, Kirsch U, Lierse W, Pokar H, Polonius MJ,

Rodewald G (1975) Induced ischemic cardiac arrest: clinical and experimental results with magnesium aspartate procaine solution (cardioplegin). J Thorac Cardiovasc Surg 16: 470–8
16. Janke J, Fleckenstein A, Hein B, Leder O, Sigel H (1975) Prevention of myocardial calcium overload and necrotisation by magnesium and potassium salts or acidosis. Recent Adv Stud Card Struct Metab 6: 33–40
17. Poliment PI, Page E (1973) Magnesium in heart muscle. Circ Res 33: 367–374
18. Holden MP, Ionescu MI, Wooler GH (1972) Magnesium in patients undergoing open-heart surgery. Thorax 27: 212–219
19. Raab W, Bajusz E, Kimura H, Herrlich HS (1968) Isolation stress, myocardial electrolytes and epinephrine in rats. Proc Soc Exp Biol Med 127: 142–14
20. Replogle RL, Levy M, DeWall Ra, Lillehei RC (1962) Catecholamines and serotonin response to cardiopulmonary bypass. J Thorac Cardiovasc Surg 44: 638–648
21. Tan C, Glisson SN, El-Etr AA, Ramakrishnaiah KB (1976) Levels of circulating norepinephrine and epinephrine before during and after cardiopulmonary bypass in man. J Thorac Cardiovasc Surg 71: 928–31
22. Raab CO (1969) Myocardial electrolyte derangement; crucial feature of pluricausal so-called coronary disease. Ann NY Acad Sci 147: 627–86
23. Potter LT, Axelrod J (1963) Properties of norepinephrine storage particles of the rat heart. J Pharmacol Exp Ther 142: 299–305
24. Holden MP (1982) The value of magnesium therapy during open heart surgery. In: Nutrition and heart disease, ch 15. N.A.I.T.O. S.P. Medical and Scientific, New York

Calcium Flux Across the Myocardial Cellular Membrane During Cardioplegic Cardiac Arrest*

E. Anyanwu, E. R. Krefting, C. P. Parali, T. Bwakura, and H. Dittrich

Introduction

Because of its role as a mediator of information between the cellular membrane and the sarcoplasm during the action potential, which leads to muscle contraction, and in its capacity as a regulating factor for the actin-myosin interaction [3], calcium (Ca) occupies a central position in the electrophysiology of myocardial contraction – especially in the electromechanical coupling. Ca is predominantly an extracellular cation partly bound to the myocardial cellular membrane (Ca pools). Following an action potential, an inward Ca current corresponding in time with the plateau of the action potential occurs. The influx of Ca ions across the membrane into the sarcoplasm proceeds via the so-called slow Ca channels. The Ca ions effect a progressive release of "free" sarcoplasmic Ca^{++} ions from the intracellular depots (sarcoplasmic reticulum and the mitochondria), and an increased binding of Ca ions to troponin C – a decisive step in the electromechanical coupling. During muscle relaxation, Ca ions are withdrawn from the sarcoplasm into the intracellular depots and out of the cell. These physiological Ca shifts in the living cell maintain a normal intracellular Ca concentration of about 0.1–1 μmol [6]. Ischemia causes myocardial injuries which may result in pathological Ca shifts with a tendency towards a high intracellular Ca accumulation during reperfusion [4, 5, 8, 9], the extent of Ca accumulation being dependent on the severity of the ischemic injury sustained. The goal of myocardial protection is the preservation of myocardial ultrastructure and function. The restoration of the intracellular ions following reperfusion to the control values is a sine qua non of normal cellular function.

In a previous study, we used electron probe X-ray microanalysis on human myocardial biopsies processed for the electron microscope to assay the intra- and extracellular myocardial Ca content during cardioplegic cardiac arrest and following reperfusion. We showed that during ischemia, intracellular Ca depletion was associated with interstitial Ca pooling and during reperfusion, the reverse was the case [2].

The present investigation makes use of shock-frozen sections, thus eliminating the time-consuming intermediate steps involved in the previous study. On the other hand, because of the small-ness of the interstitial space in shock-frozen sections, the interstitial Ca assay cannot be reliably carried out. We therefore concentrated on the intracellular Ca content before cardiopulmonary bypass, during ischemia and after reperfusion.

* Supported with funds from the Sonderforschungsbereich SFB 104, Teilprojekt B2 Dittrich

Materials and Methods

During elective cardiac surgery, myocardial biopsies were taken from the apex of the left ventricle on nine patients before cardiopulmonary bypass (control), after the planned cardiac procedure just before unclamping the aorta (during ischemia), and 15 min after unclamping the aorta, during which time all the hearts had resumed normal function and the cardiopulmonary bypass was discontinued (after reperfusion). Ca was not administered until the last myocardial biopsy was made. The biopsies were processed and analyzed as described in chapter p. 58. From the same hearts, biopsies were taken at the same time for ultrastructural studies. The biopsies were processed and morphologically evaluated in accordance with the methods and criteria already described [1]. For the Ca assay, only the wavelength dispersive system was employed. Cardioplegic cardiac arrest followed our standard procedure [2].

Table 1. Ca assay following cardioplegic cardiac arrest

	n	MV	SD	MV[a]	SD[a]
BI	20	0.035	0.012	0.037	0.013
DI	18	0.014	0.006	0.015	0.006
FR	18	0.019	0.007	0.020	0.007
BI	8	0.044	0.025	0.047	0.027
DI	8	0.012	0.006	0.013	0.006
FR	8	0.016	0.007	0.017	0.007
BI	58	0.034	0.021	0.036	0.022
DI	49	0.028	0.014	0.030	0.015
FR	49	0.027	0.012	0.029	0.013
BI	119	0.021	0.013	0.022	0.014
DI	112	0.015	0.006	0.016	0.006
FR	77	0.013	0.006	0.014	0.006
BI	10	0.005	0.002	0.024	0.006
DI	8	0.003	0.001	0.015	0.003
FR	12	0.004	0.002	0.017	0.008
BI	9	0.005	0.002	0.023	0.008
DI	8	0.003	0.001	0.012	0.004
FR	8	0.002	0.001	0.010	0.003
BI	33	0.003	0.001	0.016	0.006
DI	33	0.002	0.001	0.010	0.004
FR	19	0.003	0.002	0.012	0.011
BI	8	0.004	0.001	0.021	0.006
DI	8	0.004	0.001	0.021	0.006
FR	14	0.004	0.002	0.021	0.008
BI	14	0.003	0.001	0.015	0.005
DI	14	0.002	0.002	0.009	0.008
FR	7	0.009	0.004	0.043	0.029

MV, mean value; SD, standard deviation; BI, before ischemia; DI, during ischemia; FR, following reperfusion.
[a] Expressed as weight percent of dry mass.

Results

The results of the Ca assay are given in Table 1 as signal-to-background ratios (*Px/W;* left column) and as weight percent of dry mass (g/100 g; right column). These two methods of expressing the results lead to the same conclusions. In this respect they are completely interchangeable.

In all of the nine patients, the mean intracellular Ca content during ischemia was lower than the corresponding control value.

Following 15 min reperfusion, the Ca concentration practically attained the control value in five patients, exceeded it in one, and remained below it in three. Table 2 shows a statistical comparison of the mean values using Student's t-test. The intracellular Ca depletion during ischemia was significant in the range of 0.1%–1% in six patients, but insignificant in three. After 15 min of reperfusion, the intracellular Ca deficit was significant at about the level of 0.1% in three patients and 5% in two patients. In one patient, the intracellular Ca content was significantly higher than the control value, at the 1% level. Considering the results collectively, the intracellular Ca depletion during ischemia was statistically significant at the 1% level, whereas the differences between the control and the reperfusion values were not statistically significant.

Ultrastructurally, all the hearts suffered little ischemic injury. The myofilaments demonstrated normal ultrastructure with a few areas of intensive contraction in comparison with the biopsies taken before the cardiopulmonary bypass (Figs. 1 a, 2 a). The sarcoplasmic reticulum and the T tubules were mostly unchanged. In two patients however they showed slight distention because of edema. The nuclei showed varying degrees of accumulation of ribosome-sized granules during ischemia. Aside from increased matrix density and the loss of normal mitochondrial granules following ischemia, the mitochondria suffered no severe injury. The inter-

Table 2. Ca Assay. Comparison of any two mean values (Student's t-test)

	BI/DI	BI/FR	DI/FR
1.	+3	+3	−1
2.	+2	+1	−
3.	+	+1	+
4.	+3	+3	+1
5.	+2	+	−
6.	+2	+3	+
7.	+3	+	−
8.	(=)	(=)	(=)
9.	+	−2	−2

Results tabulated in the same order as in Table 1
Range of significance: 1=1–5%; 2=0.1–1%; 3=less than 0.1%. Plus sign before digit: mean value before virgule significantly higher than that with which it is being compared. Minus sign: mean value after virgule significantly higher than that before it. +1, −1, +, −, (=): not significant

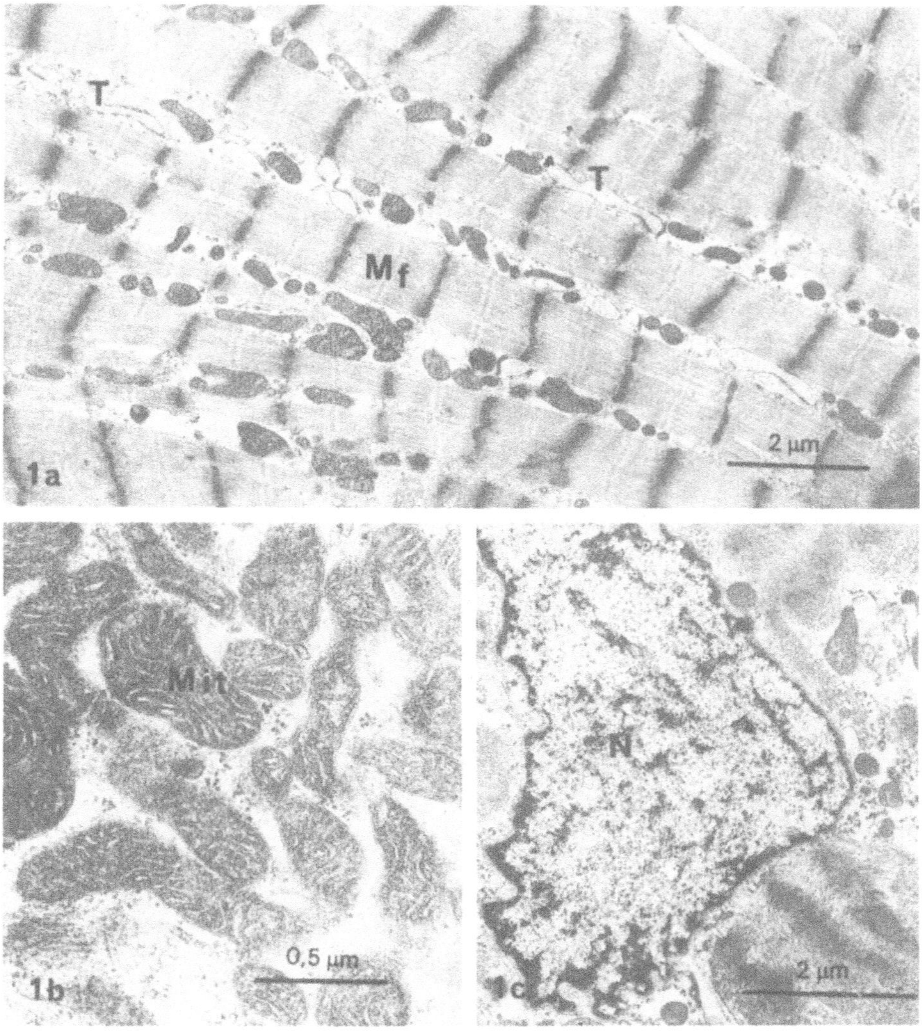

Fig. 1. Ultrastructure of the myocardium of a 50-year old man (coronary bypass surgery) before cardiopulmonary bypass. (a) Myofilaments *(Mf)* in a state of contraction, the T tubules *(T)* appear normal. (b) The mitochondria *(Mit)* present normal ultrastructure, but normal granules are lacking, (c) *N*, nucleus

calated discs were intact (Figs. 3 a–c; 2 a, b). Thus the hearts scored below 1.5 on the ischemic injury scale [1]. All the hearts recovered completely 15 min after the release of the aortic clamp. Occasionally, one observed widened sarcoplasmic reticulum (Fig. 3). Generally, the grade of injury on the recovery scale was 0–1 [1].

Discussion

The results of the Ca assay in the canine myocardium during pure ischemia have been discussed in the previous chapter. Since calcium metabolism in the dog heart

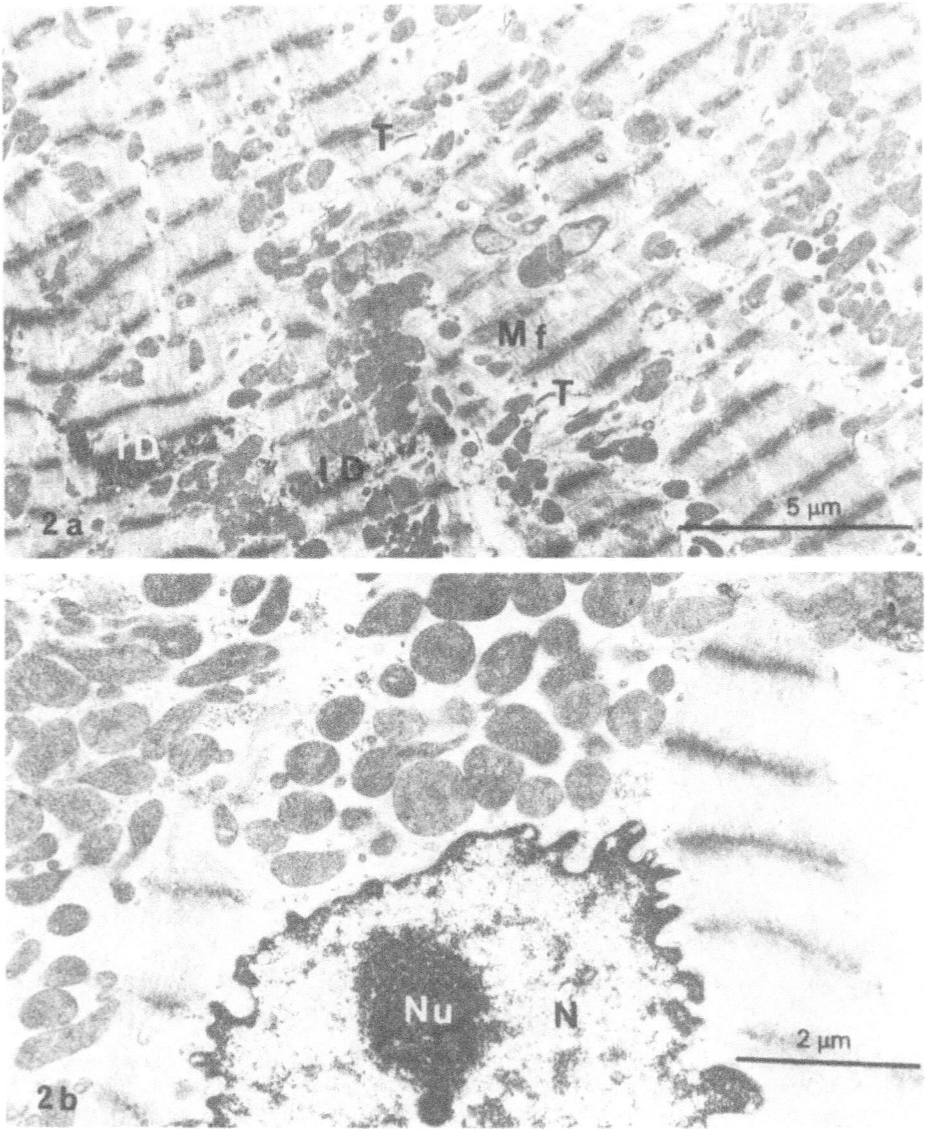

Fig. 2. Same heart as in Fig. 1, following 63 min ischemia. (a) Myofilaments *(Mf)* slightly rarefied and in a state of intense contraction. T tubules *(T)* and sarcoplasmic reticulum show no signs of edema. The intercalated discs *(ID)* are intact. (b) The mitochondria present a dark matrix and lack normal granules. The nucleus *(N)* is normal in appearance. Nu, nucleolus

is identical with that in humans, the results obtained in the former may be considered to be in agreement with the expected results in humans. As far as Ca is concerned, the deciding difference between pure ischemic and LK 352-induced cardioplegic cardiac arrest is the intracellular Ca depletion in the latter during ischemia, whereas in pure ischemia Ca accumulates intracellularly with time. This calcium ac-

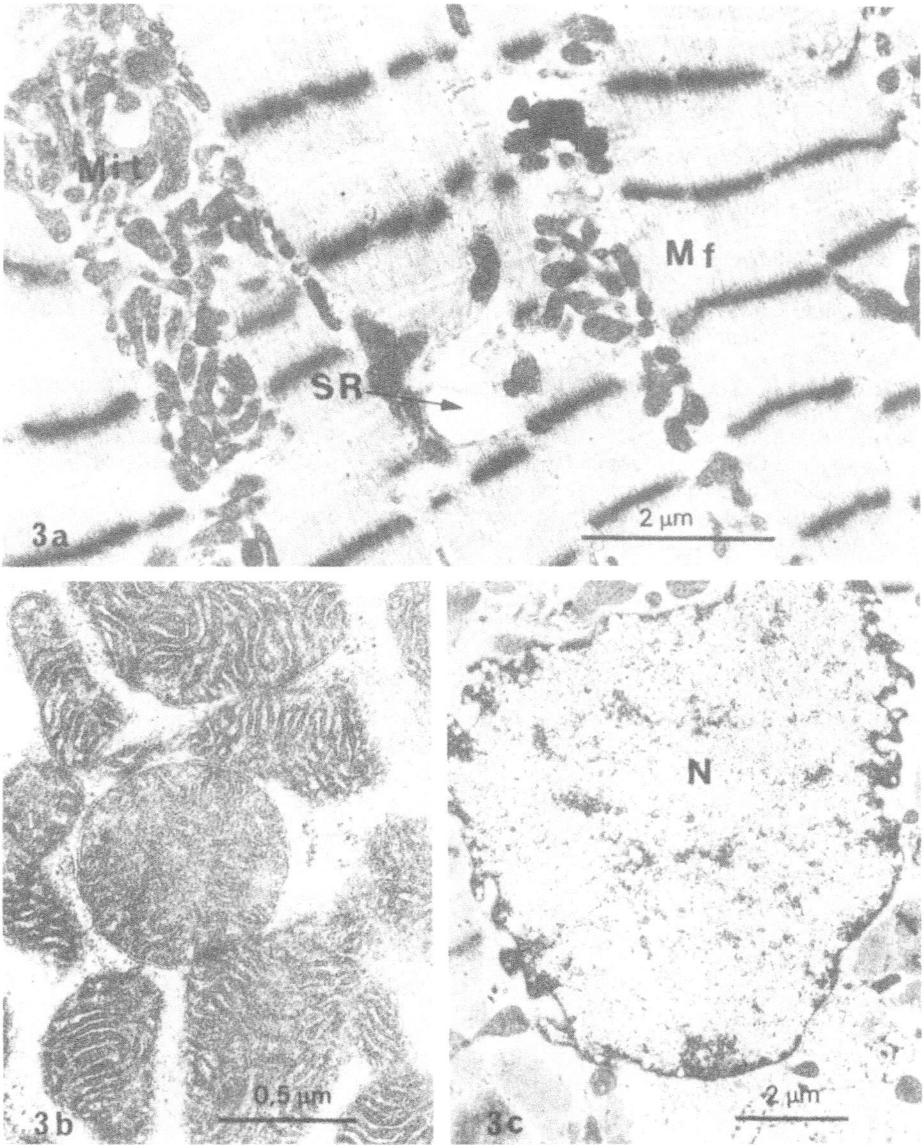

Fig. 3. Same heart following 15 min of reperfusion. Complete ultrastructural recovery. (a) Occasionally, the sarcoplasmic reticulum *(SR)* is widened because of edema. (a, b) Normal mitochondrial granules are not yet evident. (c) Mit, mitochondria; Mf, myofilaments; N, nucleus

cumulation is temperature dependent – as has been shown in the canine experiments. Cardioplegic cardiac arrest allwos Ca efflux from the myocardial cell during ischemia and Ca influx during reperfusion. This result obtained from shock-frozen sections concurs with that from specimens processed for the electron microscope [2]. After reperfusion, no excessive intracellular Ca accumulation was recorded.

This is considered a proof that the myocardial cells sustained reversible ischemic injury [4, 7, 9].

References

1. Anyanwu E, Konermann Ch, Klinke F, Dittrich H (1983) The influence of non-coronary collateral blood supply on the electively arrested heart during ischemia and reperfusion. Res Exp Med (Berl) 182: 111–126
2. Anyanwu E, Krefting ER, Dittrich H (1983) Myocardial intra- and extracellular calcium changes following cardioplegic cardiac arrest. Res Exp Med (Berl)
3. Fleckenstein A (1980) Steuerung der myocardialen Kontraktilität, ATP-Spaltung, Atmungsintensität, und Schrittmacherfunktion durch Calcium-Ionen – Wirkunsmechanismus der Calcium-Antagonisten. In: Fleckenstein A, Roskamm H (eds) Calcium-Antagonismus. Springer, Berlin Heidelberg New York, pp 1–28
4. Jennings RB, Ganote CHE (1974) Structural changes in myocardium during acute ischemia. Circ Res 34/35 (Suppl 3): 156–168
5. Hagler H, Burton K, Buja L (1981) Electron probe X-ray microanalysis of normal and injured myocardium: methods and results. In: Hutchinson TE, Somlyo AP (eds) Microprobe analysis of biological systems. Academic, New York, pp 127–155
6. Haynes RC Jr, Murad F (1980) Agents affecting calcification: calcium, parathyroid hormone, calcitonin, vitamin D and other compounds. In: Gilman AG, Goodman LS, Gilman A (eds) The pharmacological basis of therapeutics, 6th edn. MacMillan, New York, pp 1524–1550
7. Shen AC, Jennings RB (1972) Myocardial calcium and magnesium in acute ischemia. Am J Pathol 67: 417–440
8. Trump BF, Mergner WJ, Kahng MW, Saladino AJ (1976) Studies on the subcellular pathophysiology of ischemia. Circulation 53 (Suppl 1): 17–25
9. Whalen D, Hamilton D, Ganote CE, Jennings RB (1974) Effect of a transient period of ischemia on myocardial cells. I. Effects on cell volume regulation. Am J Pathol 74: 381–398

Intracoronary Nifedipine in Patients Suspected of Perioperative Coronary Spasm

R. A. E. Dion, M. Nijsen-Karelse, G. Jambroes, G. Bastianen, and J. F. Hitchcock

Introduction

Perioperative coronary artery spasm has recently attracted growing attention [1–12].

By describing in detail a group of 13 patients in whom this condition was suspected and treated as such, we hope to contribute to early recognition and both prompt and adequate treatment of this threatening complication.

Materials and Methods

In all coronary patients, moderate hypothermia (25°–28 °C) is used. After aortic cross clamping, cardioplegic solution (per liter: 77 mmol NaCl, 25 g dextrose, 30 mmol KCl, 29 mmol $NaHCO_3$, 2 mg propranolol, 0.1 mmol $CaCl_2$) is instilled in the aortic root for 2.5 min at a physiological pressure and repeated in the event of

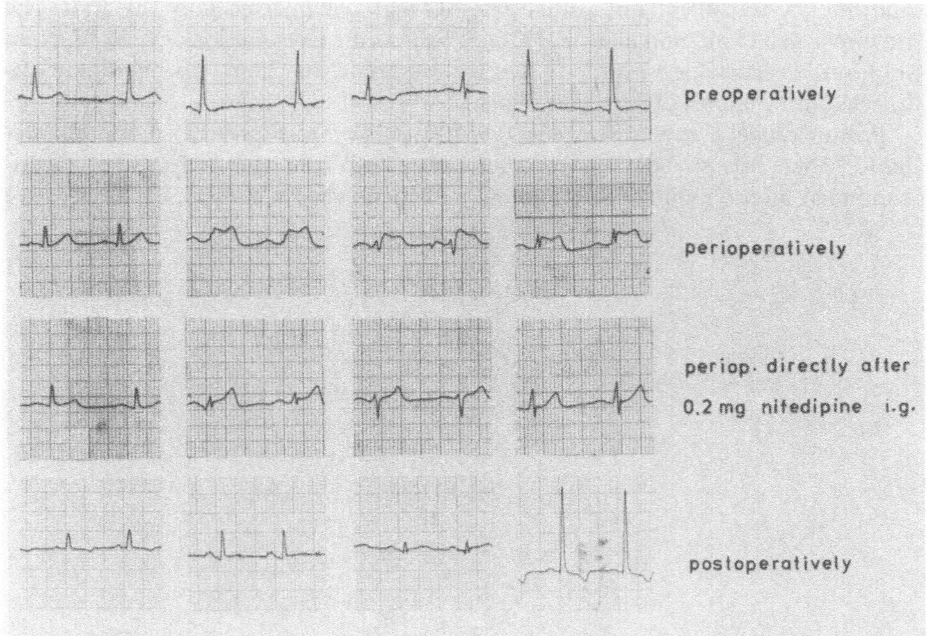

Fig. 1. Patient M. J. C., 63-year-old male. ST segment elevations during coronary bypass operation. Improvement after injection of nifedipine (0.2 mg) directly into the venous bypass graft

myocardial activity returning. Coronary bypasses are performed using reversed long saphenous vein segments, preferably taken from the lower leg.

Before protamine is given, the flow through the bypass graft is systematically measured using a Gould-Statham SP-2204 flow meter, serial number 386 (flow probe Gould-Statham SN-79549).

The 13 patients were operated on between October 1980 and April 1983. The mean age at operation was 56 years. Aortic cross-clamp time ranged from 10 to 91 min (mean 56 min) for a mean of 3.5 distal anastomoses. Eleven patients were operated on for unstable angina pectoris. None of them was known to have variant angina preoperatively.

The following two case reports are examples of the specific problems which might be encountered when dealing with suspected perioperative coronary spasm.

Case Report 1

Patient M.J.C., a 63-year-old male known to suffer from severe angina pectoris, was admitted with unstable angina despite extensive medical treatment. Heart catheterization showed severe triple coronary vessel disease. At operation five distal anastomoses were performed: two jump grafts, one with two distal anastomoses to the left anterior descending coronary artery (LAD) area, and one with three distal anastomoses to the right coronary artery (RCA) and the circumflex coronary artery (CX) area. The aortic cross-clamp time was 84 min. On termination of cardiopulmonary bypass (CBP), cardiac output was low and ST segment elevations were noticed in leads II, III, AVF and V5. The flow in the venous jump graft to the RCA and the CX was 40 ml/min; nifedipine (0.2 mg) was injected into this graft. The flow rose to 115 ml/min and the ECG as well as the left ventricular (LV) function improved spectaculary (Figs. 1, 2). During closure of the chest 1 mg nifedipine was injected intravenously by the anesthetist.

Postoperatively, oral nifedipine (4 × 10 mg/24 h) was prescribed for maintenance. There was no recurrence of symptoms or ECG changes. Nifedipine was discontinued after 3 months. At 9 months postoperatively, a stress test was negative

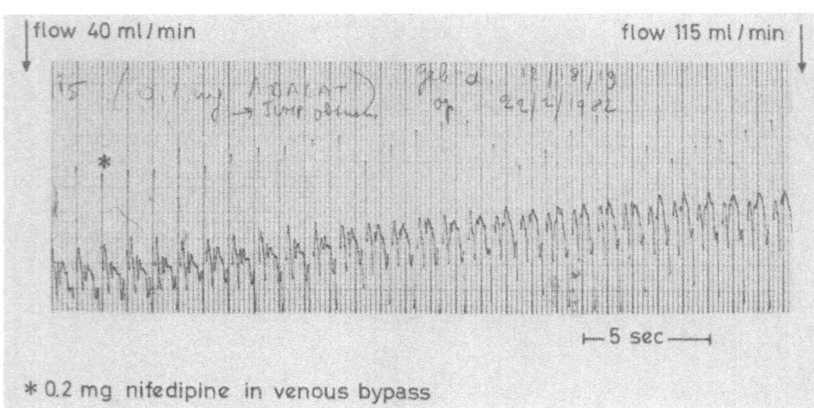

Fig. 2. Patient M.J.C., 63-year-old male. Improvement of flow after injection of nifedipine (0.2 mg) into venous bypass graft

(modified Bruce protocol). An elective recatheterization showed the patency of both jump grafts; the ergonovine provocation test was negative. The patient remains symptom-free 18 months after surgery.

Case Report 2

Patient G. J. O., a 55-year-old male known to suffer from severe chronic angina pectoris, arterial hypertension, and intermittent claudication of the left leg was admitted to undergo a coronary artery bypass operation prior to an aortic-left femoral artery bypass operation.

Heart catheterization showed diffuse triple coronary vessel disease. At operation seven distal anastomoses were performed: a single venous bypass graft to the RCA, a triple jump bypass to the LAD area and another triple jump to the CX area. The aortic cross-clamp time was 110 min. On termination of the CPB there were no ECG or hemodynamic abnormalities, but the coronary flows were extremely low in all bypasses: 23 ml/min for the RCA, 30 ml/min for the jump to the LAD area, and 52 ml/min for the jump to the CX area.

The flows improved spectacularly but temporarily after 0.1 mg nitroglycerine had been injected in each venous bypass.

The patient was extubated 6 h after surgery. At 18 h postsurgery, chest pain, acute ST elevations in leads II, III, AVF and V5 (Fig. 3), multiple VE's, severe hypotension (70/30 mmHg) and cardiogenic shock developed simultaneously. No improvement was achieved by rapid infusion of calcium chloride, dobutamine, or adrenaline bolus. While the operating theater was prepared, a bolus of nifedipine (1 mg i. v.) was tried in spite of the severe hypotension: the ECG started to improve, and before his emergency reintubation the patient could tell us that he had less chest pain. Within the next 25 min, nifedipine (1 mg i. v.) was repeated 3 times and a continuous infusion of nitroglycerine (5 mcg/kg per min) was started. After 10 min, the hemodynamics and the ECG were improved to the point that emergency reoperation was canceled. After 25 min, all parameters were normal again. After 1 h varying ST elevations in the same leads were again noted, and disappeared again after another bolus of nifedipine (1 mg i. v.). An emergency recatheterization showed the patency of all anastomoses and grafts. We did not dare to perform an ergonovine provocation test so shortly after these dramatic events. Nitroglycerine infusion was continued and nifedipine protocol was instituted.

There was no further recurrence of symptoms or ECG changes. The heart enzymes remained normal. The patient was extubated 2 h after recatheterization. An acute respiratory distress syndrome (ARDS) developed 48 h later, and the patient died 12 days postoperatively from septic shock and multiple organ failure. Postmortem examination was refused.

Electrocardiographic and/or hemodynamic abnormalities related to ischemia were seen in 10 patients immediately after termination of the CPB (Table 1). These problems were most probably induced by a localized coronary spasm, as injection of nifedipine (0.1 to 0.2 mg) into the venous bypass supplying the myocardial area corresponding to the ECG changes immediately restored the situation to normal. Interestingly, at the very beginning of our trial the same result was obtained by a rapid i. v. infusion of MgCl (25 mmol) in another patient, a 58-year-old female who could not be weaned from CPB in view of recurrent verticular tachycardia and ven-

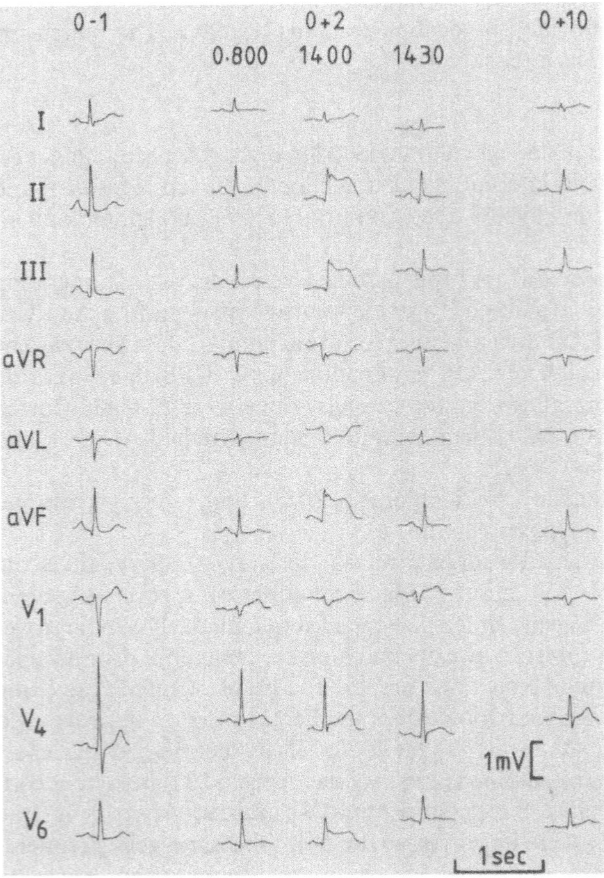

Fig. 3. Patient G.J.O., 55-year-old male. Coronary artery spasm 18 h postoperatively: improvement of ECG after nifedipine i.v.

tricular fibrillation (VT and VF) not responsive to any antiarrhythmic agent (e.g., K^+, lidocaine, bretylium). None of these patients had electrocardiographic evidence of perioperative infarction and all had a normal postoperative course. Six of them were electively recatheterized at 3 to 12 months postoperatively; only one had a positive ergonovine provocation test (Fig. 4).

The other two patients experienced chest pain, dramatic hypotension, and ischemic ECG changes, are at 12 and one at 18 h post surgery. One of them was described in case report 2.

Discussion and Conclusions

The coexistence of anatomically patent grafts and anastomoses, low flows and/or unsatisfactory flow curves, hypotension (not explainable by volume depletion or by drugs), and ECG changes (ST elevations, AV block, ventricular arrhythmia), and the simultaneous restoration of these parameters after intragraft injection of nifedipine, lead us to suspect that coronary spasm plays a major role in some early and otherwise unexplainable complications or fatalities.

Table 1. Effect of intragraft injection of nifedipine (0.2 mg)

Patients	sex/age	Grafts at operation	Before nifedipine		After nifedipine	
			Hemodyn. – ECG	Cor. flows (ml/mm)	Cor flows (ml/mm)	Hemodyn. – ECG
1	♂ 63	RCA, (small) MO3 – MO2 D2 – LAD	VE's – VT – VF end CPB ST↑II, III, AVF	–	MO3 – MO2:101	N
2	♂ 49	MO2 – MO1 LAD, RCA	VE's – VT – VF a few min. post-CPB	RCA:30	130	N
3	♀ 56	AVR+LAD D1, MO2	VE's – VT – VF ST↑I – AVL – V5 30 min post-CPB	D1:30	80	N
4	♂ 46	LAD	Severe hypotension ST I – V5 – AVL VE's 30 min post-CPB	LAD:50→12	140	N
5	♂ 63	LAD – D1, RCA – MO2 – MO1	Severe hypotension ST↑II, III, AVF	RCA–CX:40	115	N
6	♂ 56	LAD	Severe hypotension AV block ST↑I, V5	LAD:45	135	ST. N. immediately SR } Later Hemodyn. } Later
7	♂ 49	MO2, D1 LAD	Moderate hypotension Low c.o. ST↑II, III, V5	MO2:10	80	N
8	♀ 40	RCA LAD Mo2	Moderate hypotension Low c.o. ST↑II, III, AVF, V5 ST↑II, III, AVF, V5	MO2:30	80	N
9	♂ 58	MO3 – MO2 – MO1 LAD – D1	Moderate hypotension Low C.O. ST↑II, III, AVF, V5	CX:48	123	N
10	♂ 67	MO3 – MO2 RCA LAD	Moderate hypotension Low C.O. ST↑I, AVL	LAD:20	85	N

Abbreviations: Cor. flows, coronary flows; MO1, MO2, MO3, (first, second, and third) obtuse marginal coronary arteries; LAD, left anterior descending coronary artery; D1, D2, first and second diagonal coronary arteries; CX, circumflex coronary artery; RCA, right coronary artery; N = normal; AVF = atrioventricular flutter; VE = ventricular extrasystole; CPB = cardiopulmonary bypass; VT = ventricular tachycardic; VF = ventricular fibrillation

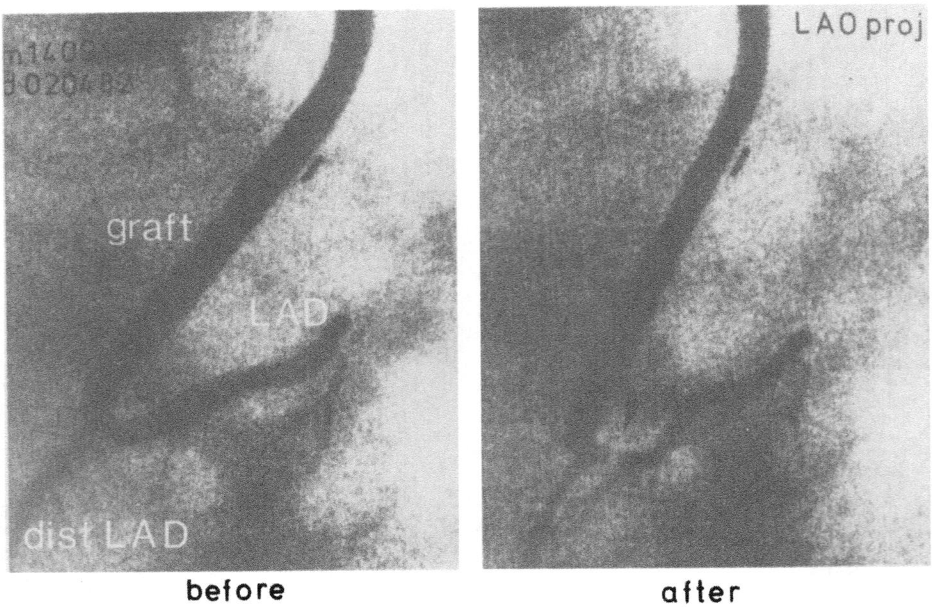

Fig. 4. Patient J. S., 63-year-old male. Postoperative elective angiography: ergonovine provocation test. The *arrow* shows a spasm in the native LAD induced by the ergonovine provocation test

None of these patients presented a similar episode later than 24 h after surgery, even after interruption of the nifedipine oral maintenance. Mechanical stimulation at operation seems a main causal factor, but other elements are probably relevant, e.g., the type of myocardial protection, the severity of coronary disease, and the quality of the distal coronary tree and the collateral circulation.

In the presence of unsatisfactory coronary bypass flows together with hemodynamic or ECG changes, we first exclude technical problems (checking patency and adequacy of grafts and anastomoses). We then inject nifedipine (0.1 mg) directly into the coronary bypass graft, while continuously recording the ECG and flow curve. If rapid normalization of flow and ECG occurs, 0.1 mg nifedipine is again injected into the venous bypass, followed by 0.8 mg nifedipine i. v. over the next hour. A continuous infusion of nitroglycerine (ca. 5 μg/kg per min) is given for 12 h postoperatively, together with 1 mg nifedipine every 6 h i. v.

An oral maintenance dose of nifedipine (4 × 10 mg daily) is instituted as soon as possible and continued for 3 months.

We realize that discussing coronary spasm in terms of flow measurement and ECG changes without simultaneous angiographic evidence is equivocal. Yet coronary angiography during such dramatic events, even if performed by experienced physicians, is usually hazardous.

We are of the opinion that extensive circumstantial evidence exists to support our theories and we hope that this report will be of use in alerting the cardiac team to the possibility of this threatening complication.

References

1. Pichard AD, Ambrose J, Mindich B, Midwall J, Gorlin R, Litwak RS, Herman MV (1980) Coronary artery spasm and peri-operative cardiac arrest. J Thorac Carciovasc Surg 80: 249–254
2. Buxton AE, Goldberg S, Harken A, Hirshfeld J Jr, Kastor JA (1981) Coronary artery spasm immediately after myocardial revascularization. N Engl J Med 304: 1249–1253
3. Buxton AE, Hirshfeld JW Jr, Untereker W, Goldberg S (1982) The natural history of perioperative coronary spasm. Am J Cardiol 49: 969
4. Klaus AP (1981) Early coronary graft thrombosis following surgery for Prinzmetal's angina: treatment with nifedipine and thrombolysis. Am Heart J 101: 110
5. Wilkinson CG, Sanders JH Jr (1980) Massive doses of nitroglycerin in a patient with variant angina. Anesth Analg 59: 707–709
6. Lewis BA, Muller JE, Rutherford J, Mudge GH, Collins JJ (1982) Nifedipine for coronary artery spasm after revascularization. (Letter to the Editor). N Engl J Med 306: 992–993
7. Ginsburg R, Stinson EB, Bristow MR, Schroeder JS (1981) Coronary artery spasm after revascularization. N Engl J Med 305: 699
8. Singh RN (1981) Editorial: Role of vasospasm in vein graft occlusion. Cathet and Cardiovasc Diagn 7: 97–100
9. Nijsen-Karelse M, Dion RAE, Jambroes G (1982) Nifedipine in cardiac operation. J Thorac Cardiovasc Surg 84: 145
10. Zeff RH, Iannone LA, Kongtahworn C, Brown TM, Gordon DF, Benson M, Phillips SJ, Alley RE (1982) Coronary artery spasm following coronary artery revascularization. Am Thorac Surg 34: 196–200
11. Kopf GS, Riba A, Zito R (1982) Intraoperative use of nifedipine for hemodynamic collapse due to coronary artery spasm following myocardial revascularization. Am Thorac Surg 34: 457–460
12. Cohen DJ, Foley RW, Ryan JM (1983) Intraoperative coronary artery spasm successfully treated with nitroglycerin and nifedipine. Am Thorac Surg 36: 97–100

Myocardial Protection with Cardioplegia in Patients with Severe CAD

J. Mulch, H. H. Scheld, H. Kölbel, G. Fraedrich, and F. W. Hehrlein

Homogeneous cardioplegic perfusion and rapid cooling of the myocardium are mandatory for effective myocardial protection during induced cardiac arrest. In addition the aortic root pressure during cardioplegic perfusion should not exceed 50 mmHg when the heart is arrested. In clinical practice cardioplegia is most frequently used in patients with coronary stenoses, in whom problems in cardioplegia distribution and rate of cooling have been proven. The attempt to achieve higher flow of cardioplegia past coronary stenoses and thereby a better distribution by increasing the driving pressure may cause regional edema in areas with unobstructed coronary arteries.

This study was designed to determine, by the technique of myocardial temperature mapping, if homogenous and rapid myocardial cooling in patients undergoing coronary revascularization can be realized by the use of a pressure-regulated cardioplegia delivery system which does not interfere with the operative procedure, and secondly, if the efficiency of the system is influenced by the viscosity of the solution.

Methods and Patients

Our perfusion system (Fig. 1) for cardioplegic solution consists of a roller pump with a transducer for measurement of coronary perfusion pressure (Bellco, BL-705 A), a recirculation circuit with reservoir and cooling coil (Bentley) placed in an ice bath, and the perfusion line to

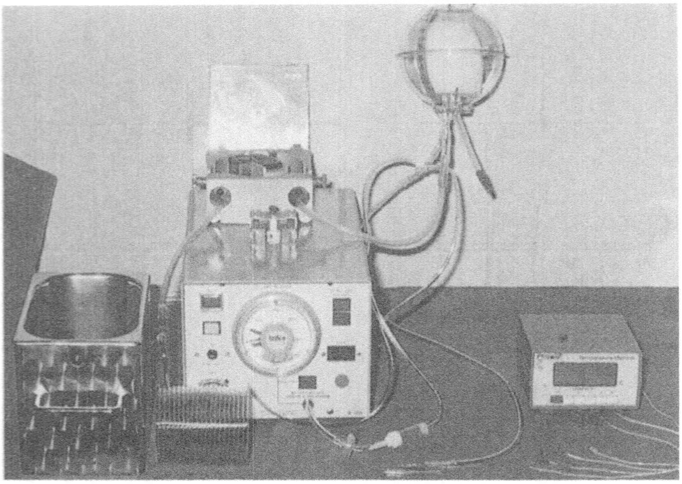

Fig. 1. Cardioplegic perfusion system with pressure-regulated roller pump and cooling coil, thermistor probes for the ventricular wall and septum

the aorta, which is cannulated by a 3.8 cm cannula (Sarns). Later on this cannulation orifice, enlarged by a punch, is used for the anastomosis with a bypass vein. Prior to cross clamping of the aorta thermistor probes (Shiley, Yellow Springs) were inserted into the mid-interventricular septum, the anterior wall in the area between the distal left anterior descending coronary artery (LAD) and diagonal branch, the lateral wall between diagonal and marginal branches, and into the posterior wall in the area between the circumflex artery and right coronary artery (RCA). Extracorporeal circulation was combined with systemic hypothermia to 26°–28 °C, the left ventricular apex was vented, and by a second vent the solution was evacuated from the right atrium.

After cross clamping of the aorta the infusion of 4 °C cardioplegic solution was started. The perfusion pressure was 100 mmHg for the first 2 min, then it was reduced to 50 mmHg for the next 5 min. No attempt was made to insulate the heart from surrounding warmer mediastinal structures. Myocardial temperature and cardioplegic flow were measured continuously. Two types of cardioplegic solution were used, the Bretschneider HTK solution (Köhler-Chemie) with low viscosity and the Fresenius solution (Fresenius KG) with its higher viscosity under these conditions.

Our studies included four groups of consecutive patients undergoing isolated aortocoronary bypass grafting. Mean age, degree of coronary artery obstruction, and rate of revascularization were similar (Table 1).

When using the Fresenius solution we could demonstrate a significant reduction of cardioplegic flow compared to the Bretschneider solution. Therefore in the third group of patients we produced coronary vasodilation by injecting dipyridamole (Boehringer) into the proximal aorta to increase the collateral flow and thereby perhaps induce a better distribution of the cardioplegic solution in the areas distal to stenoses. When the drug was distributed by some ventricular contractions, the cardioplegic perfusion was started.

In a last group of ten patients, perfusion with Fresenius solution was combined with topical hypothermia.

Results

Using our standardized cardioplegia delivery system we could document a significant greater flow rate for the HTK solution compared with the Fresenius solution; after 2 min of infusion 800 ml versus 260 ml, and 1500 ml versus 650 ml at the end of a 7-min period of perfusion. When vasodilation was induced by dipyridamole immediately before infusion with Fresenius solution the flow rate increased to 505 ml at 2 min and 1100 ml at 7 min (Fig. 2). Optimal myocardial cooling was observed in

Table 1. Profile of 40 patients undergoing myocardial revascularization

	Cardioplegia			
	Bretschneider sol. HTK	Fresenius sol. (Bleese)	Fresenius sol. + dipyridamole	Fresenius sol. + top. hypothermia
No. of patients	10	10	10	10
Mean age (yrs.)	55	52	56	53
Grafts/pt.	3.9	3.8	4.2	4.1
No. of critical stenoses (>85%)				
LAD	10	9	10	10
Diag.	9	6	8	7
Marg.	8	8	7	8
CX	5	7	8	6
RCA	8	9	9	8

Abbreviations: Diag., diagonal branches of LAD; Marg., marginal branches of LAD

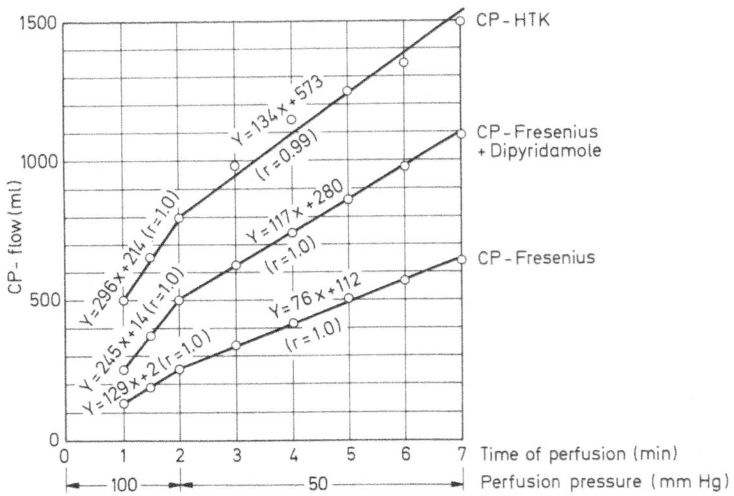

Fig. 2. Mean flow of cardioplegia *(CP)* during pressure-regulated perfusion with Bretschneider HTK solution and Fresenius solution

the Bretschneider group; after 3 min cardioplegic perfusion the mean temperature in all measured areas was lowered to the optimum range. The mean temperature of the anterior wall, which showed a certain delay in the initial phase, was reduced to less than 12 °C. Particularly in the critical posterior wall of the left ventricle rapid cooling was observed, as in the lateral wall and in the septum. At the end of cardioplegic perfusion the mean temperature difference was less than 2 °C (Fig. 3).

With Fresenius solution myocardial cooling was insufficient. The mean temperatures of the anterior and lateral walls and the ventricular septum were 18 °–19 °C, only poor cooling was observed in the posterior wall, and the mean temperature difference was nearly 5 °C.

Fresenius solution in combination with coronary vasodilation by dipyridamole showed better but still suboptimal cooling. The mean temperature difference for septum, anterior wall, and posterior walls was less than 3 °C, but a more rapid cooling could be documented in the lateral area.

Only the combination of Fresenius solution and topical hypothermia produced myocardial cooling to the optimum temperature range, but doubled perfusion time compared with HTK solution (Fig. 4).

Discussion

Critical coronary stenoses limit the distribution of cardioplegic solutions delivered into the aortic root. Both clinical and experimental studies have documented inadequate cooling and incomplete protection when using this technique [3–5] Laschinger [6] and Weisel [9] demonstrated the importance of adjunctive topical hypothermia.

In an experimental study Robertson [7] documented a higher poststenotic cardioplegic flow for blood cardioplegia compared with asanguineous cardioplegia, due

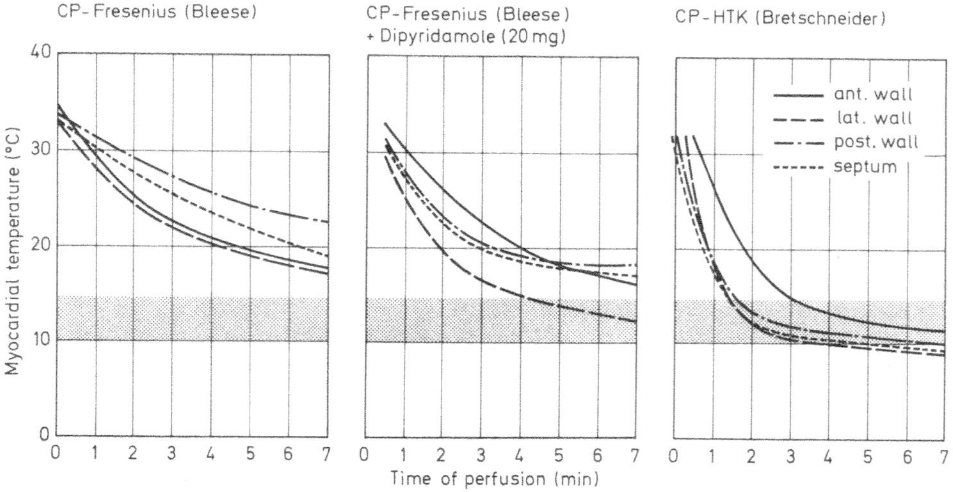

Fig. 3. Mean myocardial temperature during pressure-regulated cardioplegic perfusion for 7 min. Reduction of temperature to the optimum range (10°–15 °C) can be documented only in the Bretschneider group. *CP*, cardioplegia

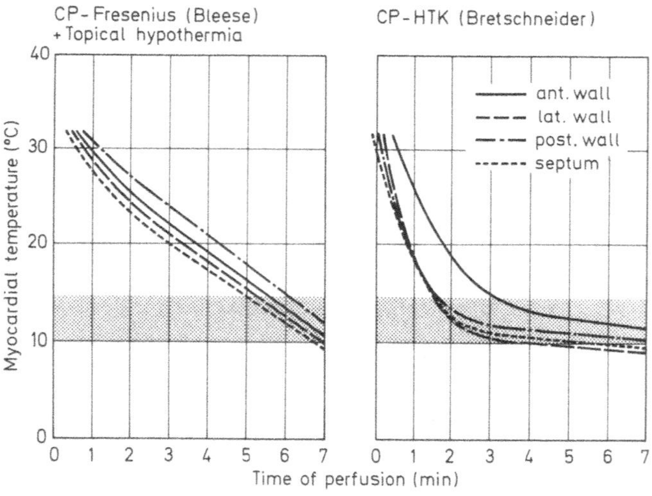

Fig. 4. Mean myocardial temperature during cardioplegic perfusion with Fresenius solution in combination with topical hypothermia and Bretschneider solution without additional cooling. *CP*, cardioplegia

to its higher viscosity. However, this effect was realized by an undesirably high aortic pressure because in his study the rate of cardioplegic delivery was fixed.

On the contrary Bretschneider [1, 2] cautions against perfusion of the cardioplegic-arrested heart with crystalloid solutions and pressures exceeding 40–50 mmHg, because this would produce myocardial edema.

Romagnoli [8] demonstrated improved distribution of cardioplegic solutions in dog hearts when papaverine was added. However in his experimental design the coronary vascular bed was not obstructed.

All patients included in this study showed severe coronary artery disease, as documented by the number of grafted vessels (3–7 grafts, mean 4.0, per patient. The most effective myocardial cooling could be realized by use of the Bretschneider solution. As could be expected, the coronary flow and accordingly the rate of temperature reduction of the Fresenius solution with its higher viscosity was significantly reduced when the perfusion pressure of the delivery system was regulated to 50 mmHg. When using the Fresenius solution additional topical hypothermia was necessary for sufficient myocardial cooling.

Addition of a vasodilator to the Fresenius solution to abolish autoregulation can perhaps reduce cardioplegic flow beyond fixed stenoses while augmenting flow to nonobstructed coronary arteries, because of variable resistance, as could be seen in our experiments by the distinct regional temperature difference, to the benefit of the lateral ventricular wall. These effects perhaps result in distribution of cardioplegia away from the areas in greatest need of protection, and therefore become dangerous in patients with critical coronary stenoses.

In conclusion, a crystalloid cardioplegic solution with low viscosity seems to be preferable for myocardial protection in patients undergoing myocardial revascularization. By use of a pressure-regulated cardioplegia perfusion system with moderate perfusion pressure a relatively high delivery rate can be achieved, which is necessary for equilibration processes in the interstitium. Additional maneuvers of topical hypothermia which may interfere with the operative procedure are not necessary.

References

1. Bretschneider HJ (1977) Physiologische und biochemische Grundlagen des künstlichen Herzstillstandes. Arbeitsgespräch über die technische Durchführung der Infusionskardioplegie, 28–29 January 1977, Göttingen
2. Bretschneider HJ, Hübner G, Knoll O, Lohr B, Nordbeck H, Spieckermann PG (1975) Myocardial resistance and tolerance to ischemia: physiological and biochemical basis. J Cardiovasc Surg 16: 241–260
3. Dagett WR, Jacocks MA, Coleman WS, Johnson RG, Lowenstein E, Vander Salm TJ (1981) Myocardial temperature mapping. J Thorac Cardiovasc Surg 82: 883–888
4. Grondin CM, Hélias J, Vouhé PR, Robert P (1981) Influence of a critical coronary artery stenosis on myocardial protection through cold potassium cardioplegia. J Thorac Cardiovasc Surg 82: 608–615
5. Landymore RW, Tice D, Trehan N, Spencer F (1981) Importance of topical hypothermia to ensure uniform myocardial cooling during coronary artery bypass. J Thorac Cardiovasc Surg 82: 832–836
6. Laschinger JC, Catinella FP, Cunningham JN, Knopp EA, Nathan IM, Spencer FC (1982) Myocardial cooling: beneficial effects of topical hypothermia. J Thorac Cardiovasc Surg 84: 807–814
7. Robertson JM, Buckberg GD, Vinten-Johansen J, Leaf JD (1983) Comparison of distribution beyond coronary stenoses of blood and asanguineous cardioplegic solutions. J Thorac Cardiovasc Surg 86: 80–86
8. Romagnoli A, Koska AJ (1981) Coronary dilators and cardioplegia. Cardiovasc Dis 8: 467–474
9. Weisel RD, Hoy FBY, Baird RD, Ivanor J, Hilton JD, Burns RJ, Mickle DAG, Mickleborough LL, Scully HE, Goldmann BS, Relaughlin PR (1983) Comparison of alternative cardioplegic techniques. J Thorac Cardiovasc Surg 86: 97–107

Enhanced Myocardial Protection by Means of Maintained β Blockade and Preoperative Carbohydrate Infusion

H. Berggren, E. Berglin, R. Ekroth, A. Waldenström, and G. William-Olsson

Introduction

Ischemic myocardial injury is the main cause for myocardial dysfunction after open-heart surgery and the main cause for ischemic damage is imbalance between energy demand and energy supply before, during, and after aortic cross clamping [1, 2]. The major steps taken to prevent myocardial injury are cooling and cardiac arrest. In patients with ischemic heart disease uneven distribution of cold cardioplegic solution will occur, resulting in impaired cooling of poststenotic areas, as shown by thermography [3]. Ischemia induces liberation of catecholamines from the nerve endings in the myocardium [4], which together with the raised sympathetic activity during cardiopulmonary bypass [5] increases the metabolic rate, with resulting energy depletion and increased ischemic damage. The energy supply during the ischemic period relies to a great extent on glycolysis or glycogenolysis.

In this study we examined whether myocardial damage could be reduced by counteraction of β-adrenergic activity or/and increase of intramyocardial energy stores.

Patients and Methods

Twenty-seven patients scheduled for valvular surgery were randomly divided into two groups. One group received 1000 ml of 10% glucose, 20 units of fast-acting insulin, and 60 mmol of potassium during the 12 h before surgery. During the 15–20 min prior to aortic cross clamping 0.6 g glucose/kg body wt. was given in a central venous line. The other group fasted overnight.

In another study 29 patients on chronic treatment with β blockers who were to undergo aortocoronary bypass grafting were randomly divided into two groups. One group continued on β blockers until the evening before operation and were in addition given 100 mg metoprolol (Selokén, Hässle, Sweden) 2 h before surgery. The other group had the β blockers withdrawn 3 days preoperatively. In a third study 28 patients, who were to undergo aortocoronary bypass surgery with a planned minimum of three peripheral anastomoses and were on chronic treatment with β blockers, were allocated at random into two groups. Both groups maintained their β blockade until the evening before operation and were additionally given 100 mg metoprolol (Selokén, Hässle, Sweden) 2 h before surgery. One group was given 1000 ml of a carbohydrate solution (Nutradex, Pharmacia, Sweden) intravenously during 12 h before surgery.

In all studies blood was sampled for serial determination of creatine kinase (CK B) and subunit B (S-CK B) activity in serum before aortic cross clamping, immediately after declamping, 30 min later, and then after 1, 3, 8, 12 and 19 h. The mean areas below the S-CK B curves were calculated for intragroup comparison.

Results

The patients were compared within the study groups and there were no significant differences as regards age, relative heart volume, left ventricular ejection fraction, mean V_{CF}, aortic cross-clamp time, number of peripheral anastomoses, or postoperative serum creatinine.

The patients who received preoperative carbohydrate infusion had a significantly lower release of CK B compared to the patients fasting overnight (Fig. 1). They also had a significantly higher myocardial glycogen content which was inversely correlated to the accumulated activity of S-CK B.

The patients undergoing aortocoronary bypass surgery with maintained plus additional β blockade had a significantly lower release of CK B compared to the patients with withdrawn β blockers (Fig. 1).

Patients with maintained plus additional β blockade who also received preoperative carbohydrate infusion had a significantly lower release of CK B compared to the patients with maintained β blockade alone (Fig. 1).

Although no statistical comparisons have been made between the different study groups it appears that coronary bypass patients have a larger release of CK B than patients undergoing valvular surgery and that the coronary patients in the third study had a larger release of CK B than the coronary patients in the second study. These intergroup differences are expressions of the difficulties in obtaining homogenous delivery of cardioplegic solution distal to coronary obstructions. The mean number of peripheral anastomoses was higher in the third study compared to the second as an expression of the more pronounced ischemic disease and subsequent poorer cooling.

Conclusions

We conclude from these studies that it is possible to create increased myocardial glycogen stores by giving glucose-insulin-potassium infusions preoperatively, and that this results in decreased myocardial damage in patients operated for valvular disease.

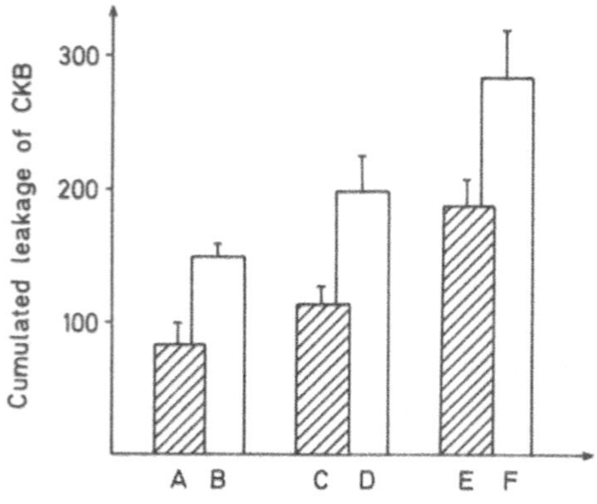

Fig. 1. Cumulative activity of S-CK B after *A*, Preoperative carbohydrate infusion; *B*, Fasting overnight ($p < 0.005$); *C*, β blocker maintained; *Δ*, β blocker withdrawn ($p < 0.01$); *E*, β blocker maintained plus carbohydrate infusion; *F*, β blocker maintained ($p < 0.05$)

Preoperative maintenance of β blockade and also the combination of maintenance of β blockers with preoperative infusion of carbohydrate solution result in reduced myocardial damage during coronary bypass surgery. These procedures should be performed complementary to cold cardioplegia to reduce myocardial damage. They are of special importance when heterogenous delivery of cardioplegia occurs during coronary bypass surgery.

References

1. Buckberg GD (1979) A proposed "solution" to the cardioplegic controversy. J Thorac Cardiovasc Surg 77: 803–815
2. Olin CL, Bomfim V, Bendz R, Kaijser L, Ström SJ, Sylvén CH (1981) Myocardial protection during aortic valve replacement. Comparison of different methods by intraoperative coronary sinus blood sampling and postoperative serial serum enzyme determinations. J Thorac Cardiovasc Surg 82: 837–847
3. Ekroth R, Berggren H, Südow G, Wojciechowski J, Zackrisson BF, William-Olsson G (1980) Thermographic demonstration of uneven myocardial cooling in patients with coronary lesions. Ann Thorac Surg 29(4): 341–345
4. Wollenberger A, Shahab L (1965) Anoxia-induced release of noradrenaline from isolated perfused heart. Nature 207: 88
5. Hoar PF, Stone JG, Faltas AN, Bendixen H, Head RJ, Berkowitz BA (1980) Hemodynamic and adrenergic response to anaesthesia and operation for myocardial revascularization. J Thorac Cardiovasc Surg 80: 242–248

Establishing Safe Parameters for the Administration of Clear Cardioplegia in Humans*

J. E. Molina, C. Maduro, and J. Marks

An evaluation of the mechanical and physical parameters involved in the injection of cardioplegia was undertaken in patients undergoing coronary artery bypass operations in whom the same cardioplegic solution was used. The purpose of this report was to investigate ideal flow patterns, pressures, time to arrest, and temperature changes obtained in the administration of clear cardioplegia. Reestablishment of spontaneous normal cardiac rhythm and elevation of cardiac isoenzymes were also investigated.

Materials and Methods

Thirty patients undergoing coronary bypass surgery with multiple grafts (3–4 grafts) and similar periods of ischemia, i.e. 50–82 min (mean 60.7) were selected for this study to enable us to compare the groups. Group I (14 patients) had the cardioplegia delivered into the root of the aorta by a cannula of 2.8 mm internal diameter (ID) (16 French). In group II (8 patients) a cannula of 1.6 mm ID (10 French) was used and in group III (8 patients) a cannula of 1.0 mm ID (14 Stubs = 5 French) (Table 1). These three sizes were chosen as those most commonly used in clinical practice in adults. Cannulas were connected by tubing to the cardioplegic solution bag placed in a pneumatic injector system set a 300 mmHg pressure (Fig. 1). Table 1 shows the cannula specifications.

Cardioplegic Solution

Plegisol (Abbott Laboratories, North Chicago, Illinois, 60064, U.S.A.), also known as St. Thomas II solution, was the cardioplegic solution used. It was provided in plastic bags connected to a tigon tubing clamped on the operative side, and the solution was delivered by releasing the clamp at the desired times (Fig. 1).

Table 1. Equivalent diameters of cardioplegia cannulas

Diameter	Scales	Sizes		
	French	16	10	5
Outer	Stubs*	–	–	14
(OD)	mm	5.33	3.33	2.1
Inner (ID)	mm	2.80	1.6	1.0

* Stubs scale used for hypodermic needles (Abbocath catheters used for this study). French size cannulas USCI manufactured

* Supported in part by a grant from the American Heart Association, Minnesota Affiliate, Inc.

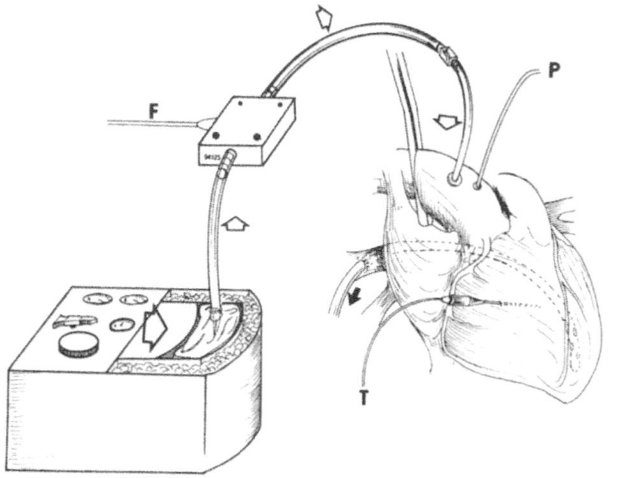

Fig. 1. Cardioplegic infusion system. *F*, electromagnetic flowmeter probe; *P*, aortic root pressure monitoring line; *T*, temperature probe

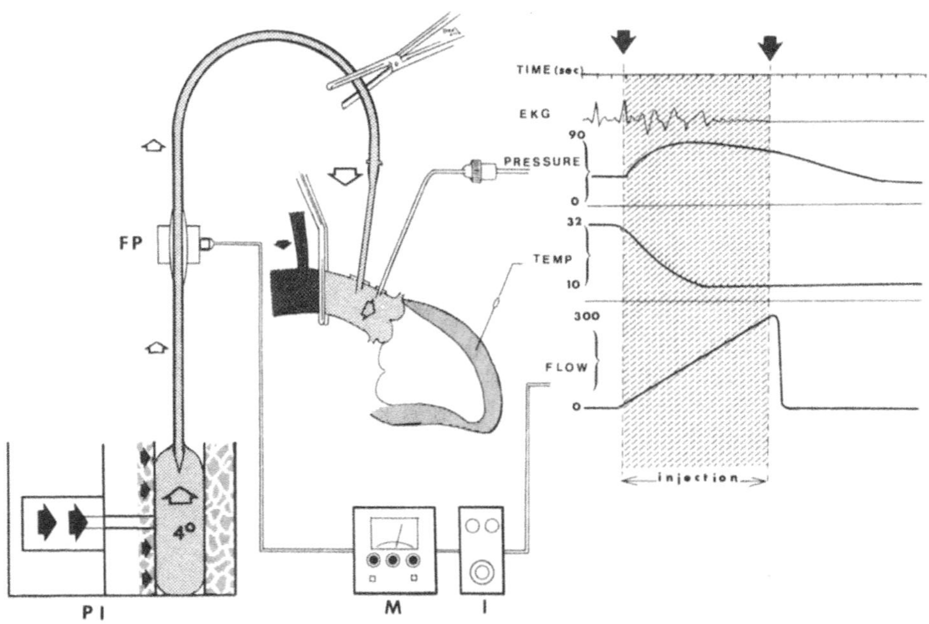

Fig. 2. Display of data and recording system; *shaded area* corresponds to the time of cardioplegia injection

Monitoring System

Aortic root pressure was measured directly. An electromagnetic flowmeter probe was connected in the cardioplegic line and zeroed at 4 °C. The flow measured was integrated into the recording unit to obtain simultaneous peak flow, flow rate, and total flow simultaneously. The patient's EKG was patched into the recording system in order to precisely observe the time during cardioplegia injection when cardiac activity stopped (Fig. 2). The same monitoring system was used to determine when cardiac activity resumed following the period of ischemia. Myocardial temperature was monitored by a needle probe positioned in the septum. Serum CK-MB and $LDH_{1,2}$ isoenzymes were monitored at 2, 24, 48, and 72 h after surgery in all patients.

Degree of Coronary Obstruction

Flows and pressures in the aortic root were compared with the degree of coronary artery obstruction present on the angiogram to determine the influence of proximal (type I) versus more distal disease (type II) (Fig. 3). Type I included patients who had significant obstruction within 2 cm of the coronary artery origin. In the left coronary system, it included patients with left main obstruction or obstruction of left anterior descending and circumflex arteries within 1 cm beyond the bifurcation. Significant obstructions present beyond that level were considered type II. In combined cases with proximal and distal obstruction, the patient was included in the group where the majority of lesions were present. Only obstructions greater than 50% of the lumen were considered significant.

Enzyme Monitoring

Elevation of enzymes (CK-MB, $LDH_{1,2}$) following cardiac surgery was monitored to assess myocardial injury. Normal values for CK-MB are <3 IU/liter; for LDH_1, up to 26.5 IU; and LDH_2, up to 39.9 IU.

Results

Time of Arrest

In group I the heart came to complete standstill within 7.4 ± 1.3 sec versus 18.9 ± 3.2 in group II and 65 ± 41 in group III. The rapid arrest induced by a large connula and rapid flow is consistent with the previous reports on the use of this system. The longest period to attainment of cardiac standstill occurred in group III, where the 14 Stubs Abbocath catheter was used. During that long process, the heart often went into ventricular fibrillation before coming to a complete arrest.

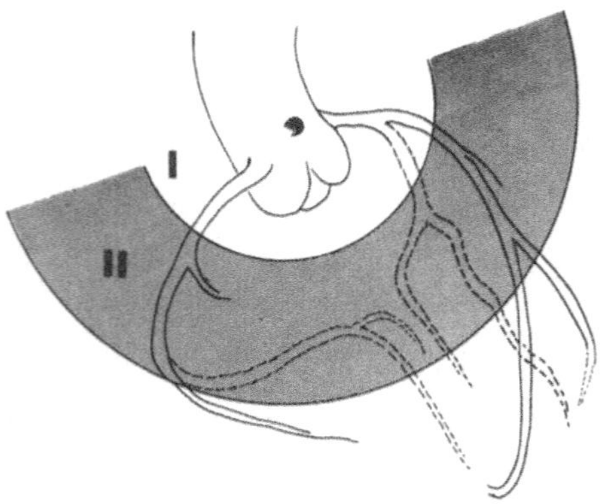

Fig. 3. Patterns of coronary artery obstruction. *I*, Proximal obstruction area; *II*, Distal obstruction zones (see text)

Cardioplegia Flows

In group I peak flows of 1133.5 ± 76.2 ml/min were reached within 2 sec from the beginning of infusion. A plateau flow was reached until the infusion was discontinued. In group II peak flow was 996.2 ± 115 ml/min, reached in 2.8 sec, and in group III the flow reached only 175.6 ml/min at 17 sec before it plateaued. Total flow per injection measured 288.7 ml in group I vs 350.4 in group II and 649.5 in group III. The infusion was stopped by the surgeon, guided by the septal temperature goal of 10 °C and by the occurrence of standstill, but without knowing at the time the amount of solution that had been injected to reach that point. With a faster flow, arrest occurred more rapidly and lower volumes were used.

Aortic Root Pressures

The aortic root pressures after cross clamping but before cardioplegic injection were identical among the three groups (51.3 ± 10.9 mmHg), however as the cardioplegic solution was injected, pressure levels varied between obstruction types I and II only when the 2.8 ID cannula was used: type I, 114.4 ± 14.6 mmHg vs type II, 84.4 ± 12.3. This difference was significant ($p < 0.01$). No difference was found between groups with the other cannulas. Group II pressures peaked at 64.5 ± 12.6 mmHg and group III at 30.6 ± 1.6.

Septal Temperatures

A myocardial temperature of 10 °C was reached in group I within 7 sec, vs 17 in group II, and 35 in group III.

Spontaneous Beat

Following the period of ischemia, a spontaneous beat in sinus rhythm was obtained in 89.9% of patients in group I; this occurred a few minutes following release of the cross clamp. It occurred in 64.3% in group II and in only 23% of group III. Electrical defibrillation was necessary in the remaining patients.

Isoenzyme Release

Levels of CK-MB were similar in all three groups at all time periods monitored. Mean CK-MB was 7.3 ± 2.1 IU/liter in group I, 9.75 ± 3.3 in group II, and 10.4 ± 2.9 in group III. At 24 h, the values were 11.43 ± 6.7 IU/liter in I, 8.25 ± 3.2 in II, and 9.5 ± 2.6 in III. At 48 and 72 h, the values were exactly the same in all three groups. No statistically significant difference was found among the groups at any time. Values of of LDH_1 and LDH_2 remained within normal limits and no difference was noted among the groups.

Arrhythmias

The most common arrhythmias on postoperative EKG were: atrial fibrillation, negative T waves, abnormalities of repolarization, and premature ventricular contractions. There was one case of abnormal repolarization observed in group I (7.1%), two cases of atrial fibrillation and premature ventricular contractions in group II (25%), and four cases of different types of arrhythmias combined in group III (50%). No EKG-detectable myocardial infarctions occurred, nor were there any deaths.

Conclusions

A system implementing high flows for administration of cardioplegia in adults seems to be preferable over a low flow and pressure system. It provides for a faster-induced cardiac arrest, lower volumes of solution administered, and rapid cooling of the myocardium. It leads to spontaneous return of normal cardiac rhythm and minimal postoperative elevation of the cardiac isoenzymes in the serum.

References

1. Molina JE, Feiber W, Sisk A, Polen T, Collins B (1977) Cardioplegia without fibrillation or defibrillation in cardiac surgery. Surgery 81: 619
2. Molina JE, Gani KS, Voss DM (1982) Pressurized rapid cardioplegia versus administration of exogenous substrate and topical hypothermia. Ann Thorac Surg 33: 434–444
3. Molina JE, Gani KS, Voss DM (1982) How should clear cardioplegia be administered? J Thorac Cardiovasc Surg 84: 762–772
4. Ellis RJ, Gertz EW, Wisneski J, Ebert PA (1979) Mild ventricular dysfunction following cold potassium cardioplegia. Circulation 60: I: 1–147
5. Coughlin TR, Levitsky S, O'Donoghue M, Williams L, Wright RN, Roper K, Feinberg H (1979) Evaluation of hypothermic cardioplegia in ventricular hypertrophy. Circulation 60: I: 164–169
6. Lolley DM, Ray JR, III, Myers WO, Sheldon G, Sautter RD (1978) Reduction of intraoperative myocardial infarction by means of exogenous anaerobic substrate enhancement. Prospective randomized study. Ann Thorac Surg 26: 515
7. Laughlin L, Bailey L, Willis W, Gaskill W, Jacobson J, Rasi A, Wareham E (1980) Myocardial preservation. A comparison of local hypothermia with and without cold cardioplegia. J Thorac Cardiovasc Surg 80: 289–292
8. Adappa MB, Jacobson LB, Hetzer R, Hill JD, Kamm B, Kerth WJ (1978) Cold hyperkalemic cardiac arrest versus intermittent aortic crossclamping and topical hypothermia for coronary surgery. J Thorac Cardiovasc Surg 75: 171

Patient Selection for Left Ventricular Aneurysmectomy

A. Hannekum, H. Dalichau, B. Herse, and W. Hügel

Both congestive heart failure due to left ventricular insufficiency and recurrent thromboembolic episodes are accepted worldwide as indications for left ventricular aneurysmectomy. On the other hand, surgical treatment for ventricular tachycardia or angina pectoris refractory to medical treatment as symptoms of inoperable multiple coronary artery disease and for left ventricular aneurysm are still controversial.

To verify our present indications for left ventricular aneurysmectomy we have reviewed our surgical data for the last 7 years.

Materials and Patient Selection

From September 1976 to September 1983 a total of 152 patients underwent left ventricular aneurysmectomy or resection of postinfarction scars at our institution. In 139 patients anterior wall resections were made, in 13 patients posterior wall resec-

Table 1. Operative procedures for left ventricular aneurysm in 152 patients (Sept. 1976–Sept. 1983)

	n	deaths
An	72	1
An + ACVG	61	10
An + ACVG + MVR	2	2
An + ACVG + VSD closure	1	
An + ACVG + EEV	4	
An + VSD closure	5	2
An + MVR	5	
An + EEV	2	1
	152	16

Abbreviations: An, isolated aneurysmectomy; ACVG, aortocoronary vein graft; MVR, mitral valve replacement; VSD, ventricular septal defect; EEV, encircling endocardial ventriculotomy

Table 2. Indications for operation

	Isolated aneurysmectomy	Combined procedure
1. Congestive heart failure	37	14
2. Angina pectoris	10	44
3. Ventricular arrhythmia	2	4
4. Thromboembolic episodes	8	0
5. Combined	15	18

tions were performed. Seventy-two patients were treated by isolated aneurysmectomy, while in the other patients, procedures concomitant to aneurysmectomy were: aortocoronary bypass grafting in 61, prosthetic valve replacement in 7, closure of ventricular septal defect in 6, and endocardial circumcision in 6 patients.

The leading indication in the group of patients with isolated aneurysmectomy was congestive heart failure (in 65%), and in the group of patients who underwent combined procedures, angina pectoris (in 75%) (Table 2).

Seventeen percent of the patients were female, 83% male. At the time of operation, 50% of the females and 26% of the males were under 45 years of age. Single-vessel disease was found in 50% of the females, with postinfarction left ventricular aneurysms, but in only 25% of the males (Fig. 1).

Almost half the aneurysmectomies were performed in patients with single-vessel disease, while procedures additional to aneurysmectomy were necessary in patients with multiple vessel disease. In the group of patients in whom isolated aneurysmec-

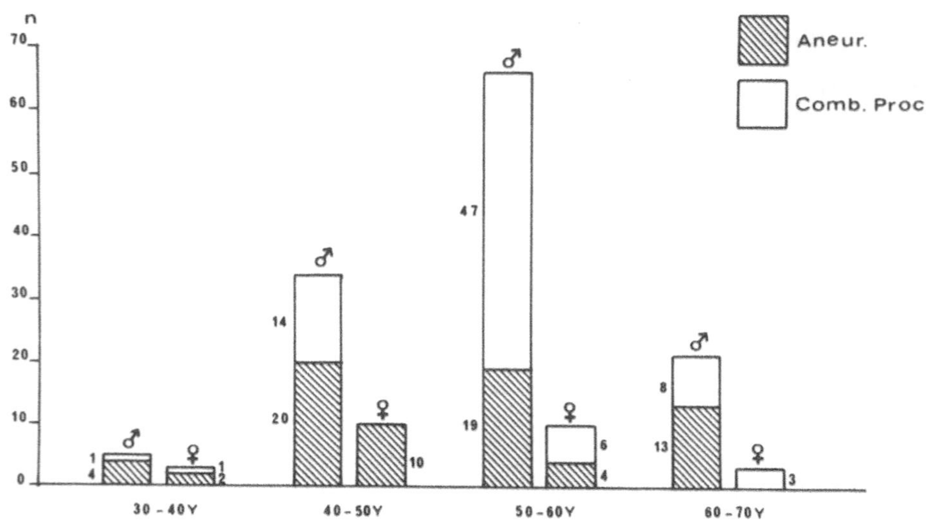

Fig. 1. Age and sex distribution of patients according to operative procedure

Table 3. Indications for operation according to extent of coronary disease

	Isolated aneurysmectomy		Combined procedure	
	n	%	*n*	%
One-vessel disease	31	43	11	13.8
Two-vessel disease	16	22	16	20
Three-vessel disease	25	35	53	66.2
	72	100	80	100

tomies were performed despite an underlying multiple vessel disease, associated bypass grafting was either not indicated or technically not possible (Table 3).

The most important angiographic criteria for patient selection for left ventricular aneurysmectomy were therefore near normal to normal function of the remaining left ventricular wall, and sufficient perfusion of the remaining myocardium.

While surgery was indicated due to recurrent thromboembolic episodes in only 5% of the patients, intraventricular thrombi could be found in 25% intraoperatively. In the majority (32) of these patients, embolic events had never occurred preoperatively.

Results

Operative mortality was 1.4% in patients with isolated aneurysmectomy and 18.5% in patients with combined procedures. The overall mortality therefore amounted to 10.5% (Table 4).

Table 4. Early Mortality

	n	Deaths	Mortality %
Isolated aneurysmectomy	12	1	1.4
Combined procedures	80	15	18.75
	152	16	10.5

Table 5. Causes of death

Cause	*n*
Low cardiac output (poor preop. LV function)	8
Sepsis	1
Arrhythmias	1
Renal and/or pulmonary insufficiency	3
Surgical reasons	2
Unknown	1

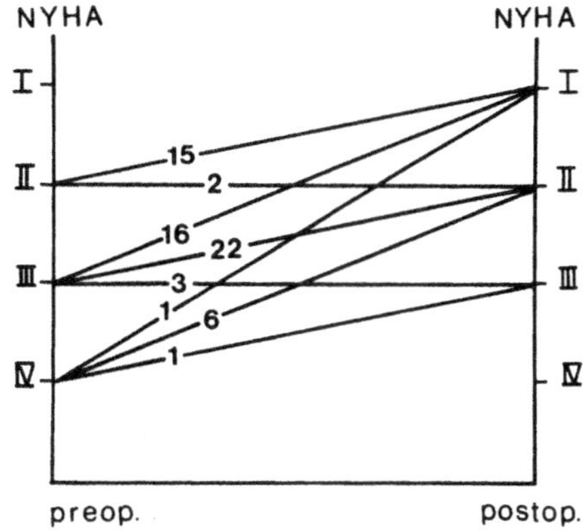

Fig. 2. Change in NYHA classification

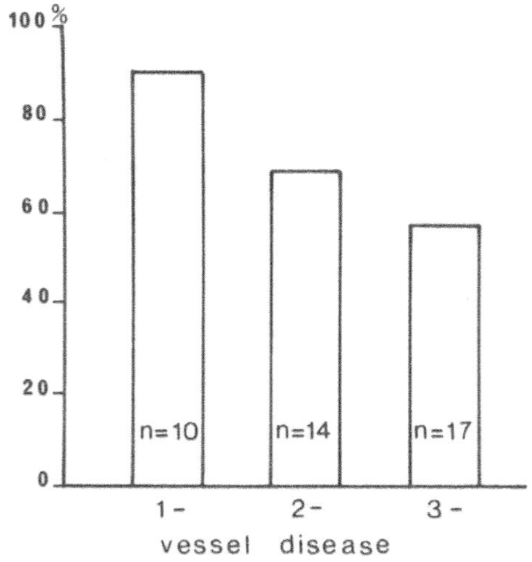

Fig. 3. Exercise capacity after aneurysmectomy (% of normal capacity) according to extent of coronary disease

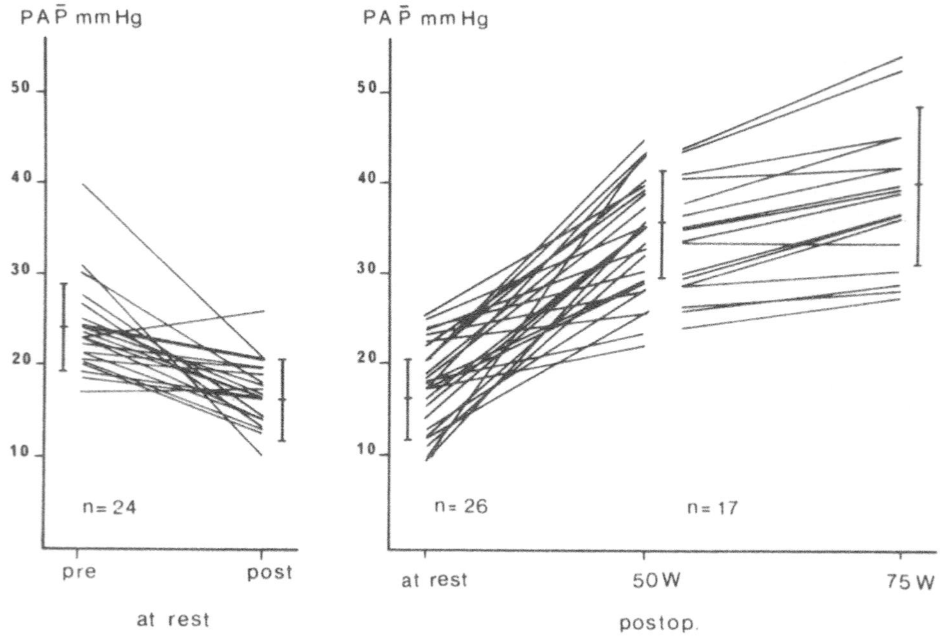

Fig. 4 a, b. Mean pulmonary artery *(PAP̄)* pressures at rest before and after aneurysmectomy (**a**) and during exercise after aneurysmectomy (**b**)

The most frequent cause of early death was postoperative low cardiac output, in eight patients with preoperative poor left ventricular function. Other causes were renal and/or pulmonary insufficiency, septicemia, tachycardia, or intraoperative technical problems (Table 5).

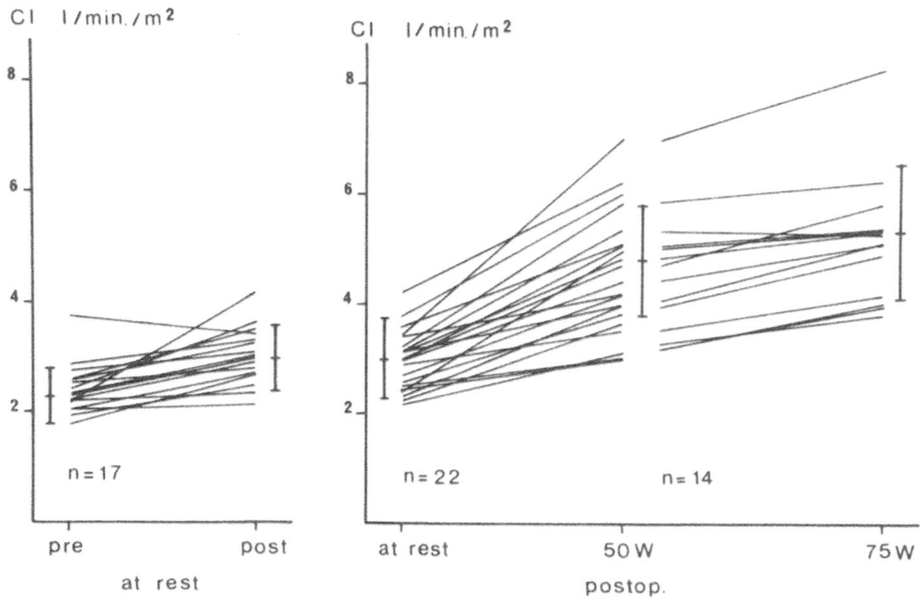

Fig. 5 a, b. Cardiac index *(CI)* at rest before and after aneurysmectomy (**a**) and during exercise after aneurysmectomy (**b**)

In only 6.2% of the patients treated surgically could no clinical improvement be found at postoperative reinvestigation. In contrast 52.8% of the patients improved by one, 30.6% by two, and one patient by three classes according to the NYHA classification. Approximately 45% of all patients were hemodynamically restudied after isolated aneurysmectomy (Fig. 2).

On exercise test, most of the patients with isolated aneurysmectomy and single-vessel disease reached 90% of the normal working capacity, while this was reduced to 70% in patients with double-vessel disease, and to less than 60% in patients with multiple vessel disease (Fig. 3).

Mean pulmonary artery pressure dropped from 26 to 17 mmHg at rest postoperatively but increased threefold during physical exercise after 6 min at 75 watts (Fig. 4).

The cardiac index increased postoperatively to 0.8 in the mean at rest and from 3 to 5.4 under exercise (75 watts). There was no relationship between exercise capacity and preoperative mean pulmonary artery pressure, left ventricular end-diastolic pressure, or cardiac index (Fig. 5).

Of 10 patients in whom isolated aneurysmectomy was performed (mainly because of angina pectoris), 9 showed remarkable improvement after the operation. However, in only 45% of the patients with preoperative ventricular tachycardia could reduction of arrhythmia could be observed postoperatively.

Conclusions

As known from previous clinical studies, life expectancy in patients with left ventricular aneurysms is much better with surgical treatment than with medical treatment. Because of these findings we have extended our indications for left ventricular aneurysmectomy in patients with isolated aneurysm to those of NYHA clinical class II. Our approach has been justified by low operative mortality and acceptable early clinical results confirmed by our hemodynamic studies. In patients with multiple vessel disease complete revascularization in addition to aneurysmectomy is indicated with regard to clinical improvement and late survival. On the other hand ventricular arrhythmias refractory to medical treatment are no longer an indication for isolated aneurysmectomy. In these patients, routine intraoperative electrophysiologic measurements are necessary to decide whether or not additional endocardial circumcision or resection should be performed.

False Aneurysm of the Left Ventricle After Myocardial Infarction

N. Goebel, R. Jenni, W. Steinbrunn, M. Turina, M. Rothlin, and Å. Senning

Rupture of the heart wall after myocardial infarction occurs in 6% of patients, mainly within the first 10 days [4]. The outcome is usually fatal, except in those cases where pericardial adhesions and paracardial tissue confine the hematoma. The formation of a false aneurysm is sooner or later followed by recurrent rupture or progressive heart failure. An early diagnosis is important, but the clinical diagnosis is often difficult. We report here our experience in 12 patients with false aneurysms.

Patients and Methods

From 1975 to 1983 the diagnosis of false aneurysm was made in 12 patients (pts), 11 men and 1 woman, with a mean age of 58 years (42–76 years). Only two pts had been transferred to our hospital because a false aneurysm had been suspected. Besides the ECG and chest X-ray, one-dimensional echocardiography was carried out in nine pts with Organon-Technica equipment (transducer, 2.25 MHz) and registered on a strip chart recorder. Two-dimensional echocardiography was performed in seven pts with a phased array sector scanner (Varian 3400) and registered on videotape together with the ECG. Parasternal long axis views, parasternal short axis views on different levels, a four-chamber view, and an RAO-equivalent view were registered. All pts were examined by heart catheterization with biplane levocardiography and selective coronary angiography.

Results

Main symptoms on admission were progressive heart failure in seven pts, new systolic heart murmur in six, and rhythm disturbances in four. One pt had only slight symptoms, one had no cardiac symptoms. He was admitted because of an abnormal heart contour (Fig. 1).

Of the pts 11 had suffered an event with severe retrosternal pain, and 5 had experienced further attacks of pain in the following days. In three pts definite symptoms of pericarditis were observed. Two pts had a holosystolic murmur with a precordial thrill, which suggested septal rupture.

The *ECG* showed inferior and/or posterior infarction in six pts and elevation of the ST segment in three, compatible with infero-posterior aneurysm. There were no signs of infarction in the ECGs of three pts. *Chest X-ray* was suggestive of an aneurysm in seven pts, but strongly suggestive of a false aneurysm [3] in only three (bulging mass projecting posteriorly in two, huge aneurysm below the apex in one). In five pts cardiomegaly was observed, because the inferiorly positioned aneurysm shifted the rest of the heart upward and outward. Eight pts had lung congestion.

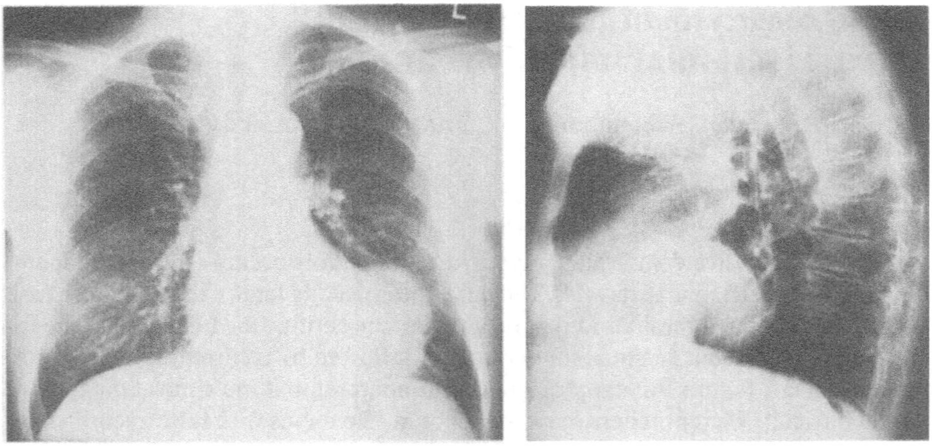

Fig. 1a, b. Typical aspects of a false aneurysm of the posterolateral wall

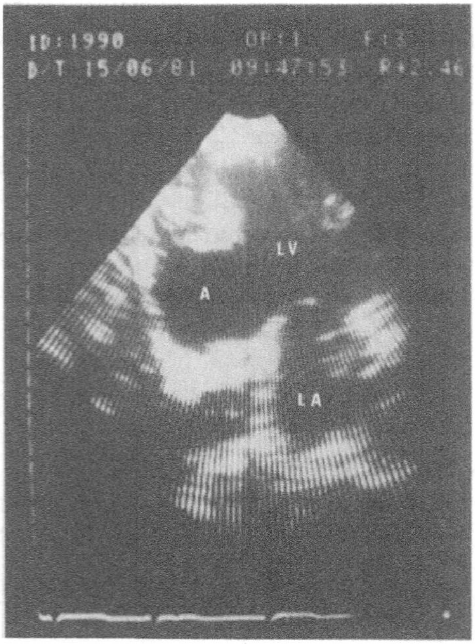

Fig. 2. Two-dimensional echocardiogram (four-chamber view): False aneurysm **A** of the inferior wall, projecting below the right ventricle. **LV,** left ventricle; **LA,** left atrium

With *two-dimensional echocardiography* [1] the diagnosis of a false aneurysm could be made in all seven pts examined, but was missed in two pts who had only one-dimensional echocardiography. Two-dimensional criteria were: an usually large saccular structure communicating with the ventricular cavity through a smaller opening, absence of myocardium in its wall, and paradoxical motions (Fig. 2).

Computed tomography which clearly delineated the false aneurysm of the posterior wall, was carried out in two pts only (Fig. 3).

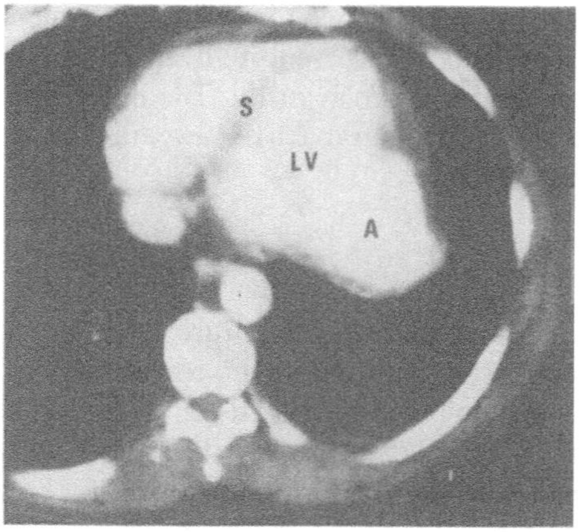

Fig. 3. Computed tomograph of false aneurysm **A** of the posterolateral wall. **LV**, left ventricle; *S*, ventricular septum

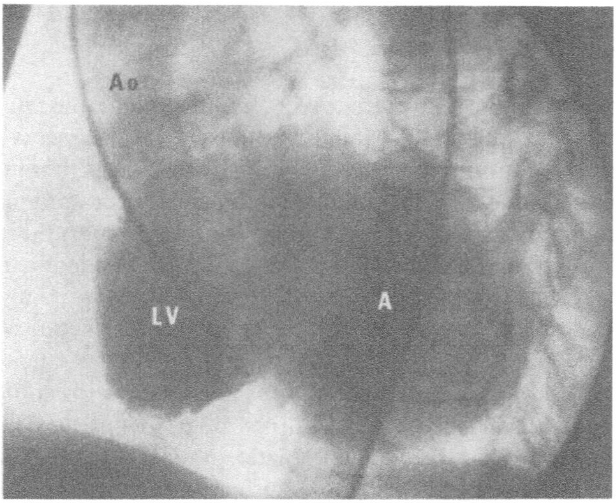

Fig. 4. Levocardiogram (LAO projection): Huge false aneurysm **A** of posterior wall. **LV,** left ventricle; **Ao,** ascending aorta

In all 12 pts the diagnosis was confirmed by *angiocardiography.* Angiographic characteristics were as in echocardiography: a saccular structure, usually bigger or at least the same size as the rest of the ventricle, communicating through a smaller opening with the left ventricle, and displaying sharp angles at the point of transition from ventricle to aneurysm (Fig. 4). The rest of the left ventricle usually showed good contractions. In 11 cases the aneurysm originated from the inferior or posterior wall. In two pts concomitant septal rupture was observed. Coronary angiography demonstrated stenoses in all pts, but six had only one-vessel disease.

In 11 pts the right or circumflex arteries were involved. The false aneurysm was resected in 11 pts, with additional closure of a ventricular septal defect in 2 and aortocoronary bypass in 5. The pt without cardiac symptoms was not operated because of concomitant dissecting aortic aneurysm. During operation pericardial adhesions were found in each case. The false aneurysms usually contained thrombi and their walls were thin. In the early postoperative period there were no deaths. Subsequently, 4–10 weeks postoperatively, three pts died; two of recurrent myocardial infarction and one of aspiration pneumonia after cerebrovascular insult. The other eight pts are symptom-free. The asymptomatic pt has also survived for 3 years without surgery.

Discussion

False aneurysms can produce the signs of progressive heart failure (7/12), new heart murmur (6/12), and rhythm disturbances (4/12), whereby the correct diagnosis is usually not made clinically. Three pts did not even have signs of infarction in the ECG. Rather typical in the chest X-ray is an enlarged heart with a protruding posterior mass [2], but this was seldom seen in our pts. The best noninvasive tool for diagnosis is two-dimensional echocardiography, but the false aneurysm may also be detected by computed tomography or scintigraphy. Resection is the treatment of choice. Long-term results are favorable: eight of the operated pts are symptom-free.

Summary

From 1975 to 1983 false aneurysms of the left ventricle were found angiographically in 1 woman and 11 men (mean age 58 years). Main symptoms were progressive heart failure in seven patients, new murmur in six, and rhythm disturbances in four. One patient (pt) had no symptoms, one had only mild symptoms. ECG showed inferior and/or posterior infarction in six pts and inferoposterior aneurysm in three pts, while three had no signs of infarction. Chest X-ray was suggestive of aneurysm in seven pts. Two-dimensional echocardiography performed in seven pts was diagnostic in all. Computed tomography in two pts also allowed noninvasive diagnosis. Angiography revealed 11 inferior and/or posterior aneurysms, one apical aneurysm, and two septal ruptures. Eleven pts were operated for aneurysm, with additional closure of ventricular septal defects in two and aortocoronary bypass in five. There were three postoperative deaths. The asymptomatic pt has survived for 3 years without surgery. In conclusion, clinical diagnosis of false aneurysm is difficult. Two-dimensional echocardiography allows noninvasive diagnosis. Early surgery is usually mandatory, but spontaneous long-term survival may be possible.

References

1. Catherwood E, Mintz GS, Kotler MN, Parry WR, Segal BL (1980) Two-dimensional echocardiographic recognition of left ventricular pseudoaneurysm. Circulation 62: 294–303
2. Gueron M, Wanderman KL, Hirsch M, Borman J (1975) Pseudoaneurysm of the left ventricle after myocardial infarction. J Thorac Cardiovasc Surg 69: 736–742
3. Higgins CB, Lipton MJ, Johnson AD, Peterson KL, Vieweg WVR (1978) False aneurysms of the left ventricle. Radiology 127: 21–27
4. Petrov K, Karalambev N, Toneva N, Vassilev C (1977) Analyse de 153 cas de rupture du myocarde. Arch Mal Coeur 70: 691–697

Clinical Experience in 445 Resections of Ventricular Aneurysms

R. Achatzy, E. Anyanwu, F. Klinke, V. Jelesijevic, H. Greve, and H. Dittrich

Of all ventricular aneurysms, 90%–95% result from myocardial infarction. The incidence of ventricular aneurysm following myocardial infarction is about 10% [1–3].

Patients

From 1973 to 1983, 445 patients (422 men and 23 women) underwent surgery for ventricular aneurysm (Table 1). Out of them 36 patients, all male, had aortocoronary venous bypass grafting at the same session.

Preoperative Findings and Clinical Symptoms

Most of the patients (86.6%) presented one to four risk factors: smoking 73%, hyperlipidemia and/or diabetes 47%, hypertension 34%, and different types of stress 44%. One-quarter of the patients had associated peripheral atherosclerotic vascular disease, especially of the lower extremities (Table 2).

The majority of the patients presented with angina pectoris (85%). Other symptoms were dyspnea following little exertion (54%), arrhythmia (33%), arterial embolism preoperatively (7%), and varying degrees of mural thrombi diagnosed during the operation (84%). Calcification of the coronary arteries was diagnosed radiologically in 17%, and calcification of the wall of the aneurysm in 3% of the patients [1, 5].

The interval between the myocardial infarction and the diagnosis of the ventricular aneurysm ranged from 6 weeks to 15 years, mean 29 months.

Surgical Approach

Following median sternotomy, pericardiotomy, and cannulation of the venae cavae and the ascending aorta, the pericardial adhesions are cut down under the protection of the extracorporeal circulation. With the patient in a head-downward position and in normothermia, ventricular fibrillation is induced, during which – with the aorta still unclamped – an incision is made at the point of greatest curvature of the aneurysm. The incision is extended under direct vision, during which time blood is superficially suctioned away from the left ventricle. Following removal of the mural thrombi which are sometimes present, the aneurysmatic sac is resected like an orange peel, leaving a fibrous rim of about 1 cm for the suture. Should fresh nonadhesive thrombotic masses be present within the sac of the aneurysm, the ascending aorta is cross clamped to avoid embolization. If reconstruction of the coronaries is planned at the same time, we incise the coronary artery at the corresponding position during partial cardiopulmonary bypass, perform resection of the

Table 1. Resection of ventricular aneurysms

Period	1973–1983
Number of patients	445
Age	23–69 yrs mean 56.8 yrs
Sex	442 m/23 f
Location of the aneurysm	
anterior	442
posterior	3
associated VSD	1
Operative procedure	
Aneurysmectomy alone	409
Aneurysmectomy + ACB	36
RCA	22
RCA + CX	8
LAD	3
CX	3

ACB, aortocoronary bypass

Table 2. Preoperative findings

Risk factors	
Smoking	73%
Hyperlipidemia/diab. mell.	47%
Hypertension	24%
Stress	44%
Atherosclerotic peripheral vascular disease	25%
Symptoms	
Angina pectoris	85%
Dyspnea	54%
Arrhythmias	33%
Thromboembolism	7%

Diab. mell., diabetes mellitus

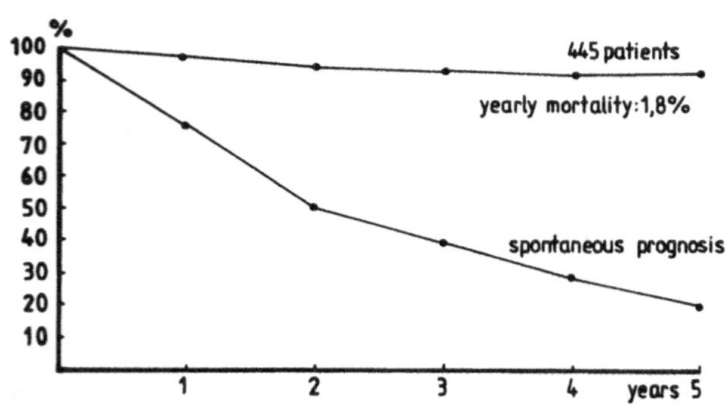

Fig. 1. Cumulative survival rate of 445 patients following resection of ventricular aneurysms

Table 3. Postoperative findings

Improvement	70%
No improvement	12%
Deterioration	18%
Reinfarction	9.8%
Continued medical management	72%
Return to profession total	28%
under 40 yrs	70%
over 40 yrs	16%

aneurysm as already described, carry out cardioplegic cardiac arrest, and perform the aortocoronary bypass grafting in total cardiopulmonary bypass [2–4].

Following careful air removal from the left ventricle and from the ascending aorta, the ventricle is closed with two rows of continuous sutures. We do not use felt routinely because hemorrhage from under the stripes of felt is difficult to control. If the myocardium is fragile, we employ felt-secured U sutures to effect hemostasis. Our average cardiopulmonary bypass time for resection of an aneurysm – without concomitant aortocoronary bypass grafting – is 14 min.

Results

Of the 409 patients who had aneurysmectomy alone, 7 (1.7%) died immediately postoperatively, and of the 36 who had concomitant coronary reconstruction, 6 (16.6%) died immediately. The long-term survival rate was 95% in the 1st year and 92% after 5 years (Fig. 1). The outcome of the operation (Table 3), as assessed by the family doctors and the patients themselves, was that 70% of the patients felt subjectively better than before. While 12% of the patients did not have any improvement of their symptoms, 18% got worse. Postoperatively 9.8% of the patients survived a new myocardial infarction, the reinfarction rate being two times higher in patients who had coronary bypass concurrently than in those who had only the resection of the aneurysm.

Postoperatively, 72% of the patients still required pharmacological treatment with nitrates, digitalis, β-receptor blockers, and calcium antagonists.

One-quarter of the patients were admitted to a sanatorium after discharge from the hospital.

Following resection of their aneurysm only 28% of the patients returned to active professional life, whereas 68% were channelled to professional pension schemes. Eventually 85% of these were permanently pensioned. Without exception, all patients beyond 60 years of age were pensioned. It is interesting to note that 70% of all the patients under 40 years of age returned to active professional life as opposed to only 16% of those beyond 40 [1, 5].

Conclusion

In view of the grave prognosis for patients with unoperated ventricular aneurysm – 50% mortality rate after 2 years, 80% after 5 years, and 100% after 10 years – resection of the aneurysm with or without reconstruction of the coronary arteries is the only alternative to extend life and improve the quality of life for most of these patients.

References

1. Emde J von der, Hacker R, Weniger J (1974) Zur Therapie des Herzwandaneurysmas. Klinikarzt 6: 170
2. Fromme A (1982) Die Chirurgie des Herzwandaneurysmas. Dissertation
3. Krause E, Satter P (1980) Die Chirurgie des Ventrikelaneurysmas. Klinikarzt 9: 880
4. Reddy SB, Cooley DA, Duncan JM, Norman JC (1981) Left ventricular aneurysm: twenty-year surgical experience with 1572 patients at the Texas Heart Institute. Cardiovascular Diseases, Bulletin of the Texas Heart Institute 8 (2): 165
5. Rudolph P (1981) Präoperative Befunde und postoperatives Befinden von Patienten mit koronarer Herzerkrankung und Ventrikelaneurysma. Dissertation

Left Ventricular Aneurysmectomy Combined with Encircling Endocardial Ventriculotomy for Treatment of Recurrent Sustained Ventricular Tachycardia*

J. Ostermeyer, G. Breithardt, M. Borggrefe, E. Godehardt, and W. Bircks

Encircling endocardial ventriculotomy (EEV) as surgical treatment for recurrent sustained ventricular tachycardia (VT) in the setting of coronary artery disease was introduced in 1978 by Guiraudon [1]. Since then this technique has proved to be a highly efficient approach to eradicating enhanced ventricular electrical vulnerability and tachycardiac rhythm disturbances of the reentry type [2–4]. The mechanism of this antiarrhythmic effect is not quite clear; interruption of reentry circuits [1] or initiation of an ischemic injury to the arrhythmogenic tissues [5] are possibilities under discussion.

The original concept of EEV was to perform a complete, deep circumcision, mostly beyond the borderline between an aneurysmatic sac and the undamaged left ventricular (LV) myocardium, at the earliest electrical activation during VT.

As we know from the research of Duke University colleagues, EEV decreases regional blood flow to the encompassed myocardium [6] and may acutely result in a significant impairment in diastolic compliance and a loss of systolic excursion of the region [7]. In addition, complete EEV may cause severe LV papillary muscle dysfunction secondary to direct or indirect impairment, and a quite number of cases have come to our attention in which mitral valve replacement became necessary after complete EEV (personal communications: O. Alfieri, Utrecht, NL; E. Kreutzer, Munich, FRG).

Keeping these potentially life-threatening disadvantages of complete EEV in mind, it seems to be mandatory to keep the incision as small as possible to eradicate the VT and to make the patient a survivor without a prosthetic mitral valve.

Between 1978 and May 1983, 50 patients with recurrent sustained VT underwent electrophysiologically guided surgery at our institution. Of these, 46 patients (92%) had severe coronary artery disease and a history of myocardial infarction. Of the recent 40 consecutive patients, 12 (30%) had a complete EEV, and 28 (70%) a partial EEV, which means the incision included 54.4% ± 2.2% of the internal LV circumference. In 22 patients (79%) of the latter group the partial incision was mainly situated in the area of the ventricular septum.

Between the two groups with different types of EEV there were no significant differences in age, sex ratio, NYHA class, coronary disease, aneurysm location, concomitant bypass grafting, and left ventricular function. Their mean age at myocardial infarction was 52.6 years. There were 35 patients (87.5%) who had an aneurysm at the LV anterior wall, mostly including septal areas. The mean tachycardia rate was 212.6 beats per min. A mean left ventricular end-diastolic pressure (LVEDP) of

* This study was supported by the Ernst und Berta Grimmke Foundation, Düsseldorf, F.R.G., and the Sonderforschungsbereich Kardiologie (SFB 30) of the Deutsche Forschungsgemeinschaft, Bonn-Bad Godesberg, F.R.G.

20 mmHg documented a significantly impaired LV function, and the NYHA classes were II, II–III, and III. The mean interval between infarction and operation was calculated to be 28.2 months, and the mean age at operation was 54.9 years. The incidences of single, double, and triple vessel disease were 20%, 30%, and 50%, respectively. In addition to the partial or complete EEV 35 patients (88%) had LV aneurysmectomy, and 30 patients (75%) underwent aortocoronary bypass grafting. Of the entire group, three patients did not survive the perioperative period; two of them could not be weaned from cardiopulmonary bypass and died intraoperatively. One patient belonged to the complete EEV group, two to the partial incision group. Statistical analysis of these data shows no significant difference between the groups regarding hospital mortality.

The 37 survivors (93%) were continuously observed postoperatively to dectect spontaneously occurring arrhythmic events, and invasive electrophysiological studies were performed about 3 weeks after surgery in all patients to determine possibly persisting enhanced ventricular vulnerability. All patients who underwent complete EEV and 24 of 26 partial EEV patients were free of spontaneous arrhythmic events after surgery. During programmed electrophysiological stimulation, a ventricular tachycardia could be initiated in three patients of the complete EEV group and in seven of the partial EEV group (Table 1). These individuals have been discharged from the hospital on antiarrhythmic drug regimens.

With respect to statistics no significant difference could be documented between the two groups, which indicates an antiarrhythmic efficacy of electrophysiologically guided partial EEV similar to that already established for the complete procedure.

On follow-up of 2 to 37 months (mean 22.6 months) for the complete EEV (CEEV) group and 0.5 to 50 months (mean 15.2 months) for the partial EEV (PEEV) patients, three individuals of group I (CEEV) died late at an average of 10 months after surgery, all due to progressive congestive heart failure (CHF). In group II (PEEV) there were also three late deaths, at an average of 27 months postoperatively, due to reinfarction after occlusion of two bypass grafts, CHF, and fulminant pneumonia. Expressing these general mortality data in terms of cumulative survival (Fig. 1), there is no significant difference between the two groups, as indicated by a *p* value of 0.36.

Regarding postoperative morbidity, first of all it should mentioned that no recurrences of VT could be documented in the follow-up. Even those patients with in-

Table 1. Antiarrhythmic efficacy of electrophysiologically guided complete versus partial EEV

	Hosp. survey	Free of spontaneous VT	70% CL	
Complete EEV	11	11 (100%)	84.2%–100%	(n.s.)
Partial EEV	26	24 (92.3%)	82.8%– 97.4%	
		Free of induced VT		
Complete EEV	11	8 (72.7%)	52.6%– 87.5%	(n.s.)
Partial EEV	26	19 (73.1%)	61.3%– 82.7%	

CL, confidence limits

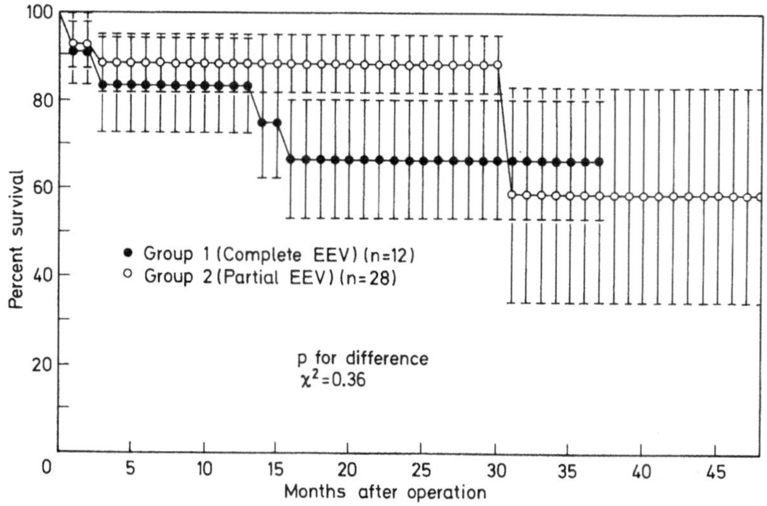

Fig. 1. Cumulative survival curves of group I (complete EEV) and group II (partial EEV) patients. The *vertical bars* enclose one standard error of the mean (i.e., approximately the 70% confidence limits)

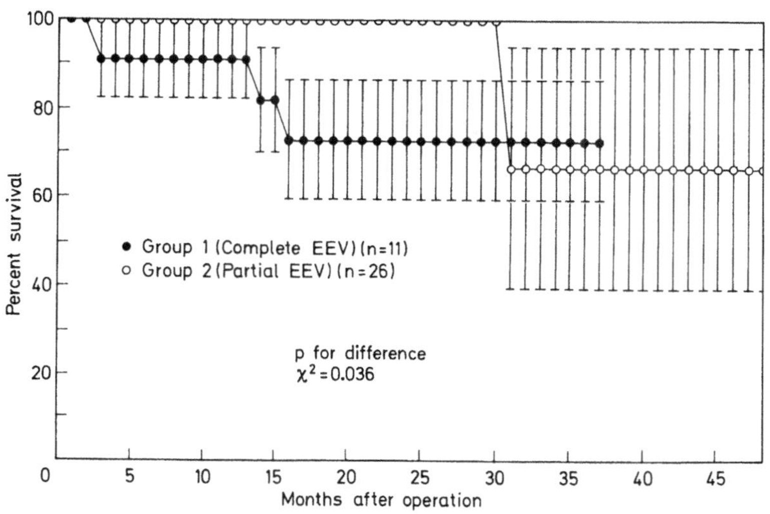

Fig. 2. "Modified" cumulative survival curves in group I (complete EEV) and group II (partial EEV) patients. In this plot the hospital deaths and all non-CHF deaths have been censored. The *vertical bars* enclose one standard error of the mean (i.e., approximately the 70% confidence limits)

ducible or spontaneous postsurgical VT have had good long-term results under the protection of different antiarrhythmic drugs. One patient has in addition an antiarrhythmic pacemaker.

In contrast to this encouraging aspect we have to indicate significant problems regarding late postoperative LV function, particularly in those patients who under-

Table 2. Incidence of late postoperative occurring LV dysfunction (clinical deterioration relative to the NYHA classification, clinical signs of progressive CHF and/or increasing LVEDP) and deaths due to CHF after complete and partial EEV

	Hosp. survey	LV Dysfunction	Death due to CHF
Complete EEV	11	5 (45.5%)	3 (27.3%)
Partial EEV	26	2 (7.7%)	1 (3.8%)
		p: 0.025	p: 0.036

went complete EEV (Table 2). The incidence of progressive LV failure relative to the preoperative state in this group was 45.5% compared with only 7.7% in the partial EEV patients ($p=0.025$). And also the role of CHF as a cause of death was significantly predominant in patients with complete EEV ($p=0.036$). In order to focus this particular problem in terms of cumulative survival in a final plot in Fig. 2, the hospital deaths and all late non-CHF deaths have been censored, which again identifies fatal LV failure as a significant late complication after complete EEV.

In conclusion: Electrophysiologically guided partial EEV as a modification of the technique introduced by Guiraudon proves to be a highly efficient approach to surgical treatment of recurrent sustained ventricular tachycardias. Complete EEV provides no significantly superior antiarrhythmic efficacy and should be avoided because of its apparent hazards to LV performance.

References

1. Guiraudon G, Fontaine G, Frank R, Escande G, Etievent P, Cabrol C (1978) Encircling endocardial ventriculotomy: a new surgical treatment for life threatening ventricular tachycardias resistant to medical treatment following myocardial infarction. Ann Thorac Surg 26: 438–443
2. Guiraudon G, Fontaine G, Frank R, Escande R, Etievent P et al. (1978) La ventriculotomie circulaire d'exclusion. Arch Mal Coeur 71: 1255–1262
3. Ostermeyer J, Breithardt G, Kolvenbach R, Borggrefe M, Seipel L, Schulte HD, Bircks W (1982) The surgical treatment of ventricular tachycardias (simple aneurysmectomy vs electrophysiologically guided procedures). J Thorac Cardiovasc Surg 84: 704–715
4. Ostermeyer J, Breithardt G, Borggrefe M, Godehardt E, Seipel L, Bircks W (in press) The surgical treatment of ventricular tachycardias (complete vs partial encircling endocardial ventriculotomy). J Thorac Cardiovasc Surg
5. Ungerleider RM, Holman WL, Stanley TE, Lofland GK, Williams JM, Ideker RE, Smith PK, Quick G, Cox JL (1982) EEV for refractory ischemic ventricular tachycardia. I. Electrophysiological effects. J Thorac Cardiovasc Surg 83: 840–849
6. Ungerleider RM, Holman WL, Stanley TE, Lofland GK et al. (1982) EEV for refractory ischemic ventricular tachycardia. II. Effects on regional blood flow. J Thorac Cardiovasc Surg 83: 850–856
7. Ungerleider RM, Holman WL, Calcagno D, Williams JM et al. (1982) EEV for refractory ischemic ventricular tachycardia. III. Effects on regional left ventricular function. J Thorac Cardiovasc Surg 83: 857–864

Surgical Treatment of Ventricular Tachycardias with Partial Endocardial Ventriculotomy

M. Vigano, L. Martinelli, G. Minzioni, C. Goggi, J. Salerno, and M. Chimienti

Introduction

Alternative surgical solutions have been proposed for some years in the face of the difficulties presented by medical treatment of ventricular tachycardia (VT) following myocardial infarction. Deeper knowledge of the electrophysiological mechanisms [2–5] of this type of tachycardia and above all the improvement of endo- and epicardial mapping techniques [6] in man have recently permitted the introduction of rational surgical techniques directed to the interruption of the reentry mechanism implicated in the pathogenesis of postinfarction VT.

In particular, two different surgical approaches have proved to be quite trustworthy both in regard to reduced perioperative mortality and the low percentage of arrhythmic recurrences. These are: endocardial encircling ventriculotomy [3], carried out with the purpose of electrically isolating the tissue responsible for the reentry, and endocardial resection, with the aim of directly eliminating the arrhythmogenic tissue [4].

The first technique, slightly modified, has been used in 16 patients affected by recurrent, sustained, life-threatening VT.

Materials and Methods

Between January 1980 and August 1983, 16 patients with recurrent VT following myocardial infarction were operated on.

The main clinical data are shown in Table 1. In particular, it must be noted that the VT was in all cases deeply incapacitating, both in its recurrence and in the symptoms evoked, comprising also cases of acute pulmonary edema and syncope. Furthermore, in all cases it has been necessary at least once to interrupt the VT with dc shock because of the hemodynamic and electrical instability of this type of tachycardia. This group of patients was selected because their VT was particularly resistant to various antiarrhythmic drugs, administered alone or in combination and in the maximum tolerable doses. Drugs have reduced the recurrence of attacks as well as the cardiac rate during VT, but they have not assured complete protection.

All patients underwent cardiac catheterization, left ventriculography, and coronary angiography. Before surgery, an endocavitary electrophysiologic study was performed in both right and left ventricles, with the aim of investigating the mechanism of VT and the possibility of inducing it with programmed pacing, as well as identifying its source and the path of electrical activation through the mapping of endocardial potentials.

Epicardial mapping was performed during the operation in all patients. In the first seven patients it was carried out manually by placing a bipolar reference elec-

Table 1. Main clinical and hemodynamic data of patients who underwent partial EEV

Age (years)	52	(±10)
Sex (M/F)	15/1	
ECG site of infarction:		
– anterior	12	
– posterior	4	
Interval between infarction and VT (months)	38	(±51)
Symptoms:		
– palpitations	16	
– severe dyspnea	10	
– syncope	4	
LVEDP	23.5	(±10.8)
LVEDV	222	(±76)
CI	3.3	(± 0.8)
EF (%)	27.8	(±11.3)

Abbreviations: LVEDP, left ventricular end-diastolic pressure; LVEDV, left ventricular end-diastolic volume; CI, cardiac index; EF, ejection fraction

trode on the epicardium of the right ventricle, while a catheter was used to explore 18–29 previously selected epicardial points on the two ventricles, using the main coronary branches as reference points. In the last ten patients we proceeded to automatic epicardial mapping, using 35 electrodes distributed over a net which is adapted to the ventricular surface and connected to a device furnished with a computer capable of reconstructing the sequence of ventricular activation on a map. Epicardial mapping (Fig. 1) was performed both during sinus rhythm and during spontaneous or electrically induced VT. In three cases intraoperative endocardial mapping was carried out over four to seven previously selected points, with an hand probe.

In all cases an endocardial ventriculotomy was performed to isolate the previously localized site of earliest ventricular activation. In the first two patients, where a positive localization was lacking, we proceeded to do an encircling ventriculotomy around the entire infarction scar along the edges of the surrounding healthy tissue, according to Guiraudon's technique [3]. In the next four patients an encircling ventriculotomy was performed, but extended to the subepicardial layers only in the area which was identified during the mapping as responsible for the onset of VT. In the last ten patients, the incision was restricted to the area of earliest activation. The incision was closed with a running suture.

Surgical Results

The operative mortality involved one patient died 2 days after surgery with low output syndrome. The postoperative course was uncomplicated in 13 patients. One patient developed clinical signs of congestive heart failure requiring chronic diuretic therapy. In another patient a recurrence of VT developed a week after the operation and the patient was discharged on antiarrhythmic treatment (amiodarone 400 mg/day).

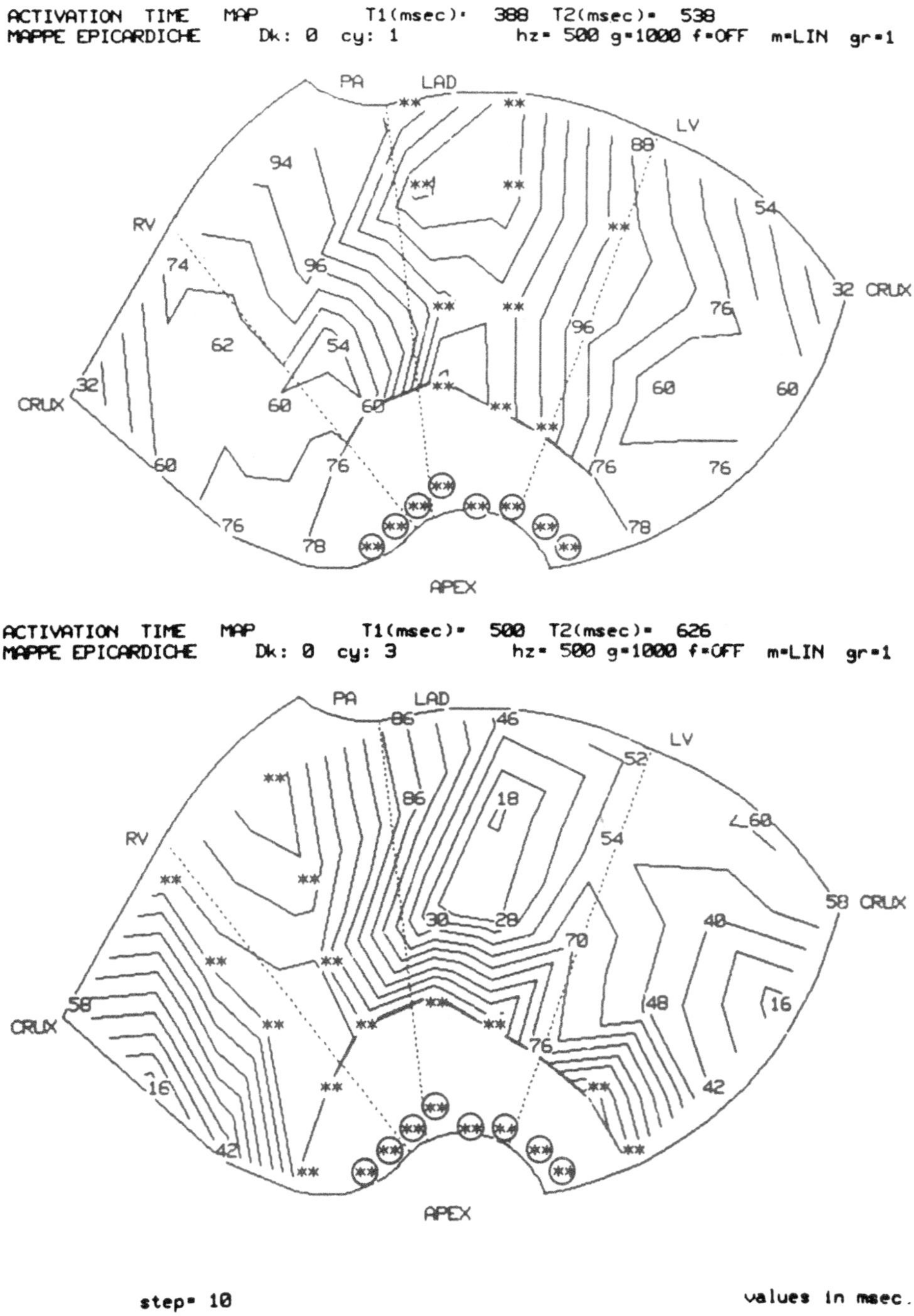

Fig. 1. Epicardial electromap determined via 35 unipolar electrodes distributed over the ventricles by means of an elastic grid. The *numbers* indicate (in ms) the time of local activation and the points at which activation occurs. *Asterisks* indicate 100 ms. The isochronic lines were traced automatically every 10 ms. *Above:* During VT, earliest epicardial activation is recorded near the crux of the heart (after 32 ms). *Below:* During sinus rhythm, delayed activation of the right ventricle was due to bundle-branch block. The difference between *T1* and *T2* indicates the duration of ventricular activation. *RV*, right ventricle; *LV*, left ventricle; *LAD*, left anterior descending coronary artery; *PA*, pulonary artery

Follow-up

The 15 patients discharged were followed (Fig. 2) for periods of between 2 and 45 months (mean 13.9±15). One patient, who had presented symptoms of heart failure in the postoperative period, developed a low output syndrome and died two months after surgery. During the follow-up period two patients had a recurrence of VT. In the first patient the VT appeared 3 months after the operation with the same electrocardiographic pattern as the previous VT. In the other patient arrhythmia recurred after a 15-month interval with different electrocardiographic aspects, at a lower heart rate, and was well tolerated. The patients were immediately given standard antiarrhythmic therapy (amiodarone 400 mg/day) with resulting complete control of the rhythm. The 11 patients clinically free from tachycardia were not given antiarrhythmic therapy. Repeated dynamic ECGs show only premature ventricular contraction in some cases.

Conclusions

The encircling endocardial ventriculotomy proposed by Guiraudon is performed at the border between the healthy endocardium and the fibrous wall, with the aim of electrically isolating this area and thus interrupting reentry circuits [3]. The major disadvantage of this technique is the negative effect that the incision has on the performance of the encompassed myocardium. In fact, the mortality usually reported is not arrhythmic, but related to low output syndrome. For these reasons we have modified the original technique, limiting the incision to around the earliest activation area. Therefore, accurate electrophysiological study is assumed to be indispensable. Intraoperative epicardial mapping performed automatically presents few technical difficulties and is a time-saving procedure. Intraoperative endocardial mapping would be more useful in investigating the origin of the VT [5], but unlike epicardial mapping it presents considerable difficulties, above all because the VT often cannot be induced or else degenerates suddenly into ventricular fibrillation.

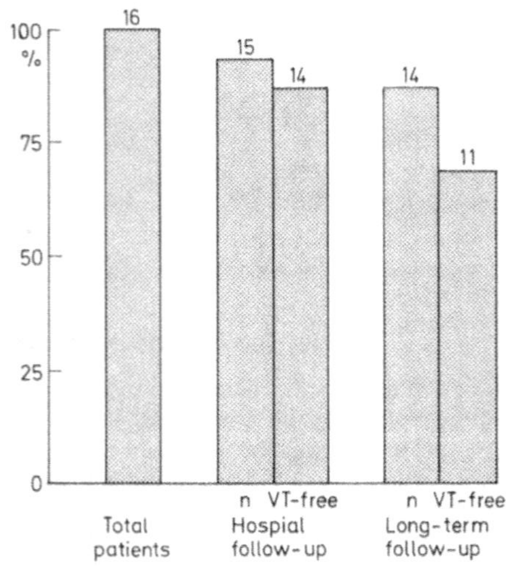

Fig. 2. Follow-up results for patients who underwent surgery for VT

In our experience the integration of the data obtained from preoperative endocardial mapping and from epicardial mapping is sufficient to localize with acceptable accuracy the arrhythmogenic area [1]. Further investigations are needed to improve the techniques of simultaneous recording of the potentials from multiple areas during preoperative and intraoperative endocardial mapping, in order to have an easy, safe and time-saving method of identifying the arrhythmogenic tissue.

References

1. Chimienti M, Salerno JA, Viganò M, Costantini M, Klersy C, Minzioni G, Pagnin A, Angoli L, Previtali M, Martinelli L, Marangoni E, Bobba P (in press) Ventricular tachycardia in chronic myocardial infarction. Electrophysiologic aspects, endocardial and epicardial mapping and surgical treatment. Giorn It Cardiol
2. Cox JL, Gallagher JJ, Ungerleider RM (1982) Encircling endocardial ventriculotomy for refractory ischemic ventricular tachycardia. IV. Clinical implications, surgical technique, mechanism of action and results. J Thorac Cardiovasc Surg 83: 865
3. Guiraudon G, Fontaine G, Frank R, Escande G, Etlevent P, Vignes R, Mattel MF, Cabrol A, Cabrol C (1978) La ventriculotomie circulaire d'exclusion. Traitement chirurgical des tachycardies ventriculaires compliquant un infarctus du myocarde. Arch Mal Coeur 71: 1255
4. Harken AH (1982) Surgery for ventricular tachycardia. The view from Philadelphia. Int J Cardiol 1: 361
5. Horowitz LN, Spear JF, Moore EN (1978) Subendocardial origin of ventricular arrhythmias in 24-hour-old experimental myocardial infarction. Circulation 53: 56
6. Josephson MF, Horowitz LN, Farshidi A, Kastor JA (1978) Recurrent sustained ventricular tachycardia. 2. Endocardial mapping. Circulation 57: 440

Ventricular Arrhythmias Before and After Aortocoronary Bypass Surgery

P. Pothen, R. Pigato, T. Rigo, C. Valfrè, V. Gallucci, and C. Dal Palù

Previous studies have shown that ventricular arrhythmias in patients with coronary artery disease are associated with an increased risk of sudden death [1–5]. More recently it has been documented that the mortality of patients with angiographically defined significant coronary artery disease is related to the grade of ventricular arrhythmia [6–7]. Callif [6] reported, in 395 patients with significant coronary artery disease, a 2-year mortality of 32% for patients who had paired premature ventricular contractions or ventricular tachycardia. If ventricular arrhythmia is related to myocardial ischemia, the hypothesis that coronary revascularization may reduce the incidence of ventricular arrhythmia by improving the perfusion defect is highly interesting. The objective of the study was to test this hypothesis.

Material and Methods

Patients (35) undergoing coronary revascularization for disabling and refractory angina were evaluated by 24-h Holter monitoring for detecting arrhythmia, before and after surgery. There were 31 males and 4 females and their mean age was 55 years. Twenty-two patients had a previous myocardial infarction, the interval between infarction and surgery varied from 1 to 10 years. Significant multivessel desease was present in 25 patients, and the remaining 10 patients had single vessel disease with stenosis of 75% or more. Twenty-four patients had asynergic left ventricular wall motion (localized hypokinesia and akinesia) and 11 patients had normal left ventricular contraction. No patient with ventricular aneurysm was included.

Nineteen patients showed a left ventricular end-diastolic pressure (LVEDP) of > 12 mmHg and the remaining 16 had an LVEDP of $\leqslant 12$ mmHg.

Holter monitoring was performed 1 week before surgery when the patients were on antianginal medication with nitrates in association with beta blockers or calcium antagonists or both. During the Holter monitoring the patients were restricted to the

Table 1. Lown's classification of ventricular arrhythmia

Grade	Type of arrhythmia
0	Without PVCs
1	Less than 30 PVCs/h
2	More than 30 PVCs/h
3	Polymorphic
4A	Pairs
4B	Ventricular tachycardia
5	R on T

ward. The first postoperative monitoring was done after 10 days: all of the patients had discontinued the antianginal medication and none of them was on antiarrhythmic drugs. The second postoperative monitoring was performed after 4 months: all of the patients except two were on beta blockers or calcium antagonists in association with antiaggregants, at dosages reduced to 40% of the preoperative levels. A two-channel portable electrocardiorecorder (model 445 Avionics) was used for monitoring. Computer-aided analysis of the ventricular arrhythmias was done using an electrocardioscanner (model Dcg VII Avionics). Lown's classification was used for evaluation of the ventricular arrhythmias, and grades 3, 4, and 5 were considered advanced grades (Table 1). The surgery was usually performed under moderate hypothermia (24°–28 °C) using cold cardioplegia.

The extracorporeal circulation time ranged from 63 to 150 min, aortic cross-clamp time ranged from 29 to 98 min, and the number of vein grafts from one to five.

Results

The frequencies of different grades of ventricular arrhythmias before surgery, after 10 days, and after 4 months are shown in Fig. 1. Before surgery 13 of 35 patients had grade 1, nine patients had grade 3, and five patients had grade 4 A ventricular arrhythmia.

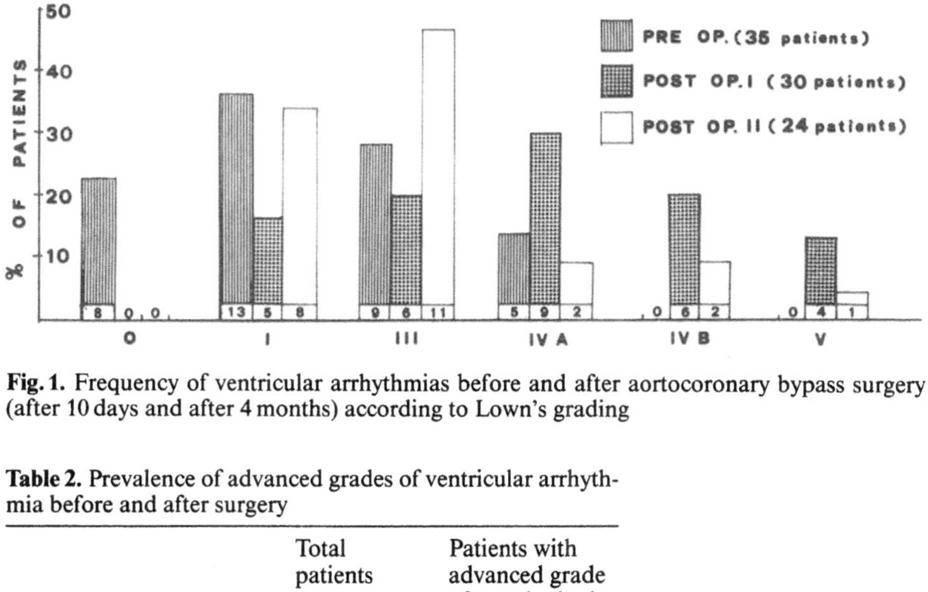

Fig. 1. Frequency of ventricular arrhythmias before and after aortocoronary bypass surgery (after 10 days and after 4 months) according to Lown's grading

Table 2. Prevalence of advanced grades of ventricular arrhythmia before and after surgery

	Total patients	Patients with advanced grade of v. arrhythmia	
		n	(%)
Before surgery	35	14	(40)
10 days after surgery	30	25	(83)
4 months after surgery	24	16	(66)

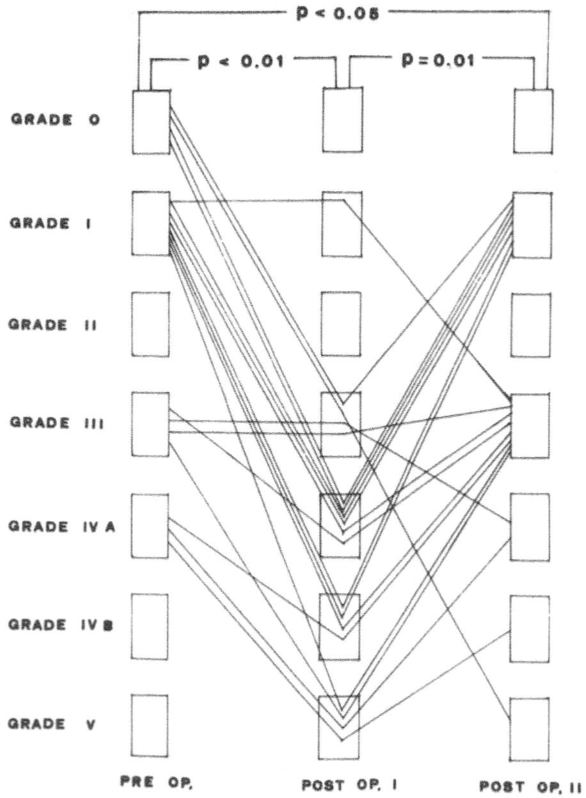

Fig. 2. Changes in the grades of ventricular arrhythmia after surgery (after 10 days and after 4 months) in 19 patients who underwent three sequential monitorings

Ten days after surgery Holter monitoring was performed in 30 patients, five of whom had grade 1, six grade 3, nine grade 4 A, six grade 4 B, and four grade 5 ventricular arrhythmia. Four months after aortocoronary bypass surgery, Holter monitoring performed in 24 patients showed grade 1 arrhythmia in eight patients, grade 3 in eleven patients, grade 4 A in two patients, grade 4 B in two patients and grade 5 in one patient. No patient had ventricular tachycardia or R on T before surgery.

Before surgery 40% of the patients had advanced grades of ventricular arrhythmia (Table 2). After 10 days 83%, and after 4 months 66% of the patients showed advanced-grade ventricular arrhythmias.

Statistical analysis using Wilcoxon's test in 19 patients who had each undergone three sequential Holter monitorings (Fig. 2), revealed that there was a significant increase in the grades of ventricular arrhythmia during the first postoperative monitoring ($p < 0.01$); nevertheless, during the second postoperative monitoring after 4 months, there was a significant reduction in the grades of ventricular arrhythmia compared to the first monitoring ($p = 0.01$).

Compared to the preoperative monitoring, there was a slight but significant increase in the grades of ventricular arrhythmia ($p < 0.05$).

In order to define those preoperative and intraoperative variables which that correlate significantly with the presence of advanced grades of ventricular arrhythmia, we used chi-square and Fisher's tests. The number of coronary arteries with significant lesion ($\geqslant 75\%$), presence of ventricular asynergy, LVEDP, previous myocardial infarction, duration of aortic clamping and extra corporeal circulation, and the extent of revascularization did not correlate statistically with the occurrence of advanced grades of ventricular arrhythmia after surgery.

Our finding that aortocoronary bypass surgery performed in patients with disabling angina does not reduce the incidence of ventricular arrhythmia within the period of 4 months, despite the marked improvement of the clinical status in the majority of the patients, is consistent with earlier studies [8–10]. We detected higher frequencies of advanced grades of ventricular arrhythmia both before and after surgery compared to the previous reports. But the studies also differ in patient characteristics, in the models of equipment used for analysis of the arrhythmias, and in the definitions of advanced grades of ventricular arrhythmia. Thus our results do not support the initial hypothesis that coronary revascularization may reduce the incidence of ventricular arrhythmia by improving the perfusion defect.

References

1. The Coronary Drug Project Research Group (1973) Prognostic importance of premature beats following myocardial infarction. JAMA 223: 1116–1124
2. Chiang BN, Perlman LV, Ostrander LD Jr, Epstein FH (1979) Relationship of premature systoles to coronary heart disease and sudden death in the Tecumseh epidemiologic study. Ann Intern Med 70: 1159–1160
3. Ruberman W, Weinblatt E, Goldberg JD, Frank CW, Shapiro S, Feldman CL (1976) Prognostic value of one hour of ECG monitoring of men with coronary heart disease. J Chron Dis 29: 497–512
4. Moss AJ, Davis HT, DeCamilla J, Bayer LW (1979) Ventricular ectopic beats and their relation to sudden and nonsudden cardiac death after myocardial infarction. Circulation 60: 998–1003
5. Vismara LA, Vera Z, Foerster JM, Amsterdam EA, Mason DT (1977) Identification of sudden death risk factors in acute and chronic coronary artery disease. Am J Cardiol 39: 821–828
6. Califf RM, McKinnis RA, Burks J, Lee KL, Harrell FE, Behar VS, Pryor DB, Wagner GS, Rosati RA (1982) Prognostic implications of ventricular arrhythmias during 24-hour ambulatory monitoring in patients undergoing cardiac catheterization for coronary artery disease. Am J Cardiol 50: 23–31
7. Bigger JT, Weld FM, Rolnitzky ML (1981) Prevalent characteristics and significance of ventricular tachycardia detected with ambulatory electrocardiographic recording in the late hospital phase of acute myocardial infarction. Am J Cardiol 48: 815
8. Grayboys TB, Lown B, Collins JJ, Cohn LH (1978) Does coronary revascularization reduce the prevalence of ventricular ectopic activity. Am J Cardiol 41: 401 (Abstract)
9. Michelson EL, Morganroth J, MacVaugh H (1979) Postoperative arrhythmias after coronary artery and cardiac valvular surgery detected by long term electrocardiographic monitoring. Am Heart J 97: 442
10. Soyza de PN, Thenabadu N, Marvin L, Murphy ML, Kane JS, Doherty JE (1981) Ventricular arrhythmia before and after aorto-coronary bypass surgery. Int J Cardiol 1: 123–130

Endocardial Resection for Ventricular Tachycardia and Ventricular Fibrillation

C. J. Hilton, R. W. F. Campbell, D. S. Reid, P. C. Adams, C. Griffiths, and D. G. Julian

Introduction

The treatment of cardiac dysrhythmias has always been primarily the concern of the physician, but despite considerable recent advances in the medical treatment of ventricular tachycardias (VT) and ventricular fibrillation (VF) there remains a proportion of patients in whom the dysrhythmia remains refractory to current drugs administered either alone or in combination. For these patients surgical treatment is an attractive alternative. The early methods of surgical treatment yielded unpredictable results [1–3]. The more recently evolved techniques of intra-operative electrophysiological mapping followed by either encircling endocardial ventriculotomy or endocardial resection have markedly improved the results in monomorphic VT [4, 5] but their role in polymorphic VT and VF remains uncertain. We will present our experience of electrophysiologically guided resection in the management of eight patients, six of whom fall into this difficult category. Prior to our first venture into the surgery of ventricular dysrhythmias we decided to use endocardial resection rather than encircling ventriculotomy as we envisaged technical problems where the areas of abnormal activation were on the septum or involved both ventricles.

Patients

Eight patients with recurrent ventricular dysrhythmias underwent surgery for control of their rhythm disorders (Table 1). Six men and one woman (ages 31–60) had coronary artery disease as the underlying cause of their dysrhythmia, while one

Table 1. Pre-operative patient data

Patient	Age/sex	Dysrhythmia	Aetiology	Drug therapy
G.R.	31 F	polymorphic VT (2)	myocardial infarction 6/12	class Ia, Ib, Ic II III IV
J.L.	58 M	polymorphic VT (2)	myocardial infarction 4/52	class Ia Ib II III
J.A.	33 F	VT/VF	unknown	class Ia Ib II III IV
J.G.	60 M	polymorphic VT (2)	myocardial infarction 4/12	class Ia Ib II III IV
W.H.R.	60 M	monomorphic VT	myocardial infarction 1 yr	class Ib III
H.G.	56 M	polymorphic VT (3)	myocardial infarction 5 yrs 8/12	class Ia Ib Ic III IV
D.H.	36 M	exercise induced VT/VF	myocardial infarction 2 yrs	–
A.M.	42 M	monomorphic VT	myocardial infarction 4/12	class Ia Ib III

woman had an anatomically normal heart. Those patients with ischemic heart disease had all suffered at least one myocardial infarction from 4 weeks to 4 years prior to surgery. Seven of the eight patients had trials of drug therapy involving multiple agents. One patient, in whom the dysrhythmia arose acutely, underwent surgery without extensive medical therapy. In seven of the eight patients the primary indication for surgery was their dysrhythmia, while the eighth patient developed a VT while awaiting left ventricular aneurysmectomy and coronary artery bypass grafting.

Pre-operative investigations in one patient (J. A.) revealed an anatomically normal heart, but all other patients had previous myocardial infarctions with or without aneurysm formation. All had varying degrees of ventricular dysfunction and coronary artery disease. In six cases this involved three major vessels while in one there was only single-vessel disease.

Electrophysiological studies showed two of the patients to have a reproducible monomorphic VT. Four patients had polymorphic VT, three showing two separate morphologies and one patient, three morphologies. Two further patients showed polymorphic VT rapidly degenerating to ventricular fibrillation or primary VF.

Techniques

Routine cardiopulmonary bypass through a median sternotomy was used in all cases. Normothermia was maintained during the mapping procedures with cardiac perfusion via a separate aortic root cannula. Hypothermia and cardioplegia were instituted once mapping was complete to facilitate additional procedures such as coronary grafting.

Epicardial and endocardial maps were constructed as described by Horowitz [6]. In five patients VT could not be sustained for sufficient time to construct complete maps. In these five patients areas of endocardium showing abnormally prolonged and fragmented electrograms were mapped while pace mapping was attempted in two. Difficulty was encountered in interpretation of the pace maps as the patients had several separate tachycardias to be identified.

In all patients areas of endocardium delineated by the above techniques were excised. In only one patient was the abnormal area excised as part of an aneurysmectomy while seven patients required specific endocardial resection. In one case the abnormal area was shown to be between the two papillary muscles and extending onto the lateral wall of the ventricle, while in the other six the area to be resected was judged to extend onto the septum. In one patient (J. G.) abnormal endocardium was removed from both right and left ventricles while another (J. A.) required total endocardial resection of the left ventricle (LV). In a further patient (H. G.) endocardial resection failed to control the dysrhythmia as the area of early activation extended onto the inferior papillary muscle. A cryoprobe was successfully used to eliminate this area.

Additional procedures were carried out in seven patients, two patients requiring coronary artery bypass grafting (CABG), two patients requiring LV aneurysmectomy and three patients undergoing both CABG and aneurysmectomy.

Results

Surgical

Of the eight patients, six survived to leave hospital (Table 2). The two deaths were not related to the dysrhythmia, one patient dying on the 9th postoperative day of a septicaemia secondary to a chest infection and one patient dying on the operating table after failing to come off bypass. This latter patient was in cardiogenic shock pre-operatively.

Of the six survivors followed up for 5–31 months, two who had pre-operative ejection fractions of < 20% suffer a degree of LV failure controlled by medical therapy.

Electrophysiology

None of the six patients has suffered a spontaneous recurrence of their pre-operative dysrhythmia. One patient (H. G.) is receiving amiodarone therapy, as a VT with a morphology unlike his natural dysrhythmia could be stimulated at postoperative

Table 2. Results of surgery in VT/VF

Patient	Operation	Result	
		Electrophysiological (EP)	Clinical
G. R.	Mapping, pace maps, and 'fragmentation' LV aneurysmectomy endocardial resection	No dysrhythmia	Excellent no drugs
J. L.	Mapping LV aneurysmectomy endocardial resection	–	Died on operating table
J. A.	'Fragmentation' mapping endocardial resection – total	No dysrhythmia	Excellent digoxin only
J. G.	Mapping, pace maps and 'fragmentation' endocardial resection LV and RV CABG × 3	Occasional VEs	Controlled LV failure no antidysrhythmic drugs
W. H. R.	Mapping and 'fragmentation' LV aneurysmectomy CABG × 3	No dysrhythmia	No antidysrhytmic drugs
H. G.	Mapping and 'fragmentation' endocardial resection cryoprobe CABG × 3	New VT on vigorous EP stimulation, no spontaneous dysrhythmia	Amiodarone mild LVF
D. H.	Mapping and 'fragmentation' endocardial resection CABG × 1 LV aneurysmectomy	No dysrhythmia	Excellent no drugs
A. M.	Mapping and 'fragmentation' endocardial resection LV aneurysmectomy CABG × 2	No dysrhythmia	Diet at nine days – septicaemia

LVF, left ventricular failure; VEs, ventricular extra beats; EP, electrophysiological

electrophysiological study. Repeat study on amiodarone failed to elicit any dysrhythmia although amiodarone had been unsuccessful in controlling his original tachycardia.

In no other patient could any significant dysrhythmia be elicited during these postoperative studies, including the patient who died at 9 days of septicaemia.

Disucssion

Electrophysiological guidance of surgery for ventricular dysrhythmia offers logical hope of increased effectiveness of the treatment of medically resistant arrhythmias. The treatment of monomorphic VT by these methods is now becoming accepted practice [7, 8]. Polymorphic VT and VF present a more challenging problem but by the use of conventional mapping techniques and attention to the morphology of the electrogram good results can be achieved.

In those patients with unmappable dysrhythmias the localization of dysrhythmic activity is more difficult. Pace mapping techniques may be of use in this regard but the matching of the morphology of the dysrhythmias may be complicated by displacement of the heart and distortion of the chest during surgery and the multiplicity of morphologies to be located. The appearance of prolonged fragmented electrograms on endocardial and epicardial mapping seems to point to abnormal areas of endocardium, the resection of which in our series controlled the patients dysrhythmias.

We preferred endocardial resection to encircling ventriculotomy for the isolation of the abnormal areas, as we anticipated difficulties in excluding abnormal areas in the right ventricle and high on the interventricular septum. We feel this proved significant in one of our patients where early activation was found on both sides of the ventricular septum. In a further patient the abnormal activity extended onto the posterior papillary muscle and a cryoprobe was used to control the tachycardia as suggested by Harrison et al. [9]. This also may be a useful technique in awkward and unresectable areas.

Conclusions

We believe that electrophysiological mapping of VT followed by endocardial resection increases the success rate in the surgery of monomorphic VT and can be successfully applied in polymorphic VT and VF.

We also feel that the paying of attention to the fragmentation of the electrogram may be of use in identifying electrophysiologically abnormal areas when sustained VT cannot be initiated at surgery and conventional mapping is therefore impossible.

Our experience with one patient with unmappable VF and no anatomical abnormality confirms our belief in 'fragmentation' maps and also suggests to us that in the absence of the facility for mapping, then extended or total endocardial resection may be a useful adjunct to LV aneurysmectomy and CABG to increase the success rate in dysrhythmia surgery.

References

1. Sealy WC, Oldham HN (1978) Surgical treatment of malignant ventricular arrhythmias by sympathectomy, coronary artery grafts and heart wall resection. In: Kelly DT (ed) Advances in the management of arrhythmias. Telectronics PTY, Sydney, pp 218–224
2. Sami M et al. (1978) Longterm follow up of aneurysmectomy for recurrent ventricular tachycardia or fibrillation. Am Heart J 96 (3): 303–308
3. Ricks WB, Winkle RA, Shumway NE, Harrison DC (1977) Surgical management of life-threatening ventricular arrhythmias in patients with coronary artery disease. Circulation 56 (1): 38–42
4. Josephson ME, Harken AH, Horowitz LM (1979) Endocardial excision: A new surgical technique for the treatment of recurrent ventricular tachycardia. Circulation 60 (7): 1430–1439
5. Giraudon G, Fontaine G, Frank R, Escande G, Etievent P (1978) Encircling endocardial ventriculotomy: A new surgical treatment for life threatening ventricular tachycardias resistant to medical treatment following myocardial infarction. Ann Thorac Surg 26: 438
6. Horowitz LN, Josephson ME, Kastor JA, Harken AH (1979) Intraoperative epicardial and endocardial mapping of ventricular tachycardia in man. Am J Cardiol 43: 401 (Abstract)
7. Horowitz LN, Harken AH, Josephson ME (1981) Electrophysiologically directed ventricular resection for recurrent sustained ventricular tachycardia. In: Harrison DC, Hall GK (eds) Cardiac arrhythmias: a decase of progress. Sunderland, Boston, Massachusetts, pp 457–473
8. Mason JW (1983) The role of surgery in the treatment of arrhythmias. In: Sinauer K, Sinauer SA (eds) Cardiac arrhythmias. Sunderland, Massachusetts, pp 124–132
9. Harrison L, Gallagher JJ, Kasell J, Anderson RH, Mikat E, Hackel DB, Wallace AG (1977) Cryosurgical ablation of the A–V node – His bundle. Circulation 55: 463–470

Hemodynamic and Angiographic Results After Left Ventricular Aneurysmectomy

V. Mühlberger, E. Knapp, R. Schistek, H. Scharfetter, and F. Unger

Left ventricular aneurysm formation occurs in approximately 5%–15% of patients with myocardial infarction [3]. Left ventricular aneurysmectomy in selected patients [5] can be performed with acceptable surgical risk [4, 9], compared to the high mortality without operation. We were interested in hemodynamic changes associated with angiographic evidence of left ventricular aneurysm resection and with symptomatic improvement after operation.

Patients and Methods

Ten consecutive patients, nine men and one woman, were selected for routine postoperative reevaluation by complete heart catheterization 15 ∓ 3 weeks after left ventricular aneurysmectomy. Mean age of the patients was 49.5 years (range 39–62).

Congestive heart failure, recurrent ventricular tachycardia, or disabling angina pectoris were the indications for aneurysmectomy. Anterior aneurysmectomy was performed in nine patients, posterior aneurysmectomy once. In five patients six additional bypass graft procedures were performed: two right coronary arteries, one left anterior descending, one circumflex artery, and in one patient two grafts to the right coronary artery and circumflex artery. In spite of postoperative mitral valve in-

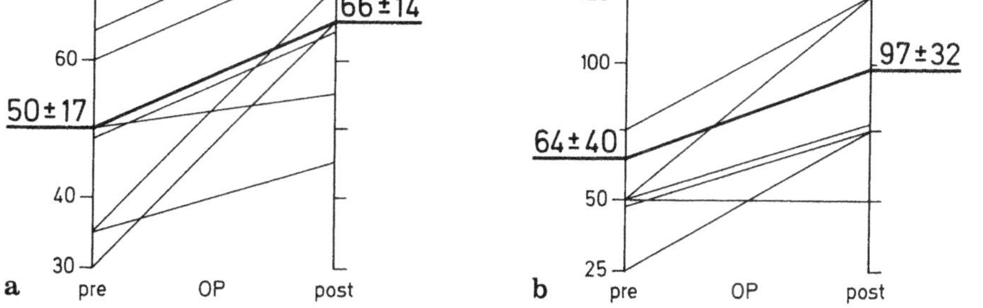

Fig. 1 a. Working capacity praeoperatively (prae OP) and postoperatively (post OP) in eight patients shows significant improvement (two patients had not been tested praeoperatively); **b** Angina pectoris free interval could be determined in seven patients and shows significant improvement postoperatively sufficiency in one patient, no further complications and no deaths occurred. Clinical, hemodynamic, and angiographic evaluations were designed prospectively and performed in the same manner preoperatively and postoperatively.

Results

Clinical Data

Mean working capacity on bicycle exercise stress test according to the Austrian Society of Cardiology improved significantly from 50% preoperatively to 66% postoperatively (Fig. 1 a) and there was an improvement in all patients. Two patients were not tested preoperatively in view of their bad condition.

Angina-pectoris-free period on the bicycle exercise stress test could be determined in seven patients preoperatively (Fig. 1 b). Angina-free working capacity increased significantly from 64 watts preoperatively to 97 watts postoperatively and there was an improvement in all but two patients.

Angiographic Data

Left ventricular end-diastolic volume decreased from 263 ml preoperatively to 163 ml postoperatively (Fig. 2 a). Only one patient showed no decrease in left ventricular end-diastolic volume (LVEDV) postoperatively and did not improve angina-pectoris-free working capacity either. All volumes were measured by biplane angiography and calculated by Simpson's rule.

Left ventricular end-systolic volume (LVESV) decreased from 177 ml preoperatively to 91 ml postoperatively (Fig. 2 b). There was a remarkable reduction in LVESV in all but one patient.

Left ventricular ejection fraction increased from 36% preoperatively to 44% postoperatively (Fig. 2 c). There was a remarkable improvement of ejection fraction in all but two patients.

Hemodynamic Results

Cardiac output, determined by the Fick principle, decreased from 6.2 liters/min preoperatively to 5.3 liters/min postoperatively (Fig. 3 a). A lower cardiac output was found in all but one patient postoperatively. The only patient with increased cardiac output postoperatively did not improve angina-free working capacity and left ventricular volumes.

Cardiac index (Fig. 3 b) decreased less than cardiac output, because most patients lose weight after surgery. But there is still a significant decrease in cardiac index from 3.4 liters/min per m^2 preoperatively to 2.9 liters/min per m^2 postoperatively. This cardiac index is even postoperatively still within normal values.

Mean aortic pressure decreased significantly as well, from 102 mmHg preoperatively to 92 mmHg postoperatively, even though five patients had no postoperative reduction in mean aortic pressure (Fig. 3 c).

Left ventricular mean working index (LVMWI), calculated from the cardiac index and mean aortic pressure, decreased from 4.70 ∓ 0.96 kp m/min per m^2 preoperatively to 3.69 ∓ 1.06 kp m/min per m^2 postoperatively ($p < 0.001$; $n = 10$).

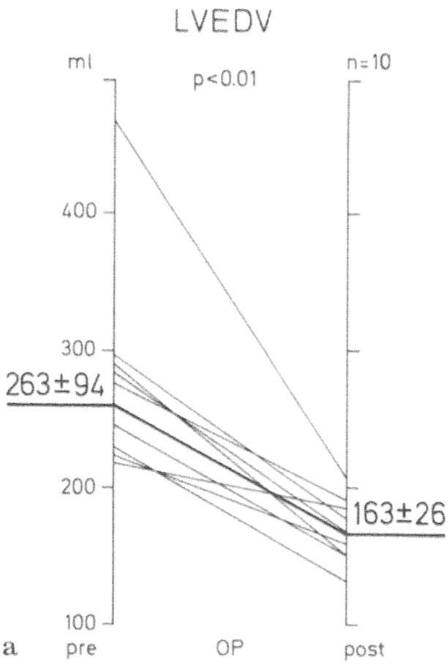

a

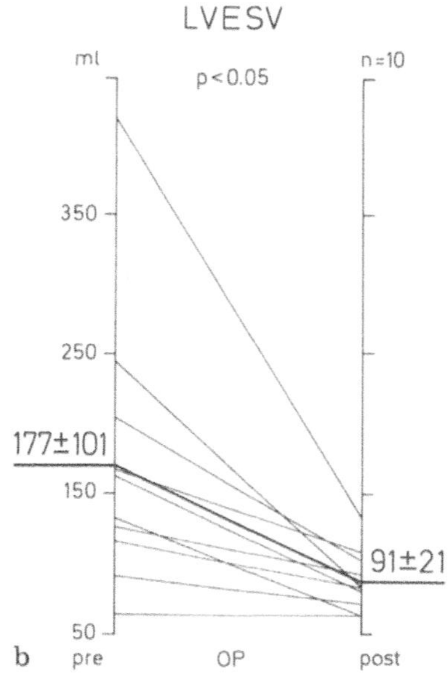

b

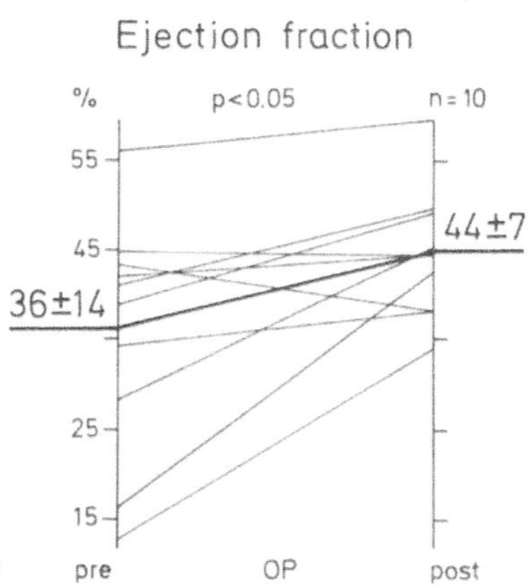

c

Fig. 2a. Left ventricular enddiastolic volume decreases after aneurysmectomy; **2b.** Left ventricular endsystolic volume decreases after aneurysmectomy as well; **2c.** Left ventricular ejection fraction increases after aneurysmectomy

No significant change could be found postoperatively for stroke volume index determined by ventriculography (SVI-Roentgen), stroke volume index determined by the Fick principle (SVI Fick), left ventricular end-diastolic pressure at rest (LVEDP rest), left ventricular end-diastolic pressure after angiography (LVEDP angio), pulmonary artery mean pressure (PA pressure), and pulmonary capillary wedge pressure (PC pressure):

		preoperative	postoperative	
		$\bar{x} \pm s$	$\bar{x} \pm s$	
SVI Roentgen	(ml/m^2)	47 ± 17	40 ± 9	n.s.
SVI Fick	(ml/m^2)	40 ± 10	34 ± 7	n.s.
LVEDP rest	(mmHg)	17 ± 6	21 ± 7	n.s.

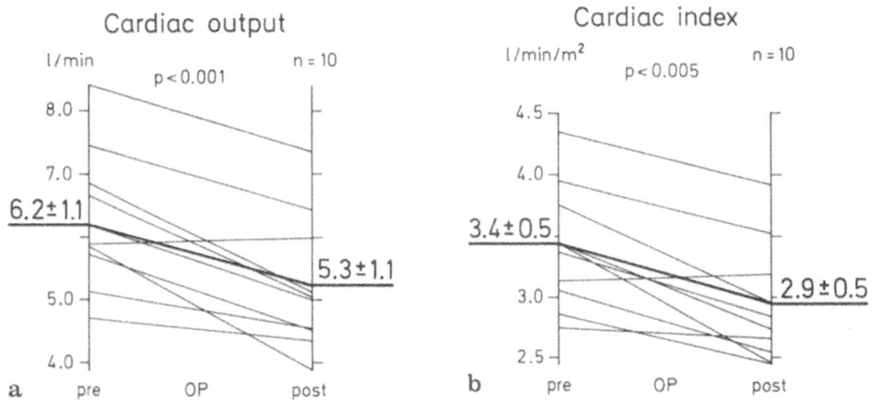

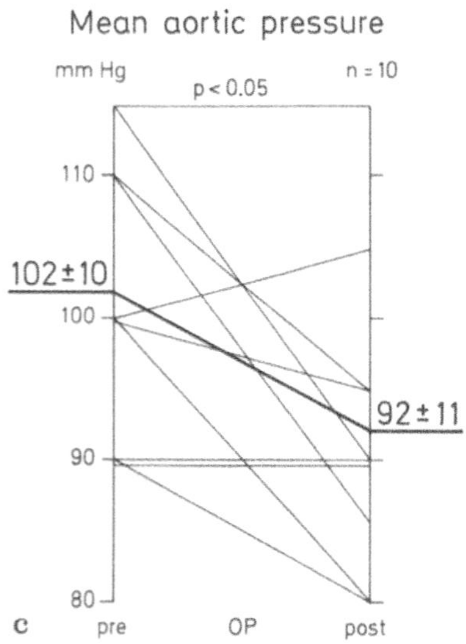

Fig. 3a. In spite of significant reduction of Cardiac Output postoperatively, values are still within normal range; **3b.** Cardiac Index shows the same reduction as Cardiac Output; **3c.** Mean aortic pressure decreases after aneurysmectomy in most patients

LVEDP angio	(mmHg)	25 ± 10	26 ± 10	n.s.
PA pressure	(mmHg)	16 ± 4	16 ± 7	n.s.
PC pressure	(mmHg)	9 ± 4	10 ± 5	n.s.

Discussion

Improved working capacity and improved angina-free interval after left ventricular aneurysmectomy are certainly results of postoperatively improved left ventricular volumes and ejection fraction. But there is still controversy about hemodynamic results after aneurysmectomy. No hemodynamic improvement of LVEDP at rest, cardiac index or wedge pressure has been reported [2, 4, 6, 7]. On the other hand an increase in ejection fraction [6, 8] and in the quotient stroke volume/left ventricular filling pressure was found [1].

Our hemodynamic changes such as decreased cardiac output, LVMWI, and mean aortic pressure are certainly not signs of impaired left ventricular function, since all data are within the normal range postoperatively. Possibly improved angina-free working capacity and improved ejection fraction are associated with a postoperatively more economical cardiac activity, and less left ventricular work is required for perfusion of coronary vessels supplying aneurysms. A greater number of patients should be investigated to confirm this hypothesis.

References

1. Björk VO, Henze A (1976) Left ventricular function at rest and during exercise before and after surgical treatment of ischemic heart disease, left ventricular aneurysm, aortic stenosis, and aortic incompetence. In: Roskamm H, Hahn C (eds) Ventricular function at rest and during exercise. Springer, Berlin Heidelberg New York
2. Blümchen G, Barthel W, Van den Bergh K, Bierck G, Brandt D, Scharf-Bornhofen E, Reidemeister SC (1980) Soziales Schicksal bei operierten und konservativ behandelten Koronar- und Aneurysmapatienten. Z Kardiol 69: 632–638
3. Diamond PS, Kowalczyk L, Pifarre R, Gunnar RM (1981) Long-term result of ventricular aneurysm repair in patients under 45 years of age. In: Roskamm H (ed) Myocardial infarction at young age. Springer, Berlin Heidelberg New York
4. Gold FL, Sharma B, Hodges M, Helseth HK (1980) Combined left ventricular aneurysmectomy, mitral valve replacement and aortocoronary bypass grafting: results of surgery. Circulation 62 (Suppl 1): 147
5. Jehle J, Heerdt M, Spiller P, Loogen F (1982) Verlaufsbeobachtungen bei Patienten mit Aneurysma des linken Ventrikels nach konservativer und chirurgischer Therapie. Z Kardiol 71: 566–575
6. Neuhaus KL, Hinck T, Tebbe U, Leitz K, Rahlf G, Kreuzer H (1982) Linksventrikuläre Funktionsänderung nach Aneurysmektomie. Z Kardiol 71: 633
7. Swan HJC, Chatterjee K, Kaushik VS, Matloff J (1976) Functional and clinical effects of surgical treatment of ventricular aneurysms. In: Roskamm H, Hahn C (eds) Ventricular function at rest and during exercise. Springer, Berlin Heidelberg New York
8. Tebbe U, Schicha H, Neumann P, Sauer G, Neuhaus KL, Emrich D, Kreuzer H (1983) Konservative und operative Therapie des Vorderwandaneurysmas: Verlaufsbeobachtungen mittels Radionuklidventrikulographie. Z Kardiol 72 (Suppl 2): 66
9. Walker WW, Stoney WS, Alford WC, Burrus GR, Glassford DM, Thomas CS (1980) Results of surgical management of acute left ventricular aneurysms. Circulation 62 (Suppl 1): 75

Combined Procedures with Aortocoronary Bypass Surgery

H. O. Vetter, B. Reichart, B. M. Kemkes, and W. Klinner

Lack of improvement in the patient's condition after heart surgery might be due to coronary artery disease. Significant lesions occur in as many as 22% [1, 2]. Therefore, all patients over 40 years of age considered for valvular surgery should have coronary angiography.

Moreover, atherosclerosis is a diffuse systemic disease which may influence several organs or tissues at the same time, e. g., the heart, the aorta, and the peripheral vessels. One-stage surgical treatment of both the coronary arteries and the carotids was introduced and recommended in early 1972 [3, 4].

This report summarizes our experiences in treating coronary artery lesions together with either significant carotid artery stenosis or valvular disease.

Patients

Between January 1978 and September 1983 a total of 2057 coronary artery bypass operations, 480 aortic valve replacements, 383 mitral valve procedures, and 119 double valve procedures (aortic valve replacement plus replacement or valvuloplasty of the mitral valve) were performed; altogether 3039 operations were completed.

Out of these 150 were combined procedures (Table 1). They include 45 patients with coronary artery bypass grafting and endarterectomy of the carotid artery, 76 patients with additional aortic valve replacement, 24 patients with additional mitral valve procedures, and 5 patients additional with double valve procedures.

Most of the patients were in clinical class III, according to the New York Heart Association classifications. There was a greater percentage of class IV patients in the valvular groups (Table 2).

The most common risk factors were smoking and hyperlipidemia, then in decreasing frequency, hypertension, diabetes mellitus, and hyperuricemia. In the group with coronary heart disease (CHD), 56% had survived a myocardial infarction and stenosis of the carotid artery, as had 28% of the patients with additional aortic valve disease and 33% of those with additional mitral valve disease.

In the group with CHD combined with stenotic carotid arteries, an asymptomatic murmur was heard in 84%, transitory ischemic attacks were reported five times, and mild stroke twice.

According to the preoperative coronary angiogram severe three-vessel disease was the predominant lesion. The patients with the most advanced atherosclerosis were those with additional carotid artery disease. As mentioned in the literature, left main coronary artery stenosis did occur more often in this group [5]; in our patients in 44% of the cases (Fig. 1).

Table 1a. Total number of coronary artery bypass graft and aortic, mitral, and double valve procedures between January 1978 and September 1983. **b** Number and age of patients having combined procedures

a

	n	♂	♀
CABG	2057	1864	193
AVR	480	306	174
MVR/vp	383	200	183
AVR + MVR/vp	119	58	61
Total	3039	2428	611

b

	n	♂	♀	Mean age (years)
CABG + carotid	45	37	8	57.8
CABG + AVR	76	62	14	58.4
CABG + MVR/vp	24	16	8	58.3
CABG + AVR + MVR/vp	5	2	3	62.6
Total	150	117	33	59.3

Abbreviations: CABG, coronary artery bypass grafting; AVR, aortic valve replacement; MVR, mitral valve replacement; vp, valvuloplasty

Table 2. Preoperative findings in patients undergoing combined procedures in aortocoronary bypass surgery

		CHD + Carotid artery ($n=45$)	CHD + aortic valve ($n=76$)	CHD + mitral valve ($n=24$)	CHD + multiple valve ($n=5$)
NYHA	II	11	10	2	–
	III	30	58	14	1
	IV	4	8	8	4
Risk factors	Hyperlipidemia	56%	44%	40%	(1)
	Smoking	65%	52%	45%	(2)
	Hypertension	44%	32%	35%	–
	Diabetes	34%	24%	20%	(1)
	Hyperuricemia	22%	37%	45%	–
Previous MI		56% (25)	28% (21)	33% (8)	–
Asymptomatic bruit		84% (38)	–	–	–
TIA		11% (5)	–	–	–
Stroke (mild)		4% (2)	–	–	–

Abbreviations: CHD, coronary heart disease; MI, myocardial infarction; TIA, transitory ischemic attack

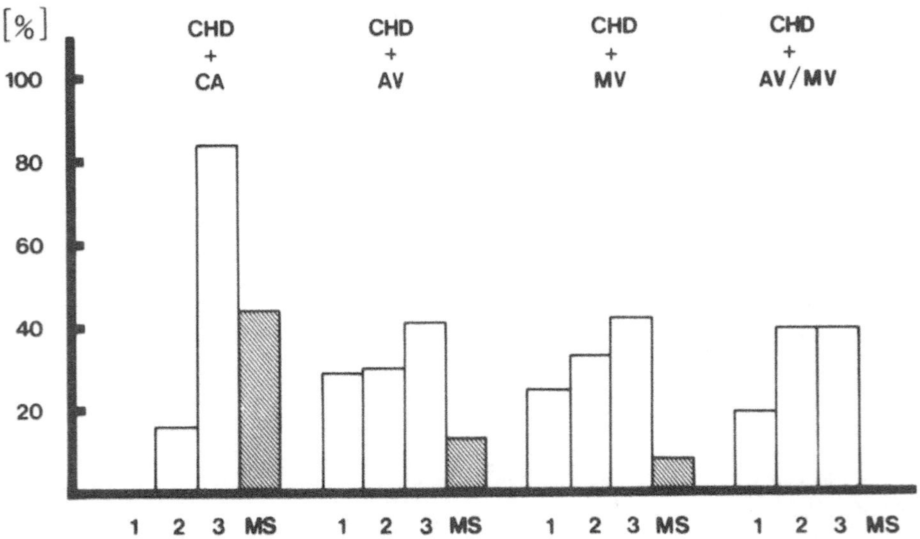

Fig. 1. Distribution of coronary heart disease *(CHD)*. In combined *CHD* and carotid artery *(CA)* disease the left main stem *(MS)* was involved in 44% of the patients. *1, 2, 3,* (single, double, triple) vessel disease; *AV*, aortic valve; *MV*, mitral valve

The preoperative ventriculograms verified a decreased ejection fraction (<60%) in 40% of the patients from the carotid group, in 55% from the aortic group, in 58% from the mitral group, and in 60% of the patients with double valve disease.

Surgical Procedures

Whenever carotid artery disease and CHD evolved, endarterectomy was carried out first. An intraluminar shunt was positioned in every case and the arterial incision closed using a piece of autologous saphenous vein. Then the median sternotomy was performed in order to proceed with the revascularization.

In all other cases – valvular disease combined with CHD – the cardiac procedure was done during aortic cross clamping, using 4 °C Bretschneider cardioplegia solution and topical cooling according to Shumway. Whenever the mitral valve had to be replaced or repaired, this procedure was done secondly in order to avoid undue stress to the mitral anulus during peripheral coronary surgery.

Postoperative Status

All surviving patients were called up within the month of October 1983 in order to establish their postoperative status.

Results

In the group with CHD and carotid artery disease, an average of 2.9 anastomoses per patient were performed (Table 3). Early mortality (death within the first 30 postoperative days) was 2.2%. There were no late deaths. Of these patients 95% were im-

Table 3. Number of anastomoses per patient, early mortality (within the first 30 postoperative days), and late mortality in combined procedures

	CHD+ carotid artery ($n=45$)	CHD+ aortic valve ($n=76$)	CHD+ mitral valve ($n=24$)	CHD+ multiple valves ($n=5$)
Anastomosis	2.9	1.6	1.5	1.0
Early mortality	2.2% (1)	18.4% (14)	16.7% (4)	– (2)
Late mortality	–	2.6% (2)	4.2% (1)	– (1)
Subjective feeling				
Better	95% (42)	80% (48)	58% (11)	– (2)
Unchanged	5% (2)	15% (9)	32% (6)	–
Worse	–	5% (3)	11% (2)	–

proved with respect to their preoperative symptoms. In only 5% was there no change in angina pectoris pain as compared to the preoperative status.

In aortic valve disease plus CHD, an average 1.6 anastomoses were performed per patient in mitral valve disease plus CHD 1.5, and in double valve disease plus CHD 1.0. Early mortality (18.4%) was much higher when compared to aortic valve replacement alone (5.5% early mortality). The same was found for valvuloplasty or replacement of the mitral valve (16.7% versus 7.2%).

Out of the 14 patients who died early after aortic valve replacement 10 had severe aortic stenosis; from the 4 patients who died early after mitral valve replacement 3 had mitral insufficiency.

The late mortality rate in the aortic valve group was 2.6%, in the mitral valve group 4.2%.

Conclusions

In our opinion, a combined one-stage procedure – carotid artery endarterectomy and revascularization – is indicated:

1. With regard to the supraaortic branches, whenever symptomatic stage II exists, filiform (≥90%) lesions are present, ulcerative plaque formation with at least 60% stenosis is verified, and both sides are involved.
2. With regard to the coronary artery system, whenever unstable angina pectoris exists, in severe triple vessel disease, left main stem stenosis, and when both the left anterior descending and the right coronary artery are involved.

One-stage procedure for valvular replacement or repair plus revascularization is also advisable. Yet, our results are somewhat disappointing. The main reason for the high perioperative mortality was a poor left ventricular function, as shown by the high percentage of low ejection fractions and preoperative class IV classifications in these groups.

In our opinion aortic stenosis or mitral insufficiency together with coronary artery disease are the most dangerous combinations.

References

1. Lacy J, Goodin R, McMartin D, Masolen R, Flowers N (1977) Coronary atherosclerosis in valvular heart disease. Ann Thorac Surg 23: 429–435
2. Loop FD, Phillips DF, Roy M, Taylor PC, Groves LK, Effler DB (1977) Aortic valve replacement combined with myocardial revascularization. Late clinical results and survival of surgically treated aortic valve patients with and without coronary artery disease. Circulation 55: 169–173
3. Faidutti B, Steichen FM, Thevoz F, Hahn CJ (1972) Coronary artery and associated aortic or major arterial atherosclerosis. Arch Surg 105: 711–714
4. Bernhard VM, Johnson WD, Peterson JJ (1972) Carotid artery stenosis. Arch Surg 105: 837–840
5. Hertzer NR, Loop FD, Taylor PC, Beven EG (1983) Combined myocardial revascularization and carotid endarterectomy. J Thorac Cardiovasc Surg 85: 577–589

Encircling Endocardial Ventriculotomy Versus Endocardial Resection for the Treatment of Drug-Refractory Ischemic Ventricular Tachycardia

J. Defauw, S. Caparrotti, N. van Hemel, and F. Vermeulen

Introduction

A variety of surgical techniques are currently available for the treatment of ischemic ventricular tachyarrhythmias (VT) refractory to pharmacological treatment. These include encircling endocardial ventriculotomy (EEV), endocardial resection (ER), and combined procedures. Since 1981 we applied serial drug testing protocols in the selection of candidates for surgical treatment of VT. Moreover, intraoperative mapping procedures were executed to delineate the earliest site of origin of VT within the ischemic border zones of the areas of myocardial infarction. Of the 51 patients operated so far, we selected the 45 patients operated upon between January 1, 1980 and March 31, 1983, in order to follow these patients up for at least 6 months after their operation.

Patients and Methods

In the above-mentioned period of time 45 patients were operated upon for intractable VT: 40 males and 5 females with a mean age of 56.8 years ± 8.6 years. All had suffered from at least one previous myocardial infarction. All patients had been treated extensively by currently available antiarrhythmic drugs including lidocaine, quinidine, procainamide, aprindine, mexithil, or combinations of these drugs, and many were treated with amiodarone as well. Except in urgent cases the patients were submitted to a standard electrophysiological study (EPS) to test the inducibility of the VT by right ventricular apical or infundibular stimulation at different cycle lengths (400, 500, 600 ms) and two, three, or four extra stimuli or with burst pacing. In some patients left ventricular catheter mapping was used to further define a septal, interior, lateral, or anterior localization of the VT, either in the proximal or distal left ventricle. The efficacy of these drugs was determined by EPS. In cases with a spontaneous recurrence of VT despite medical treatment or in cases in which serial drug testing failed, surgical treatment was carried out. All patients were subjected to a standard coronary angiography, left ventricular angiography, and left ventricular pressure determinations. In addition, ejection fractions at rest and/or at effort were determined as well, with radionuclides.

At operation the patients were subjected (except in the few emergency cases) to a standardized intraoperative mapping of the VT in normothermia with or without extracorporal circulation support. Epicardial mapping of sinus rhythm and of VT induced by epicardial electrodes or right ventricular endocardial catheter pacing was performed. A standardized epicardial grid was used to localize the earliest epicardial breakthrough of the VT. Sinus rhythm mapping was used to correlate areas with slow conduction or fractionation of potentials to the areas of earliest breakthrough of VT. Since 1981 endocardial mapping was performed as well. In the most recent cases a multielectrode intraventricular balloon was used, with the cooperation of the electrophysiological department of the University of Amsterdam [1]. We attempted to correlate the findings of the perioperative mapping with those obtained at preoperative endocardial catheter mapping of VT. Once the area of earliest activation of VT was determined, the patient's circulation was cooled, aortic cross clamping performed, and cardioplegia startet.

From January 1980 until January 1982 EEV as described by Guiraudon [3] was used. Initially the EEV incision was perpendicular and just outside the visible endocardial limits of the myocardial infarction sclerosis. Later, a more oblique incision was made following the sclerosis border zone from endocardially to epicardially and the incision was made within the limits of the border zone in order to minimize exclusion of normal myocardial tissue. From 1982 on an ER was performed electively in all cases; depending on the precision of the pre- and intraoperative localization of the VT and the quality of the left ventricle, either restricted [6] or extended peeling [10] of the endocardial fibrosis was performed. The surface area of the total endocardial scar was calculated by an endocardial surface map, dividing the heart into three sectors within each of its three endocardial surfaces (Fig. 1). Postoperatively, the patients were subjected to a control EPS by the epicardial wires left in place during the operation or were readmitted later for complete EPS. Postoperative ejection fractions were checked by radionuclides. All patients were followed closely at the outpatient department and readmitted if suspected manifestations or recurrence of VT were recorded as well in case of other events.

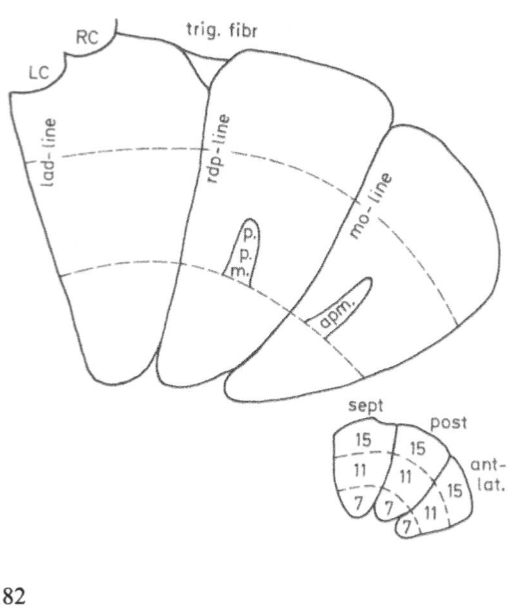

Fig. 1. Endocardial surface map: the endocardial surface is divided in three areas by the left anterior descending artery *(lad)*, right descending posterior artery *(rdp)* and the marginal obtuse artery *(mo)*. The location of the posterior papillary muscle *(ppm)* and anterior papillary muscle *(apm)* is drawn schematically; the septal *(sept)*, posterior *(post)*, and anterolateral *(ant-lat.)* areas are divided in three sectors of respectively 15% for the proximal, 11% for the middle, and 7% for the apical sector of each area

Results

The mean preoperative ejection fraction at rest was 0.22% ± 0.11%; LVEDP (left ventricular end-diastolic pressure) was 17 ± 8.0 mmHg. Preoperative EPS was not performed in the earliest ten patients and was not indicated in five patients with extremely bad left ventricles or emergency operations. Preoperative EPS brought satisfying results in 30 patients: a VT with the same QRS configuration as that of the spontaneous VT was obtained in 26 patients, and a VT with a QRS morphology different from that of the spontaneous VT was observed in 4 patients. Intraoperative mapping provided satisfying results in 34 patients in whom a sustained arrhythmia could be analyzed. In four patients only short runs of VT were obtained, but sufficient information could be collected by sinus mapping. Intraoperative mapping was not performed in two emergency cases at night and was technically unsuccessful in the remaining five patients.

The first 31 patients were subjected to EEV, the latter 14 patients to ER, of which the procedure was selective in 4 cases and complete in 10 cases.

The two techniques were compared with regard to mortality, morbidity, and long-term results. No striking differences could be found between the groups in regard to the percentage of patients with coronary artery bypass grafts: 48% (15/31) of the EEV patients and 42% (6/14) of the ER group. The percentages of left ventricular aneurysm resection (26% vs 50%) and mitral valve replacement (10% vs 7%) were also not significantly different. Hospital mortality was much higher in the first group: 10 of 31 patients with EEV died, a mortality of 32% (70% confidence limits: 23%–43%). In contrast, 1 of 14 ER patients died: mortality was 7% (70% confidence limits: 1%–22%). The causes of death were low cardiac output in seven patients and multiple organ failure in three patients of the EEV group, whereas the one patient in the ER group died due to a neurological problem.

However, some factors affected the difference between the hospital mortalities of EEV patients and ER patients. Although ejection fraction and LVEDP were not significantly different between the groups, the total area resected or encircled as determined by our surface grading map was significantly greater (39%) for those patients with an EEV who died than for those patients with an EEV who survived (31%) ($p < 0.01$) or for the patients with an ER (26%) ($p < 0.05$). The cross-clamp time was longer in the patients who underwent an EEV and died, but this may only reflect the extensiveness of the disease.

Late follow-up disclosed another seven deaths: five patients in the EEV group and two in the ER group. In the EEV group, two patients died due to congestive heart failure, one died because of recurrence of VT, one committed suicide and one died of pancreatitis. Late sudden death occurred in two patients of the ER group.

The postoperative recurrence rate of VT was not related to such factors as interval between myocardial infarction and first appearance of VT, or interval between myocardial infarction and operating date, but only to the localization of the infarction. The recurrence rate of VT was also related (but inversely) with the area of the infarction and with the preoperative ejection fraction. A spontaneous or clinical VT recurred in 6 out of 21 EEV survivors and in 4 out of 13 ER survivors. It appeared that the incidence of recurrence was not different (29% vs 31%).

However, in both subgroups there was a significant difference in the percentage of recurrences when the inferior wall and anterior wall infarctions were analyzed separately. In anterior wall infarction, VT recurred in 2 out of 13 EEV patients (13%; 70% confidence limits: 4%–29%) and in 2 out of 10 ER hospital survivors (20%; 70% confidence limits: 7%–41%). In inferior wall infarctions a significantly higher incidence of recurrence of VT was found: in four out of six patients of the EEV group and in two out of three patients of the ER group. The patients with recurrence of VT represent 67% of the patients with inferior wall myocardial infarction (Table 1).

The short-term survival curves for both groups of hospital survivors were rather similar and suggest that both types of surgical treatment are equally effective. However, we admit that the follow-up of the patients with an ER procedure has not been long enough to be able to compare both groups of patients precisely (Fig. 2).

Table 1. Spontaneous recurrence of VT in hospital survivors

	Total	*n*	%	70% CL
EEV	21	6	29	18–42
Anterior	15	2	13	4–29
Posterior	6	4	67	38–88
ER	13	4	31	16–49
Anterior	10	2	20	7–41
Posterior	3	2	67	24–95

EEV, endocardial encircling ventriculotomy; ER, endocardial resection; 70% CL, 70% confidence limits; *n*, number of patients

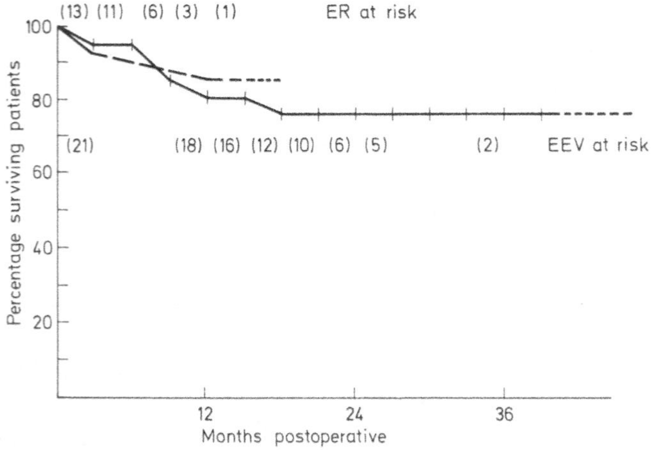

Fig. 2. Actuarial survival of hospital survivors up to 36 months in 21 endocardial encircling ventriculotomy *(EEV)* patients and 13 endocardial resection *(ER)* patients at risk

Discussion

Several procedures have been proposed for the surgical treatment of medically intractable VT. The simple aneurysmectomy has not been very effective but has an acceptable mortality [7]. Since Guiraudon [3] firstly introduced the concept of encircling the anatomical origin of VT by creating an "electrical barrier" or EEV to block the VT originating from macro-reentry circuits, still other concepts have been evolved. The ER introduced by Harken [6] is based on the concept of resecting the subendocardial Purkinje system surviving in the border zone of the myocardial infarction.

This system is supposed to be part of the reentry circuit or may constitute a source of triggering of VT. As opposed to the preoperative and intraoperative mapping-directed ER suggested by Harken, Moran [10] has recommended total ER of all fibrotic endocardial scar, presuming that nonresected areas may become arrhythmogenic after resection of the detected triggering zones. Recently, cryosurgical ablation [8] or cryosurgical encirclement [5] have been added to the available techniques.

The overall results of the individual techniques are still variable. Compared to the results of others [2, 4] ours can be classified as less favorable, but this may be due to the greater area of infarction (especially in those patients who died) and hence to a too optimistic or unrealistic choice of candidates in our early experience. Late follow-up results for EEV are in accordance with others [2] and point to an additional injury by the EEV of the already poor left ventricular function of these patients, resulting in some late pump failures. In our experience the outcome after ER can be compared to that in EEV with comparable endocardial scar areas. The late results were identical with regard to recurrence of VT. Although initially this was not clearly admitted by those who introduced the selected ER, it is now admitted by the Philadelphia group that recurrence of VT is still a real but acceptable problem [9]. Some of our surgical results, and comparison of the results of Harken and Moran, tend to show a better efficacy of the operations with a total ER in contrast to the selective ER guided by perioperative mapping. The roles of the alternative surgical methods are still to be determined.

The main observation in our experience was the far higher recurrence rates of VT arising in inferior wall infarctions. Also initially denied by the Philadelphia group (M. E. Josephson, personal communication) it was recently confirmed by these workers [9]. It is probably too early to suggest mechanisms for why surgical treatment of inferior wall infarctions fails more frequently.

Conclusions

The surgical treatment of medically intractable ischemic VT is promising regarding its efficacy in the short and medium term. It appeared that pump failure was the predominant complication of the initial vertical EEV procedure. Moreover, the success rate of surgical treatment of VT was identical in patients treated with EEV or ER. The high recurrence rate in inferior wall infarctions with both techniques still presents an important problem and constitutes a challenge to adaption of the surgical procedures.

References

1. de Bakker J, Janse M, van Capelle L (1982) Simultaneous endocardial mapping in patients undergoing resection of left ventricular aneurysm. Circulation 66 [Suppl II]: 344
2. Borggrefe M, Breithardt G, Ostermeyer J, Bircks W (1983) Long-term efficacy of endocardial encircling ventriculotomy for ventricular tachycardia: complete versus partial incision. Circulation 68 [Suppl III]: 176
3. Guiraudon G, Fontaine G, Frank R et al. (1978) Encircling endocardial ventriculotomy: a new surgical treatment for life-threatening ventricular tachycardias resistant to medical treatment following myocardial infarction. Ann Thorac Surg 26: 438–444
4. Guiraudon G, Fontaine G, Frank R, Barra J, Pavie A, Cabrol C (1982) Encircling endocardial ventriculotomy in the surgical treatment of chronic ventricular tachycardia after myocardial infarction. The endocardial approach. In: Bruschke et al. (eds) Coronary artery disease today: diagnosis, surgery and prognosis. Excerpta Medica, Amsterdam, pp 341–349
5. Guiraudon G, Klein GJ, Vermeulen FE, Yee R, van Hemel NM (1983) Encircling endocardial cryoablation: a technique for surgical treatment of ventricular tachycardia after myocardial infarction. Circulation 68 [Suppl III]: 176
6. Harken AH, Josephson ME, Horowitz LN (1979) Surgical endocardial resection for the treatment of malignant ventricular tachycardia. Ann Surg 190: 456–460
7. Mason JW, Stinson EB, Winkel RA, Griffin JC, Oyer PhE, Ross DL, Derby G (1982) Surgery for ventricular tachycardia: efficacy of left ventricular aneurysm resection compared with operation guided by electrical activation mapping. Circulation 65: 1148–1155
8. Mason JW, Stinson EN, Oyer PhE, Winkel RA, Anderson KP (1983) Arrhythmia mechanisms and outcome in surgery for recurrent ventricular tachycardia (VT). Circulation 68 [Suppl III]: 176
9. Miller JM, Kienzle MG, Flores BT, Rogers DP, Harken AH, Josephson ME (1983) Endocardial resection for ventricular tachycardia: predictors of success. Circulation 68 [Suppl III]: 177
10. Moran JM, Kehoe RF, Loeb JM, Lichtenthal PR, Sanders JH Jr, Michaelis LL (1982) Extended endocardial resection for the treatment of ventricular tachycardia and ventricular fibrillation. Ann Thorac Surg 34: 538–550

Changes in the Native Vessels After Aortocoronary Bypass Surgery

N. Goebel, N. Pfluger, K. Speiser, M. Turina, and M. Rothlin

An enhanced rate of progression of coronary stenoses has been reported after aortocoronary bypass surgery [4]. It was the purpose of our study to investigate the changes of the native vessels 3 months after aortocoronary bypass operation.

Patients and Methods

In a prospective study 238 men (mean age 53 ± 7 years) were restudied by coronary angiography 3 months after elective bypass surgery and 5 ± 1.5 months after preoperative angiography. The angiocardiographic findings in these patients (pts) were as follows: 13% and one-vessel disease, 32% two vessel disease and 55% three vessel disease. The preoperative ejection fraction of 58% ± 10% did not differ significantly from the postoperative ejection fraction of 59% ± 11%. A total of 760 bypasses had been implanted (3.2 bypasses per pt), of which 82% were patent. Patency rate was highest in the LAD (left anterior descending coronary artery) with 92% and lowest in the intermediate branch with 70% (Table 1).

The degree of each stenosis was assessed as percent narrowing of the diameter. Progression was defined as at least 20% increase of stenosis or new total occlusion. A maximum of 17 segments were evaluated in each pt (LAD three segments, every other vessel one segment). We distinguished between segments with and without bypass. A segment with bypass meant either that the segment had an anastomosis with a bypass or that a proximal segment was bridged by a parallel bypass.

Results

The *mean degree of stenosis* (i.e., the sum of disease in all segments divided by the number of segments) (Fig. 1) was, in segments without bypass, preoperatively 12.7% ± 0.72% (SEM) and postoperatively 14.3% ± 0.76%; in vessels with patent by-

Table 1. Angiographic findings in vessels with bypass

Vessel with bypass	Number	Patency rate	Progression at anastomosis		Progression proximally	
RIVA	217	92%	20	9%	89	41%
R. diag.	120	83%	23	19%	25	21%
R. intermed.	27	70%	11	41%	7	26%
RCX	183	72%	36	20%	58	32%
RCA	213	85%	33	15%	58	27%
Total	760	82%	123	16%	237	31%

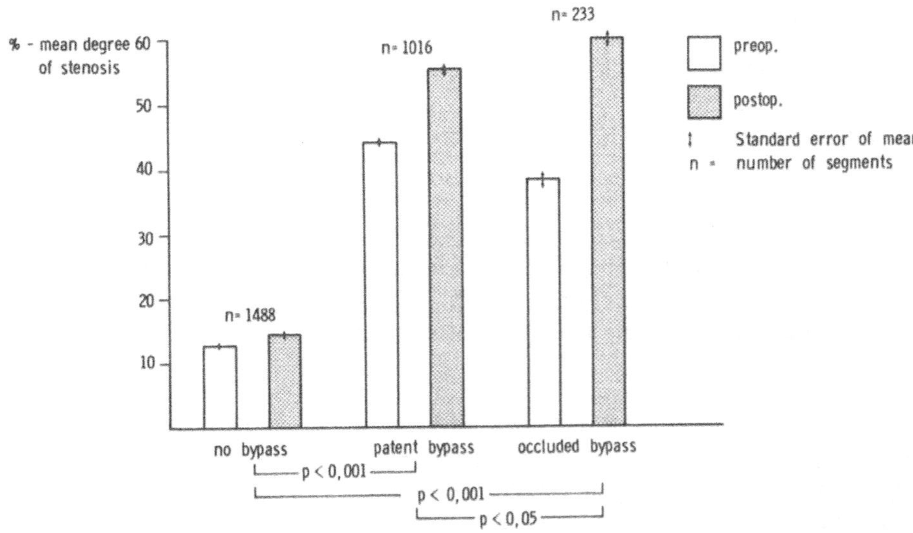

Fig. 1. Mean degree of stenosis pre- and postoperatively

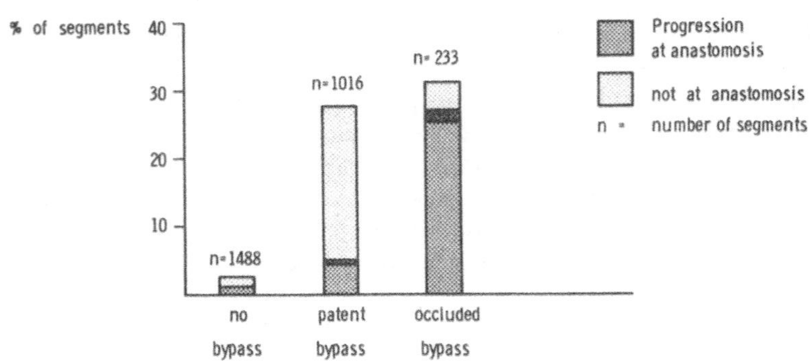

Fig. 2. Frequency of progression and location

pass, 44% ± 1.24% and 55.4% ± 1.26%; and in vessels with occluded bypass, 38.4% ± 2.58% and 60% ± 2.72%.

The relative *frequency of progression* in segments without bypass, with open bypass, and with occluded bypass is shown in Fig. 2. We differentiated between progression localized at the site of the anastomosis and that in other parts of the vessel. However, only seven segments showed progression more than 1 cm distal to the anastomosis. Segments without bypass (1488) showed progression in only 2.6% (1.1% were caused by extension of a stenosis in a neighboring anastomized segment onto the segment without bypass). With patent bypass (1016 segments) 27.7% showed progression (4.5% at the site of anastomosis, 22.8% in the rest of the vessel, 0.4% at both sites). With occluded bypass (233 segments) 31% showed progression (25.3% at the site of anastomosis, 4.3% in the rest of the vessel, 1.7% at both sites).

Progression in relation to the preoperative degree of stenosis is shown in Fig. 3. The higher the preoperative degree of stenosis, the more frequently a progression was seen ($p = 0.001$). Of the 238 pts, 92 showed a progression at the site of the anastomosis (64 pts in one segment, 20 pts in two, 6 pts in three and 2 pts in four segments; a total of 130 progressions). The mean degree of stenosis at the anastomosis was 89% ± 1.34% (SEM). Of the 130 progessions 52% were occlusions. Slight stenoses were rare (5.4%). There were 22 progressions at the anastomosis in vessels which were already occluded preoperatively. Frequency of stenosis in the anastomosis was 14.2% in end-to-side anastomoses ($n = 520$ bypasses) and 16.3% in side-to-side anastomoses ($n = 240$ bypasses) ($p = 0.45$).
Regression was found in 13 vessels with bypasses (in 12 cases caused by endarterectomy or by placing the anastomosis at the site of stenosis).

A perioperative myocardial infarction (PI) was observed in the ECG in 5% of the 238 pts. Seven pts had an anterior infarction, and five an inferior infarction. Ejection fraction in these 12 changed significantly from 61% ± 7% preoperatively to 54% ± 9% postoperatively. PI was explained by progression in the native vessels in all 12 pts and by concomitant occlusion of the bypass in 10. In 10 of the 12 pts the progression occurred at the site of the anastomosis and in only 2 did it occur proximally.

Discussion

After aortocoronary bypass surgery some investigators found no relationship between surgery and progression [2]. Most authors however described an increased progression, but some found this on vessels with patent bypass [5], some on vessels with occluded bypass [3], and others in all vessels with bypass, irrespective of patency [6]. We found that progression – measured as mean degree of stenosis – was highly significantly more frequent in vessels with bypass than without bypass ($p < 0.001$) and slightly significantly more frequent in vessels with occluded than with patent bypass ($p < 0.05$).

The progression was mainly located proximal to the anastomosis, less frequently at the site of the anastomosis, and very rarely more than 1 cm distal to the anastomosis.

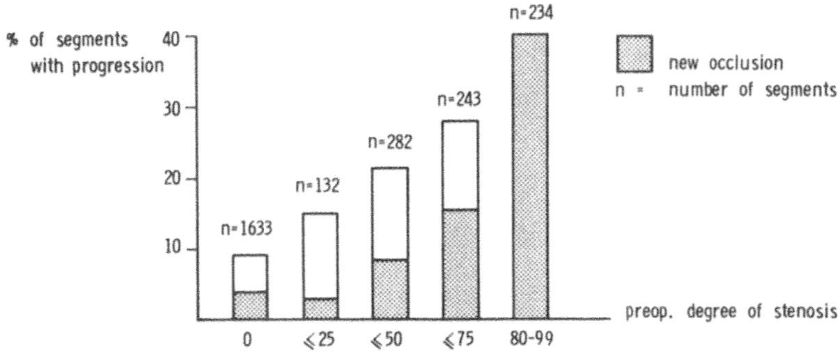

Fig. 3. Progression in relation to preoperative degree of stenosis

With patent bypass proximal progression was significantly more frequent than with occluded bypass ($p < 0.001$). With occluded bypass a stenosis at the anastomosis was significantly more frequent than with patent bypass ($p < 0.001$).

Stenoses of higher degrees showed a stronger tendency to progress than lower grade stenoses.

The different rates of progression in the various vessels with bypass (Table 1) probably reflects the different rates of patency of the grafts to these vessels.

Proximal progression usually has little relevance for the patient, the bypass being patent in most cases. The occlusion of a bypass created in several cases a new stenosis or new total occlusion at the site of anastomosis, which was the main reason for perioperative myocardial infarction.

Regression was rare and nearly always caused by surgery. In the appraisal of the accelerated early postoperative progression one must keep in mind that in follow-ups more than 5 years after surgery vessels with bypass showed only little progression compared to the early period, whereas the progression rate in vessels without bypass increased from 7% after 1 year to 41% [1].

References

1. Bourassa MG, Campeau L, Lespérance J, Grondin CM (1982) Changes in grafts and coronary arteries after saphenous vein aortocoronary bypass surgery; results at repeat angiography. Circulation 65 (Suppl 2): 90–97
2. Gensini GG, Esente P, Kelly A (1974) Natural history of coronary disease in patients with and without bypass graft surgery. Circulation 49–50 (Suppl 2): 98–101
3. Griffith LS, Achuff SC, Conti CR, Humphries JO, Brawley RK, Gott VL, Ross RS (1973) Changes in intrinsic coronary circulation and segmental ventricular motion after saphenous vein coronary bypass surgery. N Engl J Med 288: 589–595
4. Kimbiris D, Segal BL (1981) Coronary disease progression in patients with and without saphenous vein bypass surgery. Am Heart J 102: 811–818
5. Malinow MR, Kremkau EL, Kloster FE, Bonchek LI, Rösch J (1973) Occlusion of coronary arteries after vein bypass. Circulation 47: 1211–1216
6. Maurer BJ, Oberman A, Holt JH, Kouchoukos NT, Jones WB, Russel RO (1974) Changes in grafted and ungrafted coronary arteries following saphenous vein bypass grafting. Circulation 50: 293–300

Variables Influencing Patency of Coronary Artery Bypass Grafts

M. Torka and R. W. Hacker

Of 2700 consecutive patients who had coronary artery bypass surgery during the years 1974–1981, 710 patients (26%) with 1261 coronary anastomosis underwent repeat coronary angiography at a mean interval of 11.6 months after surgery. In addition, 24 patients with 49 grafts were studied at autopsy.

The group of restudied patients is not representative for all patients with respect to their postoperative functional class, in that it includes significantly more symptomatic patients than the group of patients without a second angiography (Fig. 1) [1, 10].

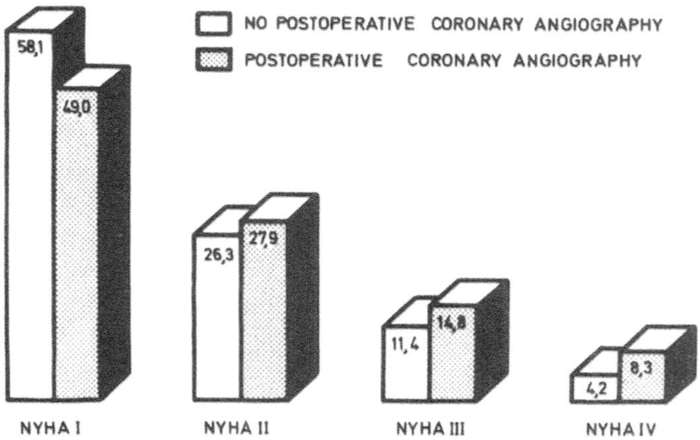

Fig. 1. Postoperative NYHA functional class in patients with postoperative angiography and in patients not restudied after surgery

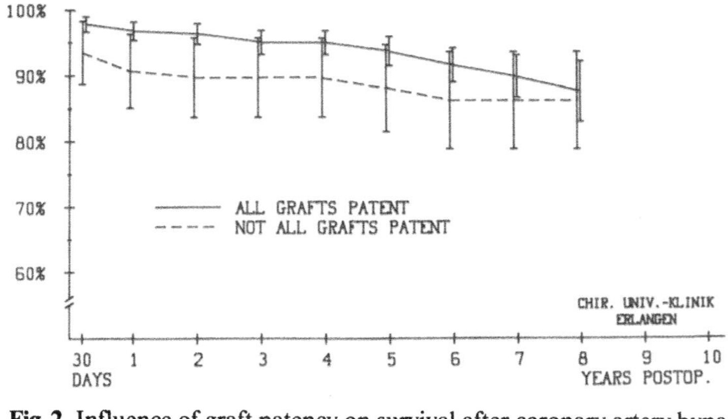

Fig. 2. Influence of graft patency on survival after coronary artery bypass surgery

Results

Graft occlusion rate was 9.2% for grafts studied angiographically and 26.5% for grafts studied at autopsy. The significance of graft patency for the risk and success of coronary artery bypass surgery can be demonstrated for all main objectives of the operation, that is, prolongation of life, prevention of myocardial infarction, and improvement of symptoms. If grafts from patients dying within the early postoperative period and examined at autopsy are included in the calculation, there is an increased early mortality in patients with occluded grafts, which influences overall survival up to 8 years after surgery (Fig. 2). The same is true for perioperative myocardial infarction, which is four times as frequent in patients with occluded grafts than in patients with all grafts patent (Fig. 3) [3, 4, 5]. The functional class is negatively influenced by graft occlusion as well, the percentage of asymptomatic pat-

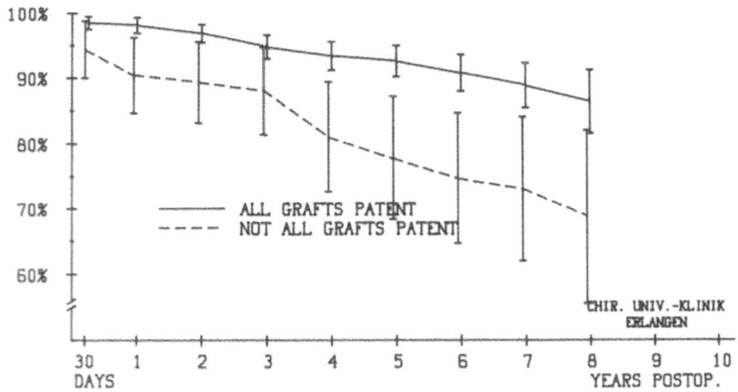

Fig. 3. Influence of graft patency on the incidence of myocardial infarction after coronary artery bypass surgery

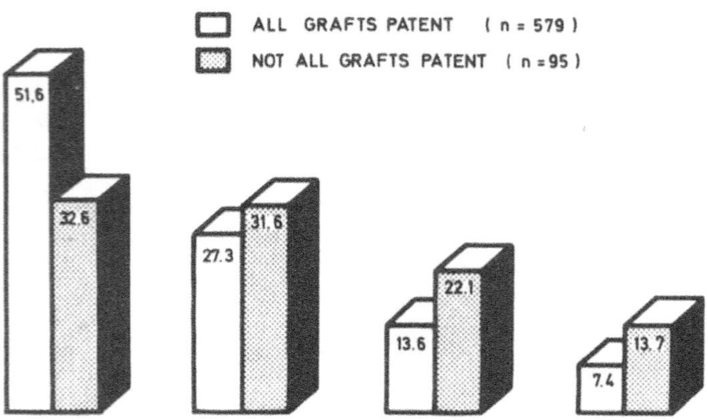

Fig. 4. Influence of graft patency on postoperative NYHA functional class

ients being less than two-thirds of what can be expected in patients with all grafts patent (Fig. 4) [6].

Preoperative parameters negatively influencing graft patency are previous myocardial infarction and excess body weight (Table 1). There seems to be a plausible explanation for more frequent graft occlusion in patients with myocardial infarction: reduced run-off through coronary arteries leading into scarred myocardium. If one examines this hypothesis by comparing the occlusion rates of grafts to coronary arteries supplying akinetic segments (4.9%) and of grafts to coronary arteries supplying normal myocardium (5.8%), there is no difference, however.

Intraoperative factors which are of major consequence to the graft occlusion rate are listed in Table 2: coronary artery luminal diameters of less than 1.5 mm at the site of the anastomosis predispose to graft occlusion, as do intraoperatively measured flow rates of less than 40 ml/min [2, 8, 10]. The recipient coronary artery has a

Table 1. Preoperative parameters vs graft occlusion

Parameter		*n*	Occlusion rate (%)
Sex	male	104/1175	8.9
	female	12/ 86	13.9
Age	≦ 40 years	7/ 91	8.0
	41–50 years	45/ 383	11.7
	51–60 years	51/ 614	8.3
	> 60 years	13/ 173	7.5
Previous MI	no	43/ 588	7.3 } $p<0.025$
	yes	72/ 648	11.1
Functional class (NYHA)	I	1/ 8	12.5
	II	27/ 246	11.0
	III	56/ 650	8.6
	IV	32/ 357	9.0
Body weight	≦normal + 10%	74/ 951	7.8 } $p<0.005$
	>normal + 10%	40/ 303	13.2
Cholesterol	≦250 mg/dl	53/ 612	8.7
	>250 mg/dl	50/ 507	9.9
Blood pressure	≦160/95 mmHg	75/ 734	10.2
	>160/95 mmHg	21/ 254	8.3
Ventricular function	normal	54/ 634	8.6
	hypokinetic segments	39/ 369	10.6
	a/dyskinetic segments	22/ 226	9.7
Ejection fraction	≦50%	5/ 47	10.6
	>50%	24/ 279	8.6
LVEDP	≦12 mmHg	44/ 382	11.5
	>12 mmHg	58/ 589	9.8
Number of >50% obstructed coronary arteries	1-vessel disease	9/ 176	5.1
	2-vessel disease	39/ 352	11.1
	3-vessel disease	55/ 494	10.0
	main stem stenosis	13/ 184	7.1

Table 2. Intraoperative parameters vs graft occlusion

Parameter		n	Occlusion rate (%)	
Luminal diameter of coronary artery	≦1.5 mm	24/ 153	15.7	$p<0.001$
	>1.5 mm	67/ 903	7.4	
Recipient coronary artery	Acd	33/ 300	11.0	
	Rda	35/ 617	5.7	
	Rdg	3/ 44	6.8	$p<0.001$
	Rcx	20/ 94	21.3	
	Rms	25/ 206	12.1	
Number of grafts/patient	1	22/ 294	7.5	
	2	56/ 593	9.4	
	3	30/ 316	9.5	
	>3	8/ 58	13.8	
Degree of revascularization	complete	65/ 718	9.1	
	incomplete	51/ 543	9.4	
Graft diameter	≦3.0 mm	15/ 156	9.6	
	=3.5 mm	21/ 217	9.7	
	=4.0 mm	27/ 347	7.8	
	=4.5 mm	3/ 75	4.0	
	≧5.0 mm	5/ 37	13.5	
Routing of grafts	directly	98/1110	8.8	
	Y	16/ 127	12.6	
	sequential graft	1/ 18	5.6	
Graft flow	1– 20 ml/min	11/ 35	31.4	
	21– 40 ml/min	20/ 86	23.3	
	41– 60 ml/min	7/ 99	7.1	$p<0.001$
	61– 80 ml/min	4/ 83	4.8	
	81–100 ml/min	3/ 68	4.4	
	> 100 ml/min	7/ 107	6.5	

distinct influence on graft occlusion. Grafts attached to the posterolateral branch of the circumflex coronary artery exhibit a significantly higher occlusion rate than grafts to all other branches [1, 6, 7, 10]. This may in part be due to the difference in luminal calibers between different coronary artery branches, since the circumflex coronary artery has the highest percentage of luminal calibers less than 1.5 mm. But even considering only grafts with luminal diameters of 1.5 mm or more, the occlusion rate remains highest (16.4%) for grafts to the posterolateral branch of the circumflex coronary artery. The greater length, and the routing of the graft along the posterior wall of the heart, which is difficult to control once the heart is put back into the pericardium, may predispose to kinking and to subsequent graft occlusion [10]. With increasing numbers of grafts per patient, there is a tendency toward higher occlusion rates. It is obvious that more grafts per patient mean a higher percentage of grafts to small-caliber vessels, which, as already pointed out, increases the likelihood of graft occlusion [7].

Size and routing of venous grafts have no significant influence on graft occlusion, although grafts with a diameter of around 4.5 mm and grafts routed directly from

Table 3. Time interval between surgery and angiography vs graft occlusion

Parameter		*n*	Occlusion rate (%)
Postop. interval	0–31 days	15/239	6.3
	31 days–1 year	37/406	9.1
	1–2 years	39/385	10.1
	2–3 years	8/ 97	8.2
	3–4 years	5/ 48	10.4
	4–5 years	5/ 42	11.9
	5–6 years	3/ 21	14.3
Postop. interval including autopsy	0–31 days	27/255	9.6
	31 days–1 year	38/374	9.2
	1–2 years	39/385	10.1
	2–3 years	8/ 97	8.2
	3–4 years	5/ 48	10.4
	4–5 years	5/ 42	11.9
	5–6 years	3/ 21	14.3

the aorta to the recipient coronary artery seem to be preferable. The small number of sequential grafts does not allow a statistical analysis with regard to the possible benefits of this technique.

All parameters influencing graft patency which have been mentioned so far should theoretically lead to early graft occlusion. There is, in fact, no significant increase in occlusion rates later than 1 month after surgery, especially when grafts from patients dying within the early postoperative period and examined at autopsy are included in the calculation (Table 3) [8, 9, 10]. This finding might not be absolutely conclusive, however, since the figures for the different postoperative intervals were derived from different patients instead of the same patients repeatedly recatheterized.

Conclusion

Graft occlusion after coronary artery bypass surgery is a potentially dangerous event, since it increases operative risk and lessens operative success. It can in part be prevented by avoiding situations through which graft flow can be compromised, especially by technical mistakes and selection of recipient coronary arteries too small to provide a sufficient run-off.

References

1. Lytle BW, Loop FD (1982) Elective coronary surgery. In: McGoon DC (ed) Cardiac surgery. Davis, Philadelphia
2. Roth JA, Cakingnan RA, Braun BG, et al. (1978) Factors influencing patency of venous grafts. Ann Thorac Surg 28: 176
3. Lim JS, Proudfit WL, Sheldon WC, Alosilla C, et al. (1978) Perioperative myocardial infarction related to coronary artery surgery. Am Heart J 96: 463
4. Morton BC, Mc Laughlin PR, Trimble AS, Morch JE (1975) Myocardial infarction in coronary artery surgery. Circulation 51/52 (Suppl 1): 198
5. Sheldon WC (1978) Factors influencing patency of coronary bypass grafts. Cleve Clin Q 45: 109

6. Sheldon WC, Rinson G, Pichard A (1974) Results of graft surgery for coronary artery disease. A progress report. Cleve Clin Consult 93: 103
7. Roskamm H, Schmutziger M, Weisswange A, et al. (1977) Ergometrische und hämodynamische Ergebnisse nach aortokoronarem Bypass bei 378 Patienten. Schweiz Med Wochenschr 107: 1888
8. Favorolo RG (1979) Direct myocardial revascularization: a ten year journey. Am J Cardiol 43: 109
9. Sheldon WC, Rincon G, Effler DB (1973) Vein graft surgery for coronary artery disease. Circulation 47/48 (Suppl 3): 184
10. McIntosh HD, Garcia JA (1978) The first decade of aortocoronary bypass grafting, 1967–1977. Circulation 57 (3): 405

Evaluation of Aortocoronary Graft Patency with Computed Thomography

B. Urbanyi, B. Wimmer, K. Wink, A. Santana, G. Spillner, and V. Schlosser

After aortocoronary saphenous vein bypass surgery a simple and relatively noninvasive method to determine graft patency would be useful for evaluating surgical results. Early postoperative angiography would be the method of choice; most patients, however, are reluctant to have this costly and invasive examination performed. Following encouraging reports [1–7] with contrast-medium-enhanced computed tomography (CECT) in evaluating graft patency, the value and limitations of the method were studied.

Materials and Methods

Between October 1981 and May 1983 a total of 400 aortocoronary saphenous vein bypass grafts in 228 patients were examined with CECT in the early postoperative period. Of these, 59.5% (238/400) were single grafts, 40.5% (162/400) were sequential grafts with two or more anastomoses, and 7.8% (31/400) were with three or more anastomoses. Computed tomography (CT) was performed without patient selection within the first 10 postoperative days in 72.8% and within 15 days in 97.8%, unless the patient refused examination or the equipment was not available.

After selection of the appropriate scan levels where the grafts were expected, CT was performed with contrast-medium enhancement, using a manual intravenous bolus injection of 30 ml Telebrix-30 into an arm vein; within 60 sec five scans were obtained using the Siemens Somatotom 2. In positive findings the contrast-medium-filled graft appeared in transverse or longitudinal section simultaneously with the opacification of the aorta, at the appropriate level and position relative to the heart, at the appropriate time, and with adequate density (in Hounsfield units). If opacification did not appear the graft was considered occluded. In patients showing graft nonvisualization an attempt was made to obtain early angiographic correlation. Angiography was also considered necessary in patients with suspected occlusion in spite of patency of the grafts in CT.

Results

In 16.4% the single grafts, and in 16.0% the sequential grafts (overall 16.3%) were not adequately identified and were considered "occluded" in CECT (Table 1). Computed tomographic patency was overall 83.7% (335/400). Single and sequential grafts showed similar occlusion rates in CT. Those grafts which were unidentifiable because of radiation scatter through artifacts were considered for this purpose to be occluded; these were 17 of the 65 nonvisualized grafts.

Of the 65 nonvisualized grafts only 7 had correlating angiographic examinations within 3 to 11 months of CT examination. In all seven the proximal segment of the

Table 1. Graft identification in CT: nonvisualized grafts

	Single	Sequential
10/81–12/82	19.0% (24/126)	16.5% (17/103)
1/83– 5/83	13.4% (15/112)	15.9% (9/ 59)
Bypass "occluded" total	16.4% (39/238)	16.0% (26/162)
Bypass patent (CT)	83.6% (199/238)	84.0% (136/162)

Table 2. CT graft visualization in relation to flow rate in bypass grafts $n = 341$

	flow in graft (ml/min)							
	-40		>40–100		>100–200		>200	
	pos	neg	pos	neg	pos	neg	pos	neg
Single graft *n*	19	1	76	28	64	4	10	3
Sequential graft *n*	4		49	4	52	10	16	1

graft was patent in angiography. In two there was a stenosis at a laterolateral anastomosis. In one patient angiography of a sequential graft showed proximal patency but occlusion of the distal segment to the outflow anatomosis.

Discussion

The utilization of CECT to determine graft patency in the postoperative period after aortocoronary bypass surgery [1–6] has been proposed, with possible use of the method to select patients for early reoperation if graft occlusion was demonstrated [7]. The results of this prospective study, however, have shown the definite limitations of this examination method.

Other factors besides graft occlusion may influence graft identification. Experience with the examination technique and accurate knowledge of the course of the graft veins of the part of the radiologist is necessary, which is borne out by the fact that graft identification rate has improved over the study period (Table 1). Biological cardiac motion is a problem with present equipment. Artifacts, particularly metal marking rings around the proximal aortic anastomoses and clips used for occlusion of the side branches in the vein graft, cause difficulty in graft identification through scatter radiation. If CT examination is contemplated plastic marking rings and side clips or ligatures should be used.

Pericardial vessels such as bronchial arteries coming directly off the aorta, the left auricle, and patent native coronary vessels may be misinterpreted as patent grafts. Identification of grafts running on the dorsal surface of the heart has been difficult in our experience. Injection of contrast medium at a period too early or late in the scan sequence may give erroneous results.

In those grafts in which intraoperative flow measurements were performed, no real correlation was found when comparing flow rates in the venous graft with visibility in CT (Table 2). In fact, even those grafts with low flow rates of up to 40 ml/

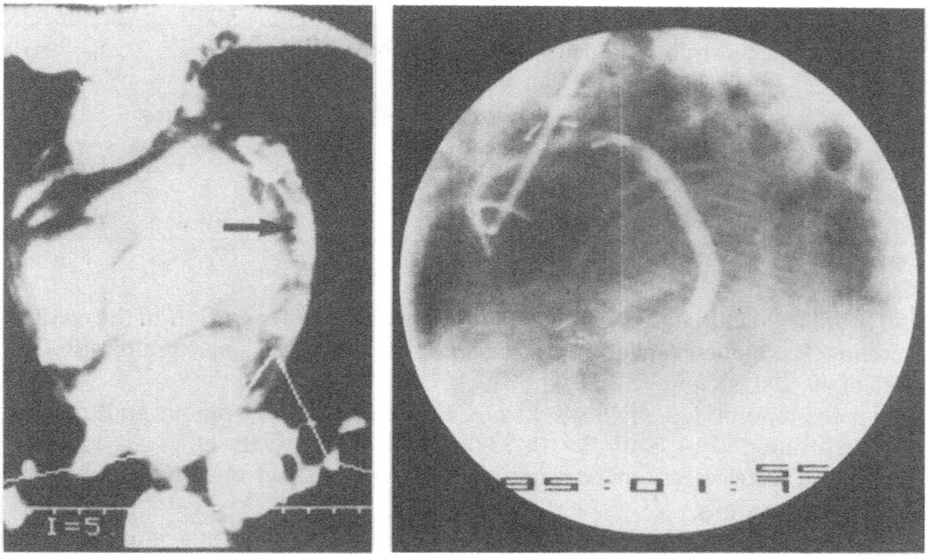

Fig. 1. Sequential aortocoronary graft. CT *(left)* indicates patency; angiography *(right)* shows occlusion in the distal segment

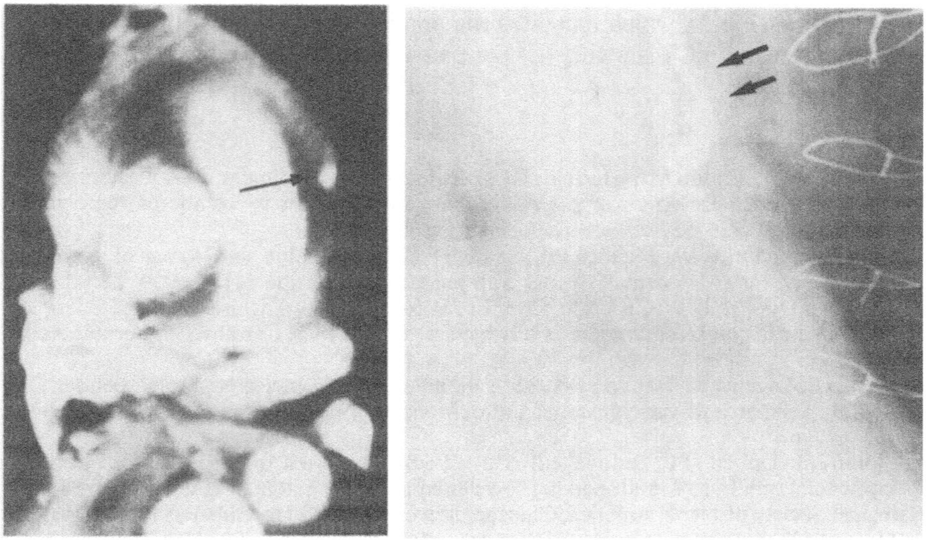

Fig. 2. Torsion of a single graft to the LAD, positively identified on CT

Table 3. Sensitivity and specificity of CECT of aortocoronary bypass grafts

	grafts with angiographic correlation *n*	CT patient *n*		sensitivity %	CT occluded *n*		specificity %
		correct	incorrect		correct	incorrect	
Brundage [1]	62	39	1	93.0	20	2	95.0
Daniel [2]	125	84	4	91.3	29	8	87.9
Heuser [4]	199	125	14	92.6	50	10	78.1

min could be identified in most cases, possibly due to poorer outflow of the contrast medium. The highest rate of nonvisualization was found in single grafts with flow rates of 40–100 ml/min.

In some reports [1, 2, 4] sensitivity of CECT in diagnosing venous graft patency has been reported to be 91.3% to 93.0%, with a specificity of 78.1% to 95.0% (Table 3). The necessary angiographic correlation was not obtained in adequate number in our study.

Problems of anastomotic stenosis or distal occlusion in sequential grafts were not picked up with CT. In one patient (Fig. 1) with a postoperative infarction demonstrated with electrocardiography and enzyme levels CT showed proximal patency of the sequential graft to the diagonal branch and left anterior descending arteries (LAD); angiography, however, revealed the bypass to be patent only up to the diagonal laterolateral anastomosis with occlusion of the segment distal to the LAD. Graft torsion (Fig. 2), which increases the possibility of early graft occlusion, was not diagnosed, with CT showing normal patency of the LAD graft.

References

1. Brundage BH, Lipton MJ, Herfkins RJ, Berninger WH, Redington RW, Chatterjee DK, Carlson E (1980) Detection of patent coronary bypass grafts by computed tomography. Circulation 61: 826–831
2. Daniel W, Döhring W, Lichtlen PR, Stender HS (1981) Value and limits of computed tomography for assessment of bypass graft patency. Circulation 64 (Suppl 4): 221–225
3. Guthaner DF, Brody WR, Ricci M, Oyer PE, Wexler L (1980) The use of computed tomography in the diagnosis of coronary artery bypass graft patency. Cardiovasc Intervent Radiol 3: 3–8
4. Heuser L, Lackner K, Hauser H (1982) Validität der Computertomographie bei der Darstellung offener und verschlossener aortokoronarer Venenbrücken. Fortschr Röntgenstr 137: 619–626
5. Lipton JM, Doherty PP, Brundage B et al. (1978) Computed tomography for evaluating saphenous vein bypass graft patency. Presented at the 64th annual meeting of the Radiological Society of North America, Chicago, November 27 to December 1, 1978
6. Moncada R, Salinas M, Churchill R, Love L, Reynes C, Demos TC, Hale D, Schreiber R (1980) Patency of saphenous aortocoronary bypass grafts demonstrated by computed tomography. N Engl J Med 303: 503–505
7. Ullyot DJ, Turley K, McKay CR, Brundage BH, Lipton MJ, Ebert PA (1982) Assessment of saphenous vein graft patency by contrast-enhances computed tomography. J Thorac Cardiovasc Surg 83: 512–518

Early Exercise Testing and Coronary Bypass Surgery Post-infarction

F. Akhras, J. Upward, J. Keates, and G. Jackson

Introduction

Following uncomplicated myocardial infarction the one-year morbidity and mortality can be predicted by early exercise testing [1, 2]. In patients with exercise-induced ST segment depression the average mortality is 19% [3] with one study revealing a one-year mortality of 27% in contrast to only 2% in those with normal exercise ECG's [1]. We have shown previously that early exercise testing has considerable potential for the early identification of coronary disease additional to that which subtends the infarcted area [4]. It is likely therefore that the morbidity and mortality is determined by the presence and degree of significant further coronary disease.

The European coronary artery bypass surgery study [5], which involved angina patients, reported increased survival in the surgical group for those with significant three-vessel or left main stem disease. Though not indicated, the presence of a previous infarction is likely in some of these patients. In the belief that the disease process is the same whether the patient has or has not previously sustained a myocardial infarction we have prospectively evaluated exercise testing and angiography as a means of identifying the at-risk patient early following his uncomplicated myocardial infarction. Once the anatomically at-risk were identified coronary artery bypass surgery was performed.

Patients and Method

Patients

Following an uncomplicated acute myocardial infarction 114 patients were studied prospectively by 12-lead maximal treadmill stress testing and by coronary angiography, at 2 and 6 weeks respectively. All patients entered the study at 2 weeks post infarct. Their clinical data is summarised in Table 1.

Patients were excluded from the study if they had residual angina needing therapy, heart failure, cardiac arrhythmia, bundle-branch block or valvular heart disease. No patient was dependent on cardiac drug and thus none had taken digoxin or beta blockers for at least 48 h before the stress test. In all patients the diagnosis of myocardial infarction was based on a diagnostic enzyme rise and electrocardiographic changes.

Exercise Testing

All patients underwent 12-lead maximal stress testing (MST) according to the Bruce protocol 2 weeks after infarction. Though the details of the test have been described previously [4] it is necessary to repeat the description with some amplification to detail the end point and criteria for a positive test. The test was terminated if there was

Table 1. Patient characteristics

	Surgical group $n = 53$	Medical group $n = 61$	p
Age (years)	50∓1	49∓1	NS
Sex (% males)	91.5	95	NS
Location of MI			
Anterior	15	36	<0.001
Inferior	38	25	<0.001
Admission SBP (mmHg)	124∓2	127∓3	NS
Admission DBP (mmHg)	78∓2	82∓1	NS
Admission HR (beats/min)	83∓3	81∓2	NS

HR, heart rate; SBP, systolic blood pressure; DBP, diastolic blood pressure; MI, myocardial infarction

Table 2. Exercise testing and coronary angiography data

	Surgical group ($n = 53$)	Medical group ($n = 61$)	p
Resting HR (beats/min)	83 ∓3	81 ∓2	NS
Peak HR (beats/min)	148.5∓2	151 ∓3	NS
Peak SBP (mmHg)	134 ∓4.2	145 ∓3.3	NS
Exercise time (min)	5.5∓0.3	7.5∓0.28	<0.001
ST segment change (mm)	2 ∓0.14	1 ∓0.17	<0.001
No. of vessels ≥70% stenotic			
1	0	30	
2	5	24	<0.0001
3	48	7	

cardiac pain, a fall in systolic blood pressure of 15 mmHg, ST segment depression of 3 mm, dyspnoea or exhaustion. Unlike our previous study [4], a test was considered positive when a net horizontal or down-sloping depression of the ST segment greater than 1 mm persisted for 80 ms after the QRS complex in a non-infarct area. The ischaemic area criteria we have described in our previous study.

Coronary Angiography

Within 4 weeks of the exercise test each patient underwent selective coronary angiography and left ventriculography. There were no complications. The anatomy was reported without knowledge of the results of the exercise test. Significant coronary artery disease was defined as a luminal narrowing of greater than 70% in any of the three major coronary arteries. The occluded artery to the infarct area was classed as one-vessel disease.

Coronary Artery Bypass Surgery

Based on the anatomy at angiography and/or symptoms, the patients with additional significant coronary artery disease were offered coronary artery bypass surgery. All patients were regularly seen during a mean follow-up of 23∓0.7 months.

Statistical Analysis

Data are expressed as mean ∓ SEM. Logarithmic analysis was used and differences between continuous variables were assessed by the unpaired t-test and chi-square test.

Results

Comparison of Medical and Surgical Subsets

The 53 patients managed surgically and the 61 patients managed medically were remarkably similar with regard to age, sex, location and extent of infarction (Table 1). However, as one would expect from our selection criteria the surgical group had significantly more ST segment depression on exercise testing at a significantly reduced exercise time (Table 2). At catheterisation they also had more coronary arteries with greater than 70% stenosis in comparison to the medical group (3.2 ∓ 0.1 vs 1.6 ∓ 0.1, $p < 0.001$). Patients with inferior infarcts had a significantly greater change of additional disease in comparison to those with anterior infarcts.

Exercise Data and Coronary Angiography Results

Sixty-three patients suffered inferior and 51 anterior infarction. Based on the ST segment change, 81 patients had a positive MST indicating additional coronary artery disease in vessels remote from the infarct area. At angiography all but two were shown to have additional coronary artery disease. The two patients with single vessel disease in whom the MST was positive in the infarct area underwent successful coronary artery dilatation and subsequently remain asymptomatic during the follow-up period.

Surgical Group

Based on the anatomy at angiography 53 (48 with three-vessel and 5 with two-vessel disease) of the 79 patients who had a true positive MST were allocated to have surgery. Of these, 47 patients underwent elective coronary artery bypass surgery. There was one perioperative death. The remaining 46 are symptom-free during the follow-up period. Five patients are receiving beta blockade and awaiting bypass surgery, being unable to resume an active life because of anginal symptoms, and one patient died following re-infarction at 4 months.

Medical Group

In 30 patients, angiography revealed single vessel coronary disease to the infarct area and this was correctly predicted by the exercise ECG in 28 (93%), i.e., there were no areas of ST depression outside the infarct area. Twenty-four patients had two-vessel coronary disease. Seven patients with positive stress tests had inoperable distal and diffuse three-vessel coronary disease and they were offered intensive medical therapy.

One has subsequently died, two are asymptomatic on treatment and four are restricted by angina or dyspnoea in spite of medical therapy. Of the 61 patients in the medical group the exercise ECG correctly predicted the anatomy in 57. In all 28 patients who had true negative stress tests for additional ischaemia, the exercise ECG correctly predicted coronary anatomy (Table 3).

Table 3. Correlation between MST and coronary angiography in both groups

Mode of therapy	Location of MI	MST				No. of vessels 70% stenotic			
		TP	FP	TN	FN	1	2	3	Total
Medical $n=61$	Anterior $n=36$	14	1	20	1	21	12	3	36
	Inferior $n=25$	15	1	8	1	9	12	4	25
Surgical $n=53$	Anterior $n=15$	15	0	0	0	0	3	12	15
	Inferior $n=38$	35	0	0	3	0	2	36	38
Total		79	2	28	5	30	29	55	114

TP, true positive, FP, false positive; TN, true negative; FN, false negative

Discussion

By exercising patients at 2 weeks following an uncomplicated myocardial infarction, mortality and morbidity can be accurately predicted [1, 2]. This has particular advantages for physicians who have more ready access to exercise testing facilities than to angiography, reducing the need for and the number of unnecessary angiograms. While it is clear that post-infarct exercise testing has considerable potential for the early identification of multivessel coronary disease, clear guide-lines for subsequent management do not exist. Recognising the high one-year mortality figure of up to 27% for those with positive exercise tests following uncomplicated infarction and an overall average one-year mortality of 10%–20% [6, 7], it is reasonable to assume that a means of identifying and modifying the anatomy may influence survival. With the proven benefits of surgery in patients with angina and in the belief that the disease process is the same, we electively referred our post-infarct patients with additional significant coronary artery disease for early surgery (6–12 weeks). Of 47 patients operated on, one died and 46 remain well at a mean follow-up of 23 months (surgical mortality 2%).

The 53 patients considered for surgery had significantly more ST segment depression on exercise testing at a significantyl shorter exercise time than the medically managed patients (2 ∓ 0.14 vs 1 ∓ 0.17 mm and 5.5 ∓ 0.3 vs 7.5 ∓ 0.28 min respectively, $p < 0.001$) and at angiography they had significantly more coronary arteries with greater than 70% stenosis than the medical group.

Thus, MST early post-infarct can predict the anatomy and has the potential to define an at-risk group with an expected mortality of up to 27%. Our overall mortality at 23 months is 3% and all deaths occurred in the high risk group – one at operation, one awaiting operation and one allocated to medical therapy because of inoperable lesions. The patient who died from re-infarction at 4 months regretably had his operation delayed by factors outside our control. Seven patients were considered unsuitable operative cases because of advanced disease; one has subsequently died, two are asymptomatic and four are symptomatic though stable on medical therapy. The remaining 54 patients in the medical group are active and symptom-free.

Though this was a prospective study we recognise the absence of a randomised control trial and the use of historical controls. We feel however, that it is difficult to justify ignoring the current anatomically based evidence of surgical benefits and the well-established high mortality rate following uncomplicated myocardial infarction for those with early abnormal stress tests. A large scale randomised trial would possibly be more definitive and we are not opposed to this idea, though past experience has shown that even randomised trials in ischaemic heart disease are impaired by several factors, including (1) the randomised population fails to be representative of all patients with the disease, e.g., the more symptomatic, more extensively diseased patients are offered surgery without randomisation; and (2) large numbers of medically allocated patients "cross over" to surgical therapy during the follow-up because of symptoms refractory to medical management [8].

We believe our strikingly low mortality of 3% overall and 6% in the high risk group is a result of early surgical intervention. Our operative mortality was 2% with no deaths in the surgical group at follow-up. Thus, of those with high risk lesions considered suitable for surgery the one-year survival is 46 of 47 patients operated on.

References

1. Theroux P, Waters DD, Halphen C, Deboisieux JC, Mizgala HF (1979) Prognostic value of exercise testing soon after myocardial infarction. N Engl J Med 301: 341–5
2. Markiewicz W, Houston N, Debusk RF (1976) Exercise testing soon after myocardial infarction. Circulation 56: 25–31
3. Epstein SE, Palmer ST, Patterson RE (1982) Evaluation of patients after acute myocardial infarction: indications for cardiac catheterisation and surgical intervention. N Engl J Med 307: 1487–1492
4. Akhras F, Upward J, Stott R, Jackson G (1982) Early exercise testing and coronary angiography after uncomplicated myocardial infarction. Br Med J 284: 1293–4
5. European Coronary Surgery Study Group (1980) Prospective randomised study of coronary artery bypass surgery in stable angina pectoris. Lancet 2: 491–495
6. Beard OW, Hipp HR, Robins M, Taylor JS, Egbert RV, Beran LG (1960) Initial myocardial infarction among 503 veterans. Am J Med 28: 871–883
7. Granath A, Sodermark T, Winge T, Volpe U, Zetterquist S (1977) Early work-load tests for evaluation of long-term prognosis of acute myocardial infarction. Br Heart J 39: 758–763
8. Hurst JW, King SB III, Logue RB, Hatcher CR Jr, Jones EL, Craver JM, Douglas JS Jr, Franch RH, Dorney ER, Cobbs BW Jr, Robinson PH, Clements SO Jr, Kaplan JA, Bradford JM (1978) Value of coronary bypass surgery. Am J Cardiol 42: 308

Short-Term Radionuclide Study of Ventricular Function After Coronary Bypass Surgery

E. Astorri, M. Busi, G. A. Contini, G. Ugolotti, E. Restori, and P. P. Ferretti

Gated radionuclide ventriculography is a rapid, safe, noninvasive and easily reproducible procedure for measuring the left ventricular performance and the hemodynamic effects of therapy in patients with coronary artery disease. Using this radionuclide method, we evaluated short-term changes in left ventricular performance after coronary artery bypass grafting (CABG).

Methods

Informed consent was obtained from 13 patients (11 males, 2 females, ages 44 to 65 years, mean 53 years), and these were studied while scheduled for myocardial revascularization. Nine patients had a previous inferior myocardial infarction, and one patient a previous anterior one. One patient had significant stenosis of one, three patients of two, and nine patients of three coronary vessels. Contrast angiography revealed normal myocardial kinesis in seven patients, and hypokinesis in six patients (five inferiorly and one anteriorly localized).

Myocardial revascularization required one (in one patient), two (in five patients), three (in five patients), and four (in two patients) CABG. All surgical procedures were performed in total cardiopulmonary bypass and general hypothermia (27° ± 2 °C), myocardial preservation was obtained by local cooling and ischemic cardioplegic arrest with hyperpotassic solution.

Gated radionuclide left ventriculography was performed in all the patients on the 2nd–3rd day before and the 5th–7th day after myocardial revascularization. After intravenous injection of 20–25 mCi ^{99m}Tc-labeled human serum albumin, the patients were examined in 35°–45° left anterior oblique projection and 15° caudal angulation, using an LFOV Searle gamma camera, interfaced to a dedicated computer (PDP 11/34 Digital Eq.Co.). Thirty frames per cycle from a total of 600 cardiac cycles, gated for the ECG, were collected and analyzed for each examination.

The global ejection fraction (EF) was determined along with the EFs of three anatomically distinct segments of the left ventricle, namely anteroseptal, apical, and inferoposterior [6]. Peak ejection and peak filling rates (PER, PFR) and their times to peak were also calculated.

Data were analyzed by the t-test using paired data and by linear regression analysis as appropriate.

Results

Before surgery all the patients had a global EF $\geqslant 50\%$. These radionuclide data were shown to correlate significantly with EF values from contrast angiography ($r = 0.75$; $p < 0.01$).

After surgery, the conditions of all the patients were satisfactory, and no ECG or humoral signs of perioperative infarction were reported. No significant EF changes were found in comparison with preoperative values, although actually EF increased slightly (Table 1, Fig. 1). Regional wall motion was changed: anteroseptal EF was observed to be reduced significantly, while apical EF was found to be only moderately increased. Inferoposterior EF showed constant, remarkable, highly significant improvements (Fig. 2). Postoperatively, the dynamic parameters PER and PFR increased in a highly significant manner (Fig. 3). The reduction of times to peak of ejection and filling rates paralleled the reduction of R-R intervals postoperatively (Table 1).

The extent and direction of the observed variations were not correlated with the duration of cardiopulmonary bypass and aortic cross clamping. When the variations observed for the various parameters were compared, the only significant linear correlation was between increase of PER and parallel increase in inferoposterior EF ($r = 0.73$; $p < 0.01$).

Discussion

After CABG left ventricular performance varied with time in checks performed with different techniques. If measured 4–8 h after myocardial revascularization EF values were shown to be clearly reduced [5], while no changes [5] or improvements [2] were detected a week after surgery. In sequential studies of myocardial wall motion using radiopaque markers [7], both decreased EF and increased circumferential shortening rate have been found a week after operation. In our study, global EF showed only limited, nonsignificant improvements.

Myocardial revascularization had variable effects with respect to regional wall motion [4]. We have observed a postoperative decrement in anteroseptal kinesis;

Table 1. Changes in left ventricular performance after myocardial revascularization

	A	B	
HR (beats/min)	64.4 ± 14.8	97.0 ± 8.6	P<0.001
MAP (mmHg)	99.6 ± 14.2	103.8 ± 8.2	NS
EF (%)	58.3 ± 12.0	61.5 ± 11.7	NS
EF-AS (%)	55.1 ± 14.4	48.2 ± 17.3	P<0.05
EF-AP (%)	64.2 ± 16.4	68.5 ± 10.7	NS
EF-IP (%)	50.0 ± 13.7	68.8 ± 13.5	P<0.001
PER (sec^{-1})	3.97 ± 1.15	6.60 ± 2.18	P<0.001
T-PER/R-R	13.01 ± 3.11	14.37 ± 4.75	NS
PFR (sec^{-1})	3.80 ± 1.57	5.90 ± 2.02	P<0.001
T-PFR/R-R	23.05 ± 7.49	26.66 ± 5.79	NS

Values expressed as mean ± standard deviation of the selected parameters determined before (A) and after (B) surgery. *Abbreviations:* HR, heart rate; MAP, mean arterial pressure; EF, global ejection fraction; EF-AS, EF-AP, EF-IP, anteroseptal, apical, inferoposterior regional ejection fractions; PER, peak ejection rate; T-PER/R-R, time to PER/R-R interval; PFR, peak filling rate; T-PFR/R-R, time to PFR/R-R interval

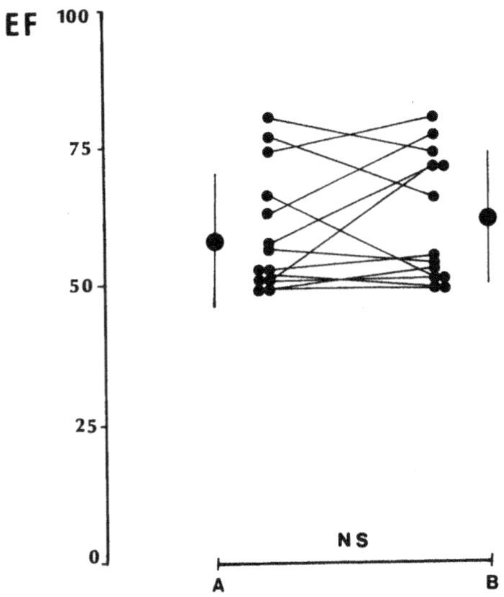

Fig. 1. Global ejection fraction % *(EF)* in each patient, before *(A)* and after *(B)* surgery. Mean values are shown with standard deviation

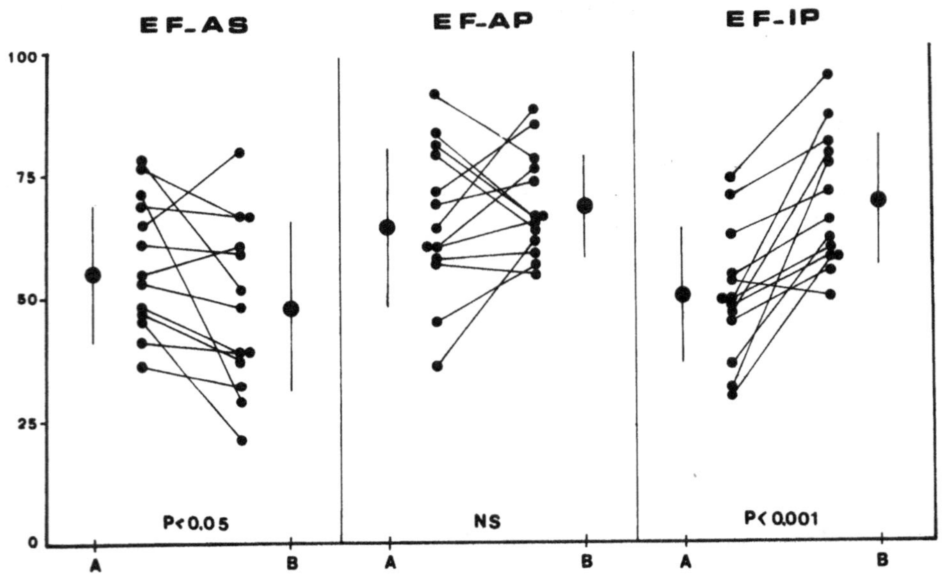

Fig. 2. Anteroseptal *(AS)* apical *(AP)*, and inferoposterior *(IP)* ejection fraction % *(EF)* in each patient before *(A)* and after *(B)* surgery. Mean values are shown with standard deviation

this result was in agreement with the angiographic and echocardiographic findings [3, 4] of a paradoxical septal motion after cardiopulmonary bypass. The different degrees and directions of changes in postoperative anteroseptal motion (Fig. 2) were dependent neither on the kind or severity of coronary artery disease, nor on the number and localization of the CABG performed.

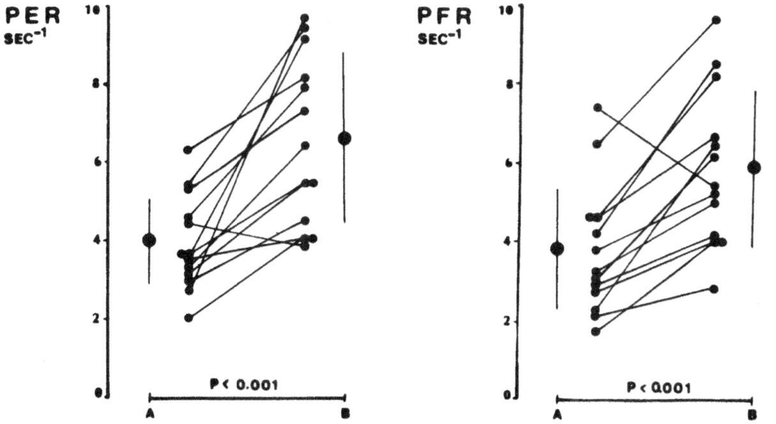

Fig. 3. Peak ejection rate *(PER)* and peak filling rate *(PFR)* in each patient before *(A)* and after *(B)* surgery. Mean value are shown with standard deviation

Posteroinferior wall motion had the greatest improvements after operation. Most of our patients had the scar of an inferior myocardial infarction and, even when maintaining a good global EF, they presented a slightly impaired inferoposterior motion before operation. The most remarkable improvements after surgery were observed in three patients who had also presented the greatest preoperative decrements in inferoposterior kinesis (Fig. 2). The tentative explanation for these data is that restored perfusion improved the performance of previously damaged ischemic areas [7].

While global EF did not change significantly after surgery, PER was remarkably increased, although they are bot parameters reflecting global ventricular performance. It is worth recalling that improvements in PER were correlated with increases in inferoposterior kinesis.

Taking into account the significant increase in heart rate, all these results are compatible with a more elevated adrenergic action in the first days after surgery [1]; we did not study this aspect of the problem.

The clear-cut increase in PFR observed after myocardial revascularization apparently pointed to a better ventricular compliance.

These data gave a first assessment of left ventricular performance during a short period following surgery. Future radionuclide angiographic measurement, which will be performed together with ergometric and pharmacological trials, should help to decide whether these preliminary data were the result of improvements in perfusion due to the surgical therapy or, instead, were a temporary outcome of any performed cardiopulmonary bypass.

References

1. Boudulas H, Lewis RP, Vasko JS, Karayannacos PE, Beaver BM (1976) Left ventricular function and adrenergic hyperactivity before and after saphenous vein bypass. Circulation 53: 802–806
2. Brundage BH, Anderson WT, Davia JE, Cheitlin MD, De Castro CM (1977) Determinants

of left ventricular function following aortocoronary bypass surgery. Am Heart J 93: 687–698
3. Burggraf GW, Craige E (1975) Echocardiographic studies of left ventricular wall motion and dimension after valvular heart surgery. Am J Cardiol 35: 473–480
4. Freeman MR, Gray RJ, Berman DS, Maddahi J, Raymond MJ, Forrester JS, Matloff JM (1981) Improvement in global and segmental left ventricular function after coronary bypass surgery. Circulation 64 (Suppl 2): 34–39
5. Levine FH, Phillips HR, Carter JE, Philbin DM, Osbakken MD, Boucher CA, Pohost GM, Okada RD, Buckley MJ (1981) The effect of pulsatile perfusion on preservation of left ventricular function after aortocoronary bypass grafting. Circulation 64 (Suppl 2): 40–44
6. Maddox DE, Holman LB, Wynne J, Idoine J, Parker JA, Uren R, Neill JM, Cohn PF (1978) Ejection fraction image: a noninvasive index of regional left ventricular wall motion. Am J Cardiol 45: 1230–1238
7. Mintz LJ, Ingels NB, Daughters GT, Stinson EB, Alderman EL (1980) Sequential studies of left ventricular function and wall motion after coronary artery bypass surgery. Am J Cardiol 45: 210–216

Stress-Radionuclide Ventriculography in the Evaluation of CABG Patients

L. Fridrich, A. Gaszner, and M. Pichler

Introduction

The noninvasive assessment of myocardial perfomrance and graft function after coronary artery bypass grafting (CABG) is important for prescribing the patient's postoperative exercise and rehabilitation program. The postoperative stress electrocardiograph (ECG) and exercise performance are often used as noninvasive tests, but are limited due to their low sensitivity and specificity for detecting graft dysfunction [4]. Thallium-201 scintigraphy offers the possibility of detecting additional reversible perfusion defects in the postoperative patient, but lacks a high sensitivity and specificity [2]. Exercise radionuclide ventriculography (RNV) is another noninvasive tool which can provide quantitative and qualitative information about cardiac performance in the postoperative phase [5].

We performed exercise ^{99m}Tc-RNV in our patients early and late in the period of postoperative rehabilitation. The aim of the study was to determine the clinical value of postoperative stress and poststress RNV as a noninvasive way to gather information about graft patency, and to investigate myocardial function during the course of rehabilitation.

Subjects and Methods

We evaluated 25 male patients (mean age 53 ± 7 years) 2–10 weeks after CABG (mean number of grafts 2.3) by supine RNV at rest, during peak exercise, and postexercise. Sixteen patients had pre- or perioperative myocardial infarction (eight posterior, eight anterior). Rest, stress, and poststress RNV was performed using standard procedure after injection of 25 mCi (93×10^4 Bq) of autologous in vivo – in vitro ^{99m}Tc-labeled red blood cells [1]. All cardioactive drugs β blockers, long-acting nitrates) were withdrawn prior to the study. Acquisition was performed in supine LAO 35°–45° position with a prototype of a Siemens cardiac gamma camera equipped with a high sensitivity collimator supporting an MDS-A^2 data system. Frame mode acquisition (16 images/cycle) was performed at rest, peak exercise, and immediately post exercise for almost 4 min within a heart frequency limit of ± 5% for each acquisition. Ejection fraction (EF) was calculated by a semiautomated computer program (normal: $57\% \pm 4.5\%$ to $66\% \pm 3.5\%$) and the semiquantiative evaluation of regional wall motion (RWM) abnormalities using a five-point scoring system was shown on the computer's video display [3].

Poststress studies were used for analysis of reversibility of RWM abnormalities.

Results

Resting EF was 51% ± 11% and did not change significantly (51% ± 15%) during exercise (heart rate 125 ± 18/min); individual responses of EF to stress are shown in Fig. 1: ten patients showed a significant increase while seven patients showed a decline of EF. In nine patients paradoxical septal movement occurred. The distribution among the groups with different stress EF responses is shown in Fig. 2: no relationship between paradoxical septal movement and EF stress response can be shown.

In 21 patients an accurate analysis of RWM during stress and resting conditions could be obtained (see Fig. 3). There was a high incidence of reversible RWM abnormalities in patients with a fall of EF during exercise; however, there was also a surprisingly high incidence of 63% in the patient group with increasing stress EF.

In 12 patients RNV stress testing could be performed in the early (2–6 weeks) and late phase of supervised rehabilitation (6–10 weeks postoperatively). Fig. 4 shows the individual responses of stress EF seen in the course of rehabilitation. Besides a higher average stress level without changes of mean stress EF and exercise heart rate (an effect of physical training), five patients showed a pronounced change of stress EF. It was higher in three patients, whereas in two individuals a decline of stress EF occurred which was obscured in the early test because of lower exercise levels. A similar effect on RWM abnormalities was seen in 6 of 12 patients.

To illustrate the diagnostic value of the RWM abnormalities analysis under stress and poststress conditions, one patient with no significant change from rest to stress

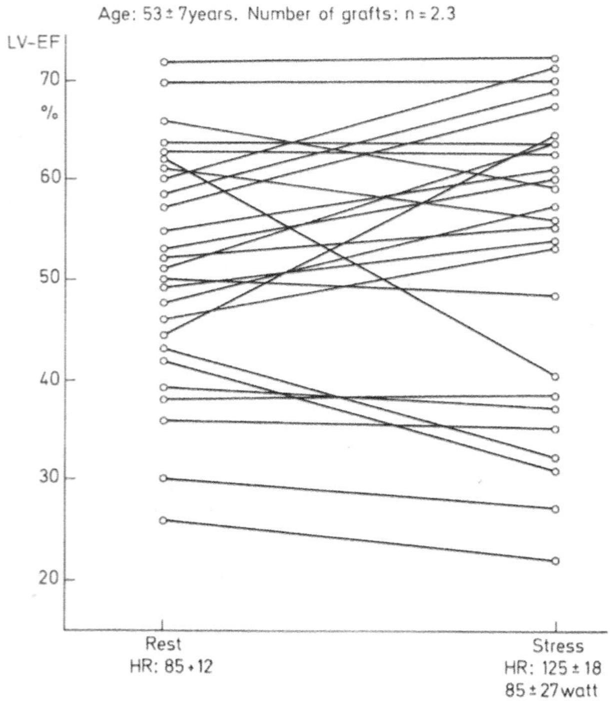

Fig. 1. Left ventricular ejection fraction *(LV-EF)* during rest and exercise in 25 CABG patients

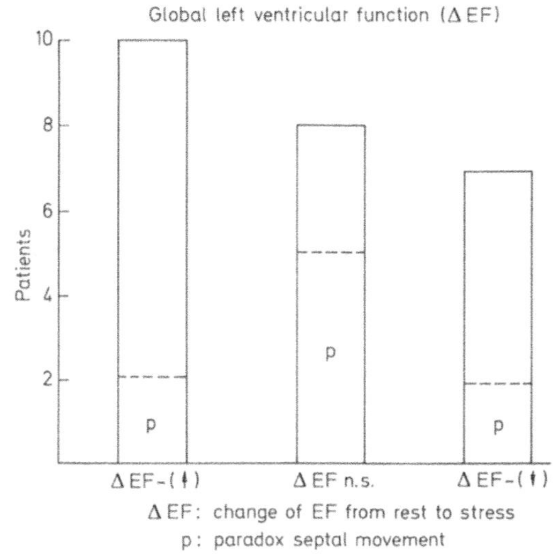

Fig. 2. Global left ventricular function *(ΔEF)* on rest and stress RNV in 25 CABG patients *p*, paradoxical septal movement

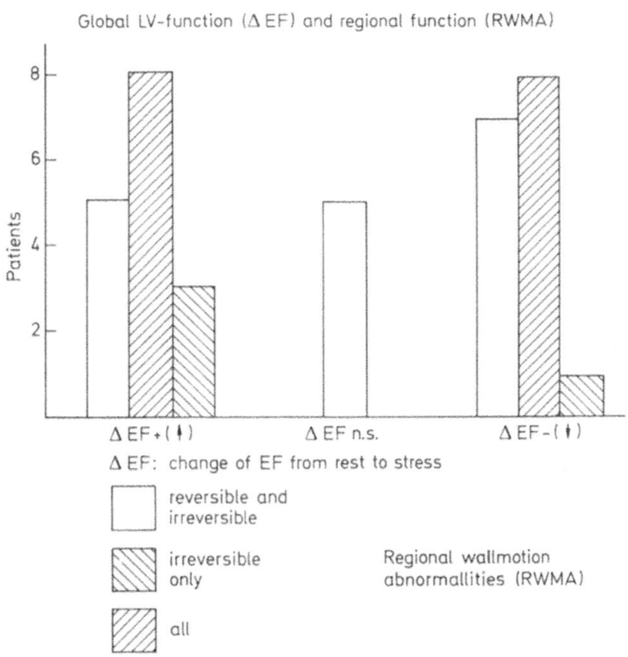

Fig. 3. Global left ventricular function *(ΔEF)* and regional function on rest, stress, and post-stress RNV in 21 CABG patients

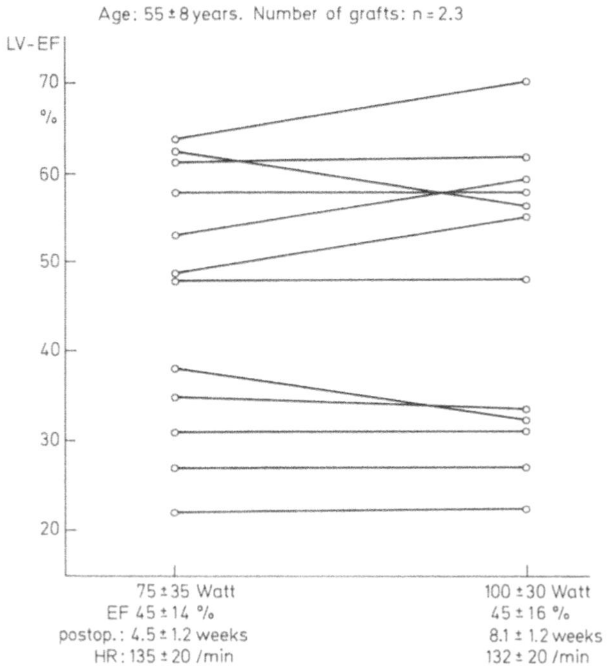

Fig. 4. Stress left ventricular ejection fraction *(LV-EF)* in 12 patients (mean age 55 ± 8 years) 4 and 8 weeks after CABG

EF (50% to 48%) will be described. RWM abnormalities analysis under resting and stress conditions revaealed only slight RWM abnormalities in the distal, septal, posterolateral, and inferoapical regions without any change, whereas in the poststress study a very good contractility in these regions was present, indicating the reversibility of the lesion. The patient was advised to undergo reangiography but he refused. He was readmitted 2 months later after extended infarction in the suspected area.

Conclusions

Rest and stress RNV after CABG is already in the early phase of rehabilitation a valuable noninvasive tool for estimation of global and regional ventricular function. It supplies valuable information for optimizing an individuals postoperative physical training. The patient with unclear symptoms and partly or totally ineffective revascularization can be recognized early by inadequate EF response to exercise and by exercise-induced RWM abnormalities, and can be managed as a risk patient.

In the late phase of rehabilitation physical efficiency can be tested through investigation of global and regional myocardial function with simultaneous judgement of graft patency, whereby stress and poststress studies are of special value.

References

1. Bauer R, Haluszczynski I, Langhammer H, Bachmann W (1983) In vivo/in vitro labeling of red blood cells with 99 m Tc. Eur J Nucl Med 8: 218–222

2. Iskandrian AS, Haaz W, Segal BL, Kane SA (1981) Exercise thallium 201 scintigraphy in evaluating aortocoronary bypass surgery. Chest 80: 11–15
3. Rozanski A, Berman D, Gray R, Diamond G, Raymond M, Prause J, Maddahi J, Swan HJC, Matloff J (1982) Preoperative prediction of reversible myocardial asynergy by postexercise radionuclide ventriculography. N Engl J Med 307: 212–216
4. Talbot S, Kilpatrick D, Oakley D (1982) Coronary artery bypass surgery. Assessment of graft patency by exercise testing. Eur Heart J 3: 348–352
5. Taylor NC, Barber RW, Crossland P, English TAH, Wraight EP, Petch MC (1983) Effects of coronary artery bypass grafting on left ventricular function assessed by multiple gated ventricular scintigraphy. Br Heart J 50: 149–156

Long-Term Results of Aortocoronary Bypass Surgery

H. Roskamm, M. Schmuziger, H. Gohlke, and C. Dorste

There are only a few studies dealing with the long-term effects of aortocoronary bypass surgery on exercise performance; reports about the influence of the degree of revascularization on these long-term effects are rare or even nonexistent.

Here we report results in 1000 patients (940 men and 60 women, mean age 51.8 years) who underwent aortocoronary bypass surgery between March 1973 and September 1979. One hundred and fourteen patients had one-vessel disease, 289 patients had two-vessel disease, and 597 patients had tree-vessel disease, including 145 patients with left main stem stenosis. All operations were performed by Schmuziger and his co-workers.

A total of 2590 grafts were constructed. Twenty-six patients died during the operation or in the course of 30 days after it; only 6 patients were lost during the (up to 6 years long) follow-up, while 33 patients died during this period.

Some details of this report have already been published in several papers from our group [1–3].

In 825 patients a second angiography was performed, mostly at 1 year after bypass surgery; according to the results of that angiography the patients were divided into four groups with different degrees of revascularization:

Group I. Complete revascularization – all vessels with a stenosis fo > 50% were provided with an open bypass;

Group II. Sufficient revascularization – all main vessels with > 50% stenosis not re-

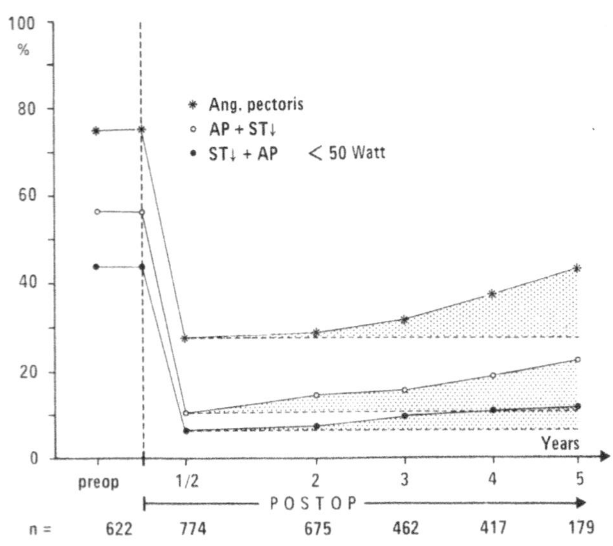

Fig. 1. Long-term follow-up of frequency of angina pectoris, angina pectoris with ischemic ST segment depression (*AP+ ST*↓), and angina pectoris below 50 watts of exercise with ischemic ST segment depression (*ST*↓ + *AP*, < *50 Watt*) in patients after bypass surgery

lated to an infarcted area were provided with an open bypass; the bypass to the left anterior descending artery (LAD) in particular is open;

Group III. Insufficient revascularization – at least one significantly stenosed main vessel (LAD or dominant right coronary artery) was not provided with an open bypass; and

Group IV. All grafts occluded.

We could follow 744 of our patients who were regularly given exercise tests (Fig. 1). Half a year after the operation 28% of the patients still experienced agina; this rate increased to 43% at 5 years after surgery. The reoccurrence rate of angina pectoris is 3.3% per year, which is comparable with the results of Campeau and coworkers [4]. Typical angina combined with ischemic ST segment depression during exercise was, half a year after surgery, persent in only 12% of the patients. Five years after surgery this had increased to 22%.

Typical angina with ischemic ST segment depression under a low work load of 50 watts – more or less the same situation as preoperatively – was reported from 5% of the patients half a year after bypass surgery. At 5 years postoperatively this rate had increased to 15%, with a reoccurrence rate of severe ischemia at low exercise levels of 2% annually.

Figure 2 shows the results of repeated exercise tests in 467 patients who were 55 years of age or younger at the time of bypass surgery [3].

Angina-free and maximum exercise tolerance increased remarkably from preoperativelly to 1 year postoperatively. There is a significant decrease from the 1st year

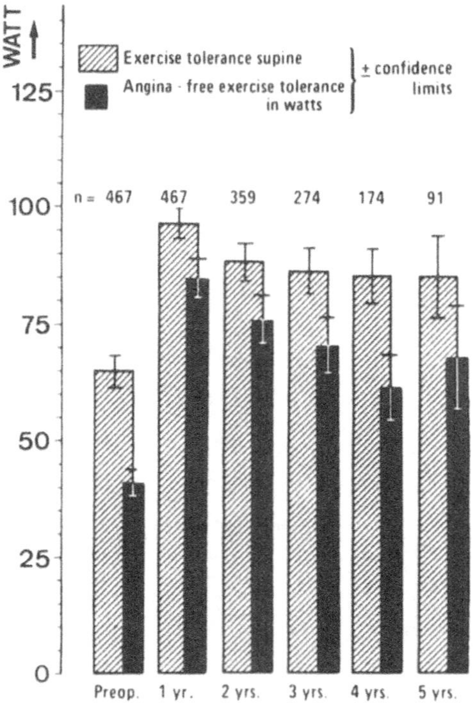

Fig. 2. Maximum exercise tolerance in supine position and angina-free exercise tolerance in watts, before and 1–5 years after bypass surgery

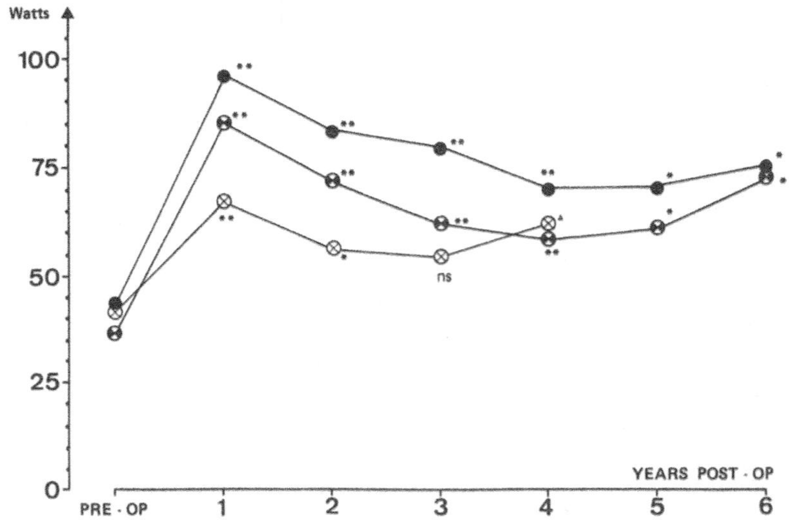

DEGREE of REVASCULARIZATION — n = No. of exercised patients

● Complete n =	178	182	155	125	113	61	49
⊖ Sufficient n =	176	176	135	116	92	33	22
⊗ Incomplete n =	57	57	45	39	25	7	7

All p - values in comparison to pre - op ** $p < 0.0005$ * $p < 0.005$ ▴ $p < 0.05$ ns = $p > 0.05$

Fig. 3. Angina-free exercise tolerance before and 1–6 years after bypass surgery in three groups with different degrees of revascularization

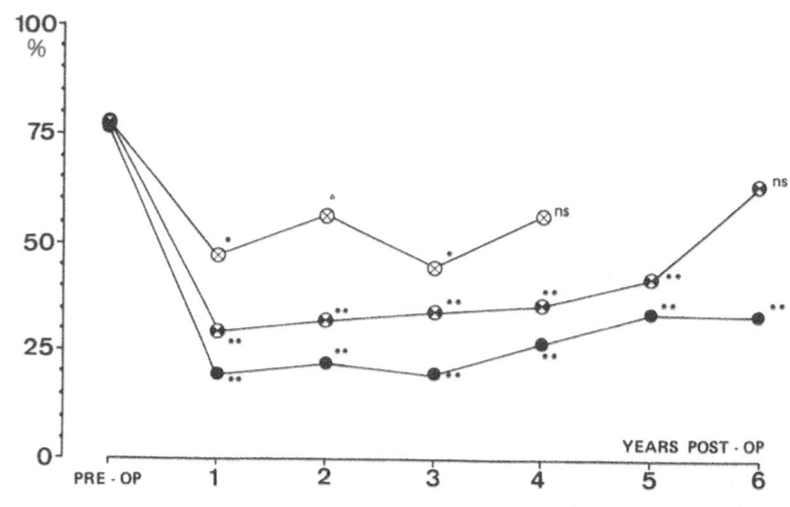

DEGREE of REVASCULARIZATION — n = No. of exercised patients

● Complete n =	178	182	155	125	113	61	49
⊖ Sufficient n =	176	176	135	116	92	33	22
⊗ Incomplete n =	57	57	45	39	25	7	7

All p - values in comparison to pre - op ** $p < 0.0005$ * $p < 0.005$ ▴ $p < 0.05$ ns = $p > 0.05$

Fig. 4. Prevalence of 0.1 mV ST segment depression before and 1–6 years after bypass surgery in four groups with different degrees revascularization to the 5th year, but at 5 years after surgery angina-free and maximum exercise tolerance is – compared to the preoperative state – still significantly improved.

To illustrate the influence of different degree of revascularization, in Fig. 3 the angina-free exercise tolerance is shown for three groups with different degrees of revascularization (group IV is not shown because the number of patients is too small).

At 1 year after surgery the angina-free exercise tolerance is improved in all three groups. Patients with complete and sufficient revascularization continued to have an improved angina-free exercise tolerance up to 6 years after surgery, whereas in group III the effect of bypass surgery on angina-free exercise tolerance is no longer significant at 3 years.

The prevalence of ST segment depression is shown in Fig. 4. Before surgery more than 75% of the patients had 0.1 mV ST segment depression during exercise. All three groups are improved after surgery. Patients with complete revascularization benefit most.

There is a slow and progressive loss of improvement for all groups; at 6 years after surgery only patients with complete revascularization had significantly less ST segment depression than before surgery.

Conclusions

In patients with complete and sufficient revascularization angina-pectoris-free exercise tolerance is still improved at 6 years postoperatively. The reoccurrence rate of angina pectoris was 3.3% per year; of severe ischemia at low exercise levels, 2% per year. Reoccurrence of angina pectoris and severe ischemia depends on the degree of revascularization.

References

1. Roskamm H, Schmuziger M, Stürzenhofecker P et al. (1981) Bestimmt die Vollständigkeit der Revaskularisation die funktionelle Verbesserung und die Überlebensdaten koronaroperierter Patienten? Ergebnisse von 1000 konsekutiv operierten Patienten. Z Kardiol 70: 590–599
2. Gohlke H, Gohlke-Bärwolf C, Samek L, Stürzenhofecker P, Schmuziger M, Roskamm H (1983) Serial exercise testing up to 6 years after coronary bypass surgery: behavior of exercise parameters in groups with different degrees of revascularization determined by postoperative angiography. Am J Cardiol 51: 1301–1306
3. Gohlke H, Schnellbacher K, Samek L, Stürzenhofecker P, Roskamm H (1982) Long-term improvement of exercise tolerance and vocational rehabilitation after bypass surgery: a 5 year follow up. J Cardiol Rehab 2: 531–540
4. Campeau L, Lesperance J, Hermann J, Corbara F, Grondin CM, Bourassa MG (1979) Loss of the improvement of angina between 1 and 7 years after aortocoronary bypass surgery. Correlations with changes in vein grafts and in coronary arteries. Circulation 60 (Suppl I): 1

Influence of Residual Disease on Late Survival After Coronary Artery Bypass Surgery

R. W. Hacker and M. Torka

Ventricular function and the number of obstructed coronary arteries are the most important prognostic parameters for the survival of medically treated patients with coronary heart disease [1–3, 6, 8, 9]. These factors seem to be of equal importance for the survival of patients after coronary artery bypass surgery [7].

Materials and Methods

To test this hypothesis, the survival data of 2700 consecutive patients were reviewed. All of them had undergone coronary artery bypass surgery, either electively or as an emergency operation, but without concomitant procedures, during the years 1974 to 1981. Preoperative data are shown in Table 1.

Left ventricular function was defined by ventriculography as being normal or impaired by hypokinetic or akinetic segments of left ventricular wall motion.

For the purpose of defining the degree of residual disease, the coronary circulation was considered to consist of four major vessel systems: the right, left main, left anterior descending, and circumflex coronary arteries. The presence of a luminal stenosis causing more than a 50% reduction in diameter in one or two of these coronary arteries without a bypass graft attached distal to it was called residual one- or two-vessel disease, respectively. Left main stenosis was considered completely bypassed only if grafts to both the left anterior descending and the circumflex coronary arteries had been placed.

Table 1. Preoperative data

	n	%
Sex (M/F)	2472/228	(91.6/8.4)
Age (years, mean ± SE)	52.9 ± 7.4	
Functional class (NYHA)		
I	23	(0.9)
II	437	(16.2)
III	1469	(54.3)
IV	771	(28.5)
Number of vessels stenosed		
1	548	(20.3)
2	793	(29.4)
3	1060	(39.2)
left main	299	(11.1)
Ventricular function		
normal	1268	(48.0)
hypokinetic segments	906	(34.3)
akinetic segments	465	(17.7)

According to this definition, 61% of all patients were completely revascularized, 34% have residual one-vessel disease, and 5% residual two-vessel disease.

Follow-up data were collected for more than 99% of all patients, mainly by telephone interviews with patients and physicians.

The survival data of different subgroups of patients relative to ventricular function and degree of revascularization were analyzed by Cutler-Ederer as well as Kaplan-Meier curves of survival probability [4].

Results and Discussion

Early mortality of the entire group was 1.1%, actuarial survival 9–10 years after surgery, as calculated by the method of Cutler and Ederer, was 83.4%, equivalent to a linearized yearly mortality rate of 1.8%.

Survival was significantly ($p < 0.001$) influenced by ventricular function (Fig. 1) and the number of obstructed yet ungrafted coronary arteries (Fig. 2).

The mortality rates of about 1% per year for patients with complete revascularization, 2% per year for patients with residual one-vessel disease, and 3% per year for

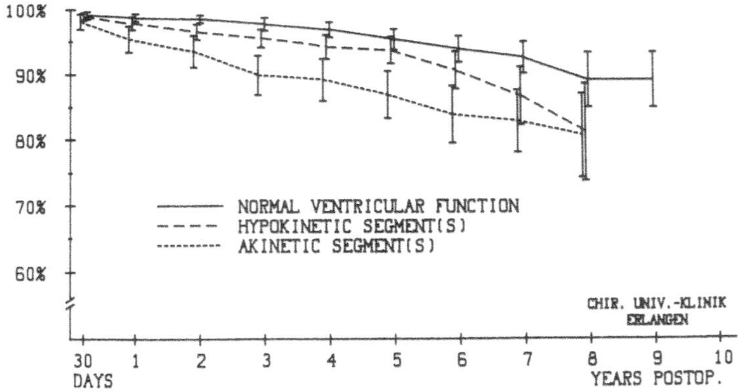

Fig. 1. Survival vs ventricular function

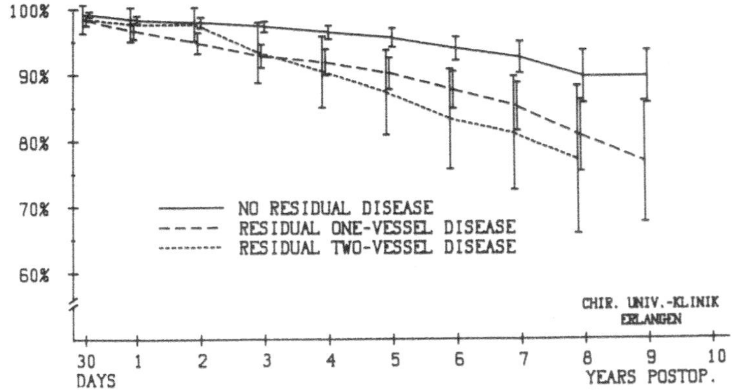

Fig. 2. Survival vs degree of revascularization

patients with residual two-vessel disease are somewhat lower than those for nonsurgical patients, which are in the range of 2%–3% per year for one-vessel and 5% per year for two-vessel disease [5]. This may be due to the fact that after surgery the important coronary arteries are usually grafted, and nonbypassed vessels are either small in size or already completely occluded and thus less likely to cause fatal myocardial infarction. On the other hand, in medically treated patients most commonly the involvement of sizeable vessels only leads to symptoms and eventually to the angiographic diagnosis of coronary heart disease.

It seems conceivable that incomplete revascularization is more likely to occur in patients with akinetic segments, because bypass grafts to vessels supplying those areas are not considered worthwhile by many surgeons. To distinguish the influence of obstructed yet not revascularized coronary arteries upon late survival from the bias of concomitant ventricular wall motion abnormalities, the parameter ventricular function was kept constant while comparing patients with different degrees of residual disease (Table 2).

Table 2. Influence of degree of revascularization on actuarial 5-year survival for subgroups with different ventricular function

Ventricular function	Degree of revascularization	Mean 5-year survival ± SE (%)
Normal	complete	96.5 ± 0.9
	residual 1-VD	93.3 ± 1.6
	residual 2-VD	93.4 ± 3.7
Hypokinetic segments	complete	96.1 ± 1.0
	residual 1-VD	90.6 ± 1.9
	residual 2-VD	89.3 ± 5.1
Akinetic segments	complete	91.2 ± 2.4
	residual 1-VD	85.6 ± 2.6
	residual 2-VD	76.1 ± 8.1

VD, vessel disease

Table 3. Influence of ventricular function on actuarial 5-year survival for subgroups with different degrees of revascularization

Degree of revascularization	Ventricular function	Mean 5-year survival ± SE (%)
Complete	normal	96.5 ± 0.9
	hypokinetic segments	96.1 ± 1.0
	akinetic segments	91.2 ± 2.4
Residual 1-VD	normal	93.3 ± 1.6
	hypokinetic segments	90.6 ± 1.9
	akinetic segments	85.6 ± 2.6
Residual 2-VD	normal	93.4 ± 3.7
	hypokinetic segments	89.3 ± 5.1
	akinetic segments	76.1 ± 8.1

VD, vessel disease

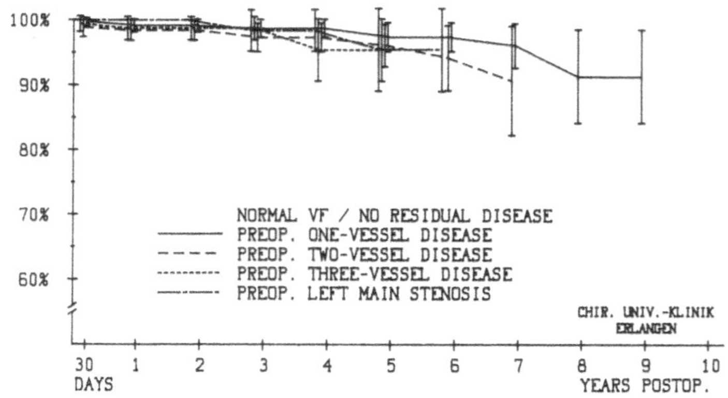

Fig. 3. Survival in patients with normal ventricular function and complete revascularization vs number of preoperatively obstructed coronary arteries

While there is no significant difference in survival when only patients with normal ventricular function are considered, there exists a significant difference in survival when patients with either hypokinetic or akinetic segments and various degrees of revascularization are compared.

The influence of ventricular function on survival, irrespective of the degree of revascularization, is already significant in the subgroup of patients with complete revascularization. This becomes even more obvious when patients with residual one- and two-vessel disease are taken for comparison (Table 3).

In summary, there is not only an independent influence of ventricular function and degree of revascularization on late survival after coronary artery bypass surgery, but the two parameters seem to potentiate each other in their effect. The worse the prognosis is, based on impaired ventricular function alone, the more obvious is the effect of the degree of revascularization on survival, and vice versa.

If we combine the best of both parameters, normal ventricular function and complete revascularization, which happens to be the case in one-third of our patients, we find a 9-year survival of 90.5%, irrespective of the number of preoperatively stenosed vessels (Fig. 3). This has not been achieved with six, seven or eight grafts per patient, including grafts to all possible secondary branches, but by concentrating on major vessels and supplying these with two to four grafts on the average. This policy makes it possible to start with an early mortality of 0.6%, thus not compromising the prognosis of surgically treated patients from the very beginning.

References

1. Bruschke AVG, Proudfit WL, Sones FM Jr (1973) Progress study of 590 consecutive non-surgical cases of coronary disease followed 5–9 years. Circulation 47: 1147
2. Bruschke AVG, Proudfit WL, Sones FM Jr (1973) Progress study of 590 consecutive non-surgical cases of coronary disease followed 5–9 years. Circulation 47: 1154
3. Burggraf GW, Parker JO (1975) Prognosis in coronary artery disease. Angiographic, hemodynamic, and clinical factors. Circulation 51: 146
4. Grunkemeier GL, Starr A (1977) Actuarial analysis of surgical results: rationale and method. Ann Thorac Surg 24: 404

5. Hacker RW, Torka M, Von der Emde J (1982) Revaskularisation des Myokards durch aorto-koronaren Bypass. Dtsch Ärztebl 79: 47/23
6. Harris PJ, Harrell FE Jr, Lee KL, Behar VS, Rosati RA (1979) Survival in medically treated coronary artery disease. Circulation 60: 1259
7. Lawrie GM, Morris GC, Silvers A, Wagner WF, Baron AE, Beltangady SS, Glaeser DH, Chapman DW (1982) The influence of residual disease after coronary bypass on the 5-year survival rate of 1274 men with coronary artery disease. Circulation 66: 717
8. Proudfit WL, Bruschke AVG, Sones FM Jr (1978) Natural history of obstructive coronary artery disease: ten-year study of 601 nonsurgical cases. Prog Cardiovasc Dis 21: 53
9. Steinbrunn W, Lichtlen PR (1977) Complete 5-year cumulative survival rates in 244 unselected, unoperated coronary patients undergoing angiography. Circulation 55/56: III-174

Survival in 1041 Patients with Consecutive Aortocoronary Bypass Operations

K. Laird-Meeter, M. M. P. Haalebos, R. v. Domburg, J. Lubsen, E. Bos, and P. G. Hugenholtz

Introduction

Aortocoronary bypass surgery performed to alleviate angina pectoris has proven to be an effective therapy [1, 2]. However, it soon became clear that operative mortality and late mortality varied considerably between institutions [3–5] and therefore influenced late results. This study was undertaken to assess both short- and long-term survival at our own institution. Also, we attempted via multivariate analysis to identify variables which might influence survival after bypass surgery.

Methods

All patients undergoing isolated aortocoronary bypass surgery between 1971 and June 1980 were studied. All suffered angina pectoris despite pharmacological therapy. A significant lesion in a major coronary artery was present when a luminal narrowing of ≥50% was seen. Ejection fraction (EF) was calculated by the area-length method adjusted for single plane view [6, 7].

Clinical characteristics of the series are presented in Table 1. Follow-up varied from 1 to 10 years, with a mean of 3.5 years. Survival probabilities were determined with the Kaplan-Meier method [8]. To study variables which might influence survival a stepwise nonlinear algorithm of the Cox proportional hazards model was used [9]. The variables were: age at operation, sex, number of preoperatively diseased vessels, preoperative EF, and number of grafts.

Table 1. Clinical profile of patients in the study

	n	%
Number of patients	1041	
males	915	88
females	126	12
Age (mean ± SD)		
males	52.6 ± 7.7	
females	55.5 ± 8.2	
Vessels diseased		
1	192	19
2	320	31
3	444	42
left main	85	8
Ejection fraction		
≥0.55	600	58
0.31–0.55	248	24
≤0.30	27	2
unknown	166	16

Results

Of the 1041 patients, 64 (6.2%) died during the follow-up period. Of these, 12 died within 28 days (1.2% operative mortality). Late mortality was 5% (52/1041). The cause of late death was in 75% cardiac (39/52).

Survival probability is shown in Fig. 1. At 5 years it was estimated at 93.5% ± 2%, at 8 years at 89.9% ± 4%. The survival probability for an age- and sex-matched Dutch population would have been 94.6% and 90.1% respectively [10].

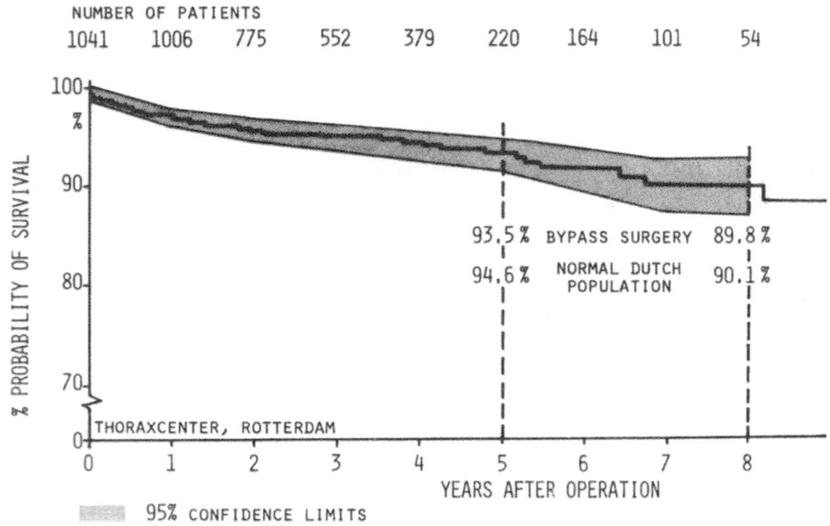

Fig. 1. The survival probability for the 1041 patients was estimated to be 93.5% at 5 years, 89.8% at 8 years. The *shaded area* is within the 95% confidence limits

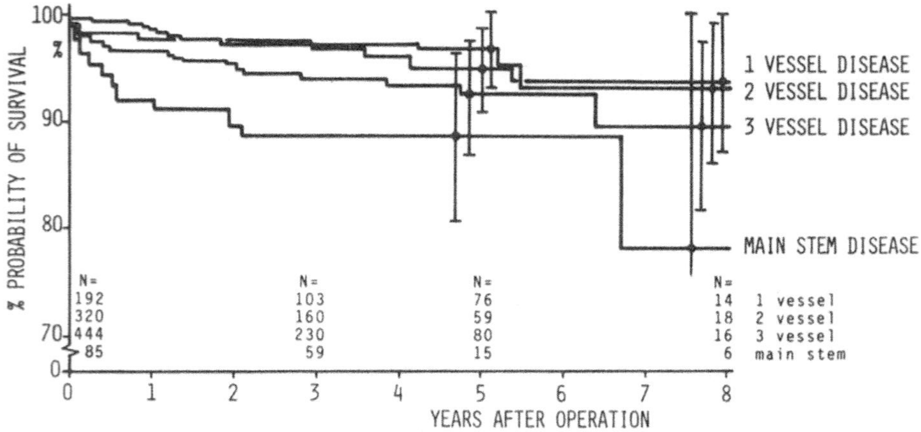

Fig. 2. The survival probability in relation to preoperative vascular disease. *N* denotes the number of patients in that group at that moment of follow-up. The *vertical bars* represent the 95% confidence limits

Survival probability analyzed according to preexisting vascular disease is shown in Fig. 2. At 5 years this was for patients with one-vessel disease 94% ± 4%, with two-vessel disease 96% ± 3%, with three-vessel disease 92% ± 4%, and with main stem disease 88% ± 6%. Preoperative EF had a more profound influence. For patients with a normal EF survival at 5 years was calculated to be 95% ± 2%, for those with a moderately impaired EF 92% ± 4% and with a poor EF 83% ± 17% (see Fig. 3).

Multivariate analysis was performed in 875 cases where all data were complete. In Table 2 is shown that, although age, female sex, and more extensive vascular disease carry an increased risk of dying, these differences are not statistically significant. Impaired EF however does influence survival significantly, expressed by a rate ratio of 2.9 in patients with a poor left ventricular function, versus 1 for those with a normal function.

Discussion

This study was not designed to prove that aortocoronary bypass surgery increases long-term survival in patients with significant coronary disease and angina pectoris. This would have required a concurrent comparable group of patients treated by pharmacological means only.

Several aspects of the results can however be used to compare with results reported in the literature. Let us consider, in turn, perioperative mortality and long-term survival for both the entire patient population and selected high-risk subsets.

Operative mortality was 1.2%, a result which compares favourably with those reported by other groups in the 1970s [3, 5].

An estimated survival probability of 90% at 8 years after surgery is the same as one would have expected for an age- and sex-matched Dutch population [10]. This is not as paradoxical as it seems. Califf et al [11] have shown that patients accepted

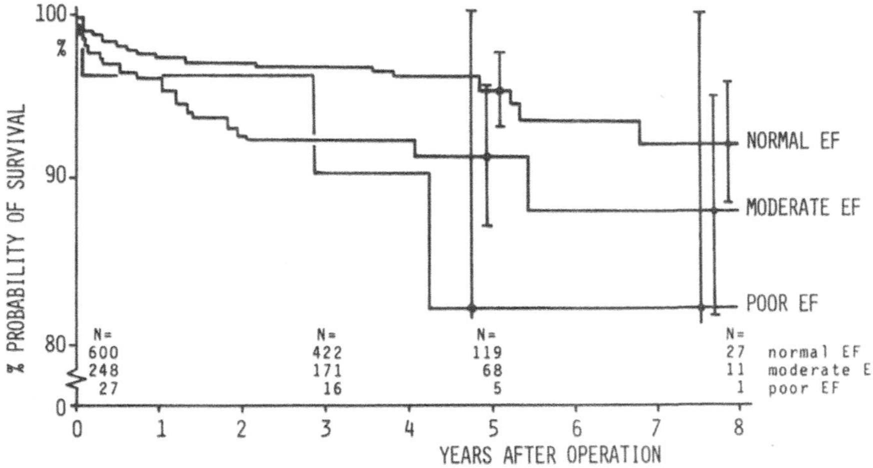

Fig. 3. The survival probability in relation to preoperative ejection fraction *(EF)*. *N* denotes the number of patients in that group at that moment of follow-up. The *vertical bars* represent the 95% confidence limits

Table 2. Rate ratios from Cox's regression analysis of survival ($n = 875$)[a]

Variable	n	Rate ratio	p
Age at operation			
< 50 yrs	321	1.0	
50–60 yrs	408	1.3	NS
> 60 yrs	146	1.7	
Sex			
female	99	1.0	Ns
male	776	0.6	
Vascular involvement			
1 vessel	161	1.0	
2 vessels	267	1.2	NS
3 vessels	374	1.9	
left main	73	2.7	
Ejection fraction			
⩾ 0.55	600	1.0	
0.31–0.55	248	1.7	0.05
⩽ 0.30	27	2.9	

/za The rate ratio is the incidence of mortality in one group divided by the incidence in the group with which the comparison is made

for coronary angiography have a better expected survival then their matched contemporaries of the general population after exclusion of expected deaths from ischemic heart disease.

It has been reported that the long-term prospects for patients with impaired left ventricular function is less good than if that function were normal [12, 13]. Neither we nor others [14] have been able to demonstrate that this fact is altered by bypass surgery.

It has also been shown that patients with left main stem disease or three-vessel disease form high-risk subsets [12, 13]. However, in our study, the survival probability in these groups was not significantly different from that of those with less extensive disease. This observation has been made by others as well [3, 5, 15]. Hence, surgery seems to reduce the dependence of the survival probability on vascular involvement. Since more than half of the patient population under study belonged to the group with higher risk, we regard this as a gratifying result of aortocoronary bypass surgery.

Summary

To assess their survival we followed for up to 10 years 1041 patients with consecutive isolated bypass operations. Surgery was performed at the same institution between 1971 and 1980. The mean follow-up time was 3.5 years. Cumulative survival was at 28 days 98.8%, at 5 years 94% ± 2% and at 8 years 90% ± 4% (95% confidence limits). For the general Dutch population matched for age and sex, this would have been 94.6% and 90.0% at 5 and 8 years respectively.

Multivariate survival analysis with the proportional hazards model did not show a significant relationship between mortality and sex or age at operation. There was a trend to higher mortality with more extensive vascular disease, however, this was not significant (rate ratio of three-vessel versus one-vessel disease 1.9, $p > 0.05$). Lowered left ventricular ejection fraction (EF) did show an association with higher death rate (rate ratio EF $\leqslant 0.30$ versus EF $\geqslant 0.55$ of 2.9, $p < 0.05$).

References

1. Hurst JW, King SB, Logue BR et al. (1978) Value of coronary bypass surgery. Controversies in cardiology part 1. Am J Cardiol 42: 308–329
2. McIntosh HD (1982) Aorto-coronary bypass grafting: an internist's perspective. Circulation 65 (Suppl 2): 77–81
3. Kirklin JW, Kouchoukos NT, Blackstone EH, Oberman A (1979) Research related to surgical treatment of coronary artery disease. Circulation 60: 1613–1618
4. Kennedy JW, Kaiser GC, Fisher LD et al. (1981) Clinical and angiographic predictors of operative mortality from the collaborative study in coronary artery surgery (CASS). Circulation 63: 793–802
5. Detre K, Peduzzi P, Murphy M et al. (1981) Effect of bypass surgery on survival in patients in low- and high-risk subgroups delineated by the use of simple clinical variables. Circulation 63: 1329–1338
6. Dodge HT, Sandler H, Baxley WA, Hawley RR (1966) Usefulness and limitations of radiographic methods for determining left ventricular volume. Am J Cardiol 18: 10–24
7. Heintzen PH, Brennecke R, Bursch JH et al. (1975) Automated video-angiocardiographic image analysis. Computer 6: 55–64
8. Kaplan EL, Meier P (1958) Nonparametric estimation from incomplete observation. J Am State Assoc 53: 457–481
9. Cox DR (1972) Regression models and life tables. J R Statist Soc (London) 34: 187–220
10. Centraal bureau voor statistiek. 's Gravenhage (1982) Maandstatistiek van de Bevolking 30: 43–44
11. Califf RM, Lee KL, Haarrell FE, Kimm SYS, Grufferman S, Rosati RA (1982) Assessment of the use of the age- and sex-specific United States population as a control group for analysis of survival in coronary artery disease. Am J Cardiol 50: 1279–1282
12. Burggraf GW, Parker JO (1981) Prognosis in coronary artery disease, angiographic, hemodynamic and clinical factors. Circulation 51: 146–156
13. Mock MB, Ringquist I, Fisher LD et al. (1982) Survival of medically treated patients in the coronary artery surgery study (CASS) registry. Circulation 66: 562–568
14. Lawrie GM, Morries GC (1982) Survival after coronary bypass surgery in specific patient groups. Circulation 65 (Suppl 2): 43–48
15. Mathur VS, Hall RJ, Garcia E, Castro CM, Cooley DA (1980) Prolonging life with coronary bypass surgery in patients with three-vessel disease. Circulation 62: 90–97

Long-Term Follow-up of Reoperation After Coronary Bypass Surgery

R. A. E. Dion, M. Feis, G. Jambroes, T. Gherli, and J. F. Hitchcock

Introduction

Coronary arteriosclerosis is a progressive disease, and angina has been reported to recur in patients postoperatively at rates of 3.5% to 7.2% per year [1, 2]. Several studies have demonstrated that coronary reoperation can be performed with an acceptable mortality rate and with good late clinical results [3–10]. In large series the rate of reoperation has been as high as 5% and appears to be increasing [3, 10].

Materials and Methods

Fifty-five (55) consecutive patients reoperated between September 1978 and July 1983 with a maximum follow-up (100%) of 5 years were analyzed. There were 46 males (84%) and 9 females (16%). The mean age at reoperation was 54.3 years (35–72 years), 15% of the patients were 45 years old or less. Twenty-eight patients (51%) had undergone their first operation at another institute. During the last year reoperations accounted for 5% of all coronary revascularizations.

At first operation a mean of 2.7 distal anastomoses per patient were performed, with a perioperative infarction rate of 9.1%. Nine patients (16%) developed postpericardiotomy syndrome: this was treated with salicylates (in one patient with corticoids). The symptom-free period ranged from 0 to 108 months, with a mean of 20 months and a median of 10 months. Thirty-five patients (64%) had recurrent symptoms within 12 months (Table 1): graft failure accounted for the majority of the recurrences, while disease progression was the cause of recurrence in 12 patients (34%). When the total group of patients is considered, progression of disease combined with other factors – graft failure or incomplete revascularization – accounted

Table 1. Cause of recurrent angina within 12 months after the first operation

	Symptom-free period (months)		
	⩽6	6–12	Total
Number of patients	26	9	35 (64%)
Cause of recurrence			
Incomplete revascularization	2	2	4
Graft failure	16	3	19[a]
Progressive disease	8 (31%)	4	12[b] (34%)

[a] Venous pathology, five patients; bad result Vineberg, one patient; bad result endarterectomy, two patients;

[b] Hyperlipidemia, six patients; hyperthyroidism, one patient; diabetes (insulin), three patients

for 60% of the recurrences. The interval between first and second operations ranged from 2 to 120 months, with a mean of 34 months and a median of 24 months. All patients were in NYHA class III or IV before reoperation, the majority had urgent reoperation for unstable angina (Fig. 1). Eighteen patients (32.7%) had poor left ventricular (LV) function, as defined by ejection fraction (EF) equal to or less than 40%, left ventricular end-diastolic pressure (LVEDP) equal to or higher than 25 mmHg, or diffuse hypokinesia with left ventricular dilatation.

At reoperation, resternotomy was used in all cases. Injuries of the innominate vein (one patient), of a previous graft (one patient), of the pulmonary artery (one patient) and of the right ventricle (one patient) could not be avoided when the pericardium had not been closed during the first operation. A dissection of the ascending aorta starting at the site of the previous cannulation was successfully managed in one patient by transsection and resuture of the ascending aorta. Cannulation of the ascending aorta was feasible in all cases. Moderate hypothermia (28°) and cold crystalloid cardioplegia were used systematically. The surgical procedures consisted of new venous grafts, patching of distal anastomoses, endarterectomies and interposition of new venous segments. Distal corrections per patient averaged 2.5. Aortic cross-clamp time averaged 63 min (11–135 min). In 4 cases the duration of cardiopulmonary bypass equalled or exceeded 180 min. The intraaortic balloon pump (IABP) had to be used in 6 patients (10.9%). The median discharge time after reoperation was 11 days.

Results

Perioperative myocardial infarction was diagnosed in 6 patients (11%). Five patients (9%) underwent resternotomy for postoperative bleeding. Inotropic agents were used in 13 patients (24%) and IABP in 7 patients (13%). Other major complications were mediastinitis (one patient), acute respiratory distress syndrome (ARDS) (one patient), acute liver failure with coma (one patient) and pulmonary embolus (one patient). The mean follow-up was 24 months (2–60 months).

There were three deaths (5.4%) within 30 days of reoperation, no late deaths. The three patients were 53, 54 and 60 years old; the intervals between first and second operation were respectively 51, 84, and 100 months. Progression of disease was the cause of recurrent angina in all. All three had been refused elsewhere for reoperation, were in NYHA class IV, and had unstable angina; one of them had an LVEDP

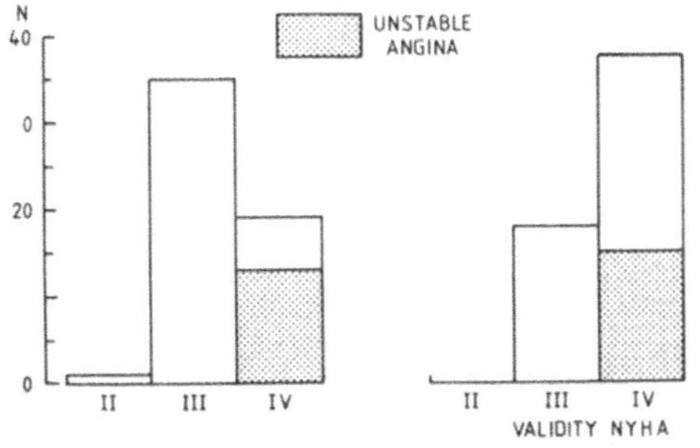

Fig. 1. Recurrent angina: NYHA class before first operation *(left)* and repeat operation *(right)*

greater than 30 mmHg, and one had moderate mitral regurgitation. Two of them died on day 3 and day 8 postoperatively from complications of myocardial infarction. One died despite technically satisfactory double saphenous vein bypass grafts to the right coronary artery (RCA) and the marginal obtusus 2 (MO2). The other died after an unsatisfactory procedure: dissection of the ascending aorta occurred at the site of previous cannulation, two coronary vessels (left anterior descending, circumflex) were not found, and the two grafted coronary vessels (posterior descending, diagonal 2) had lumina barely 1 mm in diameter. The third patient died on the table after a technically successful triple bypass graft to the left anterior descending artery, MO2, and MO3: postmortem examination revealed patent grafts, no perioperative myocardial infarction, but extensive subendocardial fibrosis of the left ventricle.

Actuarial follow-up over 5 years showed that 50% of the patients remain symptom-free while 85% improve considerably (Fig. 2). There is no correlation between the symptom-free periods after the first and the second operation (Fig. 3).

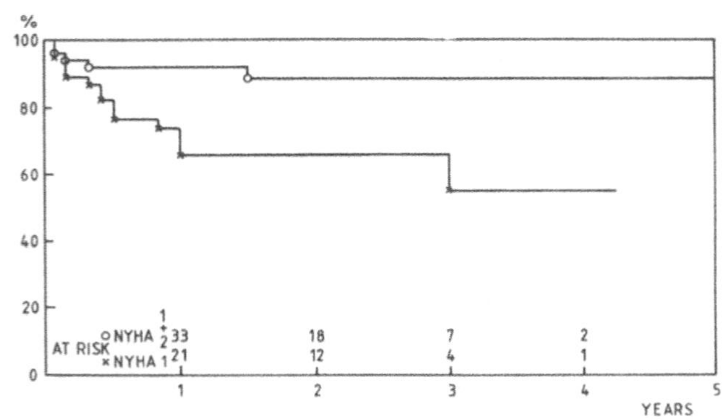

Fig. 2. Recurrent angina: actuarial curve of NYHA class after reoperation over 5 years

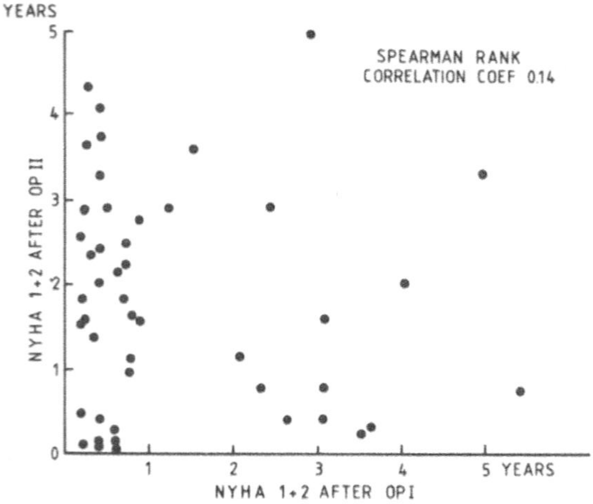

Fig. 3. Recurrent angina: improvement (NYHA classes I and II) after first operation vs reoperation

Discussion

Many studies have reported satisfactory early results from second revascularization procedures [3–11]. Operative mortality ranged from 0 to 12.5%, with the two largest series reporting hospital deaths in 4.0% and 4.8% of patients [3, 4]. Morbidity of repeat coronary operations appears to be higher than that of first operations. In our series, perioperative myocardial infarction was noted in 11% of patients. Other reports demonstrate that the rate of perioperative myocardial infarction is higher in patients undergoing reoperation [3, 5–7, 9–11]. The reoperation group demonstrated a higher frequency of perioperative myocardial infarction at their first operation (9.1%) that the group with a single operation. This has also been found by others [6].

Technical aspects of repeat operations have been discussed by Loop and colleagues [3]. We strongly recommend closure of the pericardium at the first operation to decrease the incidence of injuries at resternotomy. As can be deduced from our fatalities, our indications for reoperation are quite aggressive; but what are the life expectancy and quality of life of a patient with class IV angina pectoris and impending infarction who cannot be helped by medical treatment?

At times preoperative angiography gives only a poor idea of the graftability of a coronary vessel: for instance, in cases of total obstruction and collateral filling we would give the candidates for reoperation with unstable angina the benefit of the doubt. One of our deaths may be attributed to this policy: two vessels were not found, and the two others were hardly graftable, but other patients with similar preoperative findings who were refused elsewhere have been improved. A relationship between the symptom-free period after the first operation and the cause of recurrent angina has been discussed previously [1–11]. As did Culliford and colleagues [11] we noted that more than a third of the recurrences within a year are due to progression of disease. Unlike Schaff and colleagues [10] we have seen preoperatively that graft failure was regularly caused by new occlusive disease distal to the bypass graft.

The quality of survival for patients after reoperation in our series is comparable to that described in larger series, as 85% of the surviving patients remain in NYHA class I or II after 5 years.

Conclusions

Reoperation for recurrent angina has a higher mortality and morbidity than first operation. Of the survivors, 85% are still considerably improved after 5 years. Early recurrence of angina following first operation does not preclude successful reoperation.

We are still unable to predict the result of a reoperation by using preoperative parameters such as progression of disease and probable cause of failure of primary revascularization.

Indication for reoperation in those patients with unstable angina should be at least as aggressive as for a primary revascularization.

References

1. Cameron A, Kemp HG Jr, Shimomura S, Santilli E, Green GE, Hutchinson JE III, Mekhjian HA (1979) Aortocoronary bypass surgery, a 7 year follow-up. Circulation 60 (Suppl 1): 9–13
2. Campeau L, Lesperance J, Hermann J, Corbara F, Grondin CM, Bourassa MG (1979) Loss of improvement of angina between 1 and 7 years after aortocoronary bypass surgery. Correlations with changes in vein grafts and in coronary arteries. Circulation 60 (Suppl 1): 1–5
3. Loop FD, Cosgrove DM, Kramer JR, Lytle BW, Taylor PC, Golding LAR, Groves LK (1981) Late clinical and arteriographic results in 500 coronary artery reoperations. J Thorac Cardiovasc Surg 81: 675–685
4. Reul GJ Jr, Cooley DA, Ott DA, Coelho A, Chapa L, Eterovic I (1979) Reoperation for recurrent coronary artery disease, causes, indications, and results in 168 patients. Arch Surg 114: 1269–1275
5. Allen RH, Stinson EB, Oyer PE, Shumway NE (1978) Prediction variables in reoperation for coronary artery disease. J Thorac Cardiovasc Surg 75: 186–192
6. Krause AH, Scott Page V, Bigelow JC, Okies JE, Duncap SF (1978) Reoperations in symptomatic patients after direct coronary artery revascularization. J Thorac Cardiovasc 75: 499–504
7. Brooks N, Honey M, Cattell M, Wright JEC, Sturridge HF, Balcon R, Layton C (1979) Reoperation for recurrent angina. Br Heart J 42: 333–338
8. Qazi A, Garcia JM, Mispiretta LA, Corso PJ (1981) Reoperation for coronary artery disease. Ann Thorac Surg 32: 16–18
9. Gandjbakhch I, Pavie A, Cabrol C, Bachet J, Mussat T, Goudot B, Guilmet D (1982) Chirurgie coronarienne itérative techniques et indications. Ann Chir 36: 607–609
10. Schaff HV, Orszulak TA, Gersh BJ, Piehler JH, Puga FJ, Danielson GK, Pluth JR (1983) The morbidity and mortality of reoperation for coronary artery disease and analysis of late results with use of actuarial estimate of event free interval. J Thorac Cardiovasc 85: 508–515
11. Culliford AT, Girdwood RW, Isom OW, Krauss KR, Spencer FC (1979) Angina following myocardial revascularization. Does time of recurrence predict etiology and influence results of operation? J Thorac Cardiovasc Surg 77: 889–895

Long-Term Results After Early Revascularization for Impending Infarction

F. Vermeulen, O. Alfieri, J. Defauw, J. Ernst, R. De Geest, P. Knaepen, A. Schaepkens van Riempst, A. Schreuders

From February 1971 to January 1975, 732 patients underwent coronary artery surgery at our institution. Of these, 135 patients underwent urgent revascularization for an impending first, impending recurrent, or extending infarction. The early results after 7.5 years full follow-up are reviewed in regard to mortality, infarction rate, and recurrence of angina. The patient characteristics and early results are compared to the patient data of our recent surgical experience in 59 urgent revascularizations out of 887 patients operated upon in 1981, in order to analyze the applicability of the conclusions of our study to patient management nowadays.

Definitions

Patients with impending first myocardial infarction (II) were defined as patients with unstable angina with transient ECG changes at rest (some including transient QS patterns), normal enzyme levels, and documented significant coronary artery stenosis of 70% or more in at least one coronary artery.

The onset of these episodes had to be documented less than 1 week before the operation, the patient being operated upon for these unstable symptoms as soon as admitted to our hospital, many on weekends or at night. Patients with impending recurring myocardial infarction (IRI) presented the same clinical characteristics with the clinical history or electrocardiographic evidence of a previous myocardial infarction. Patients with extension of myocardial infarction (IEI) were defined as patients with the same clinical characteristics during recovery from an acute myocardial infarction.

Patients and Methods

The study group with late follow-up consisted of 135 patients (out of 732 coronary artery operations performed between February 1971 and January 1975) presenting with either an II, IRI or IEI.

The composition and patient characteristics of this follow-up group were compared to a sample of 887 coronary operations performed in 1981, of whom 59 patients presented the same indications for urgent operation. Differences in composition between study groups were analyzed and mortality and morbidity compared; the initial study population was followed by at least yearly controls at our outpatient clinic and reviewed after 7.5 years of follow-up in all patients. The follow-up beyond 7.5 years in the earlier group was not included as this could afford only an additional actuarial analysis. The late mortality, infarction rates, and recurrence rates for angina were analyzed.

Results

The compositions of the two populations studied did not present significant differences in regard to the male/female ratio; the early series contained 18 females and 117 males, the 1981 series 7 females, and 52 males. However, the composition in regard to admission diagnosis was significantly different, as less than 20% (24/135) of the early group were patients with impending IRI or IEI as opposed to almost 50% (29/59) of the 1981 group. This is explainable by the introduction of percutaneous transluminal coronary angioplasty (PTCA) in 1981 as the alternative treatment of

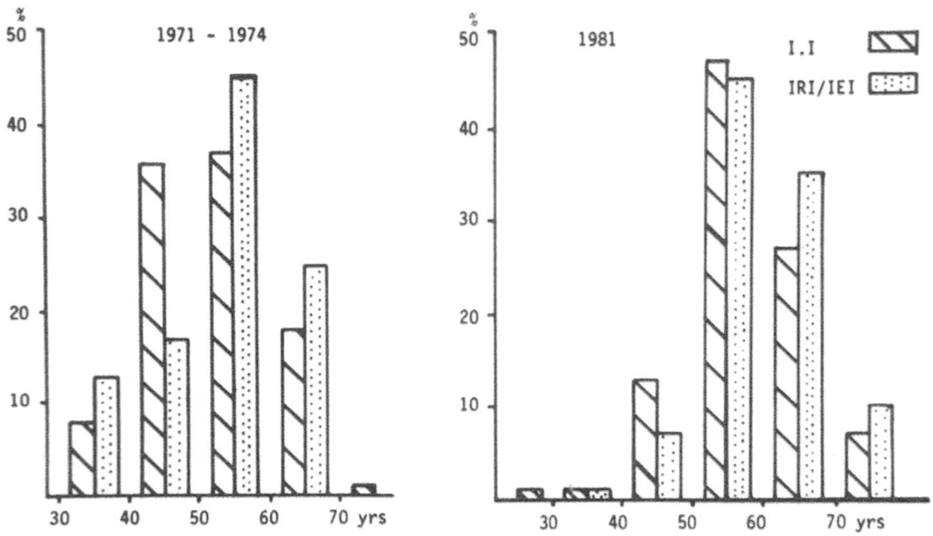

Fig. 1. Age distribution of both study groups: the *vertical bars* indicate precentages of patients

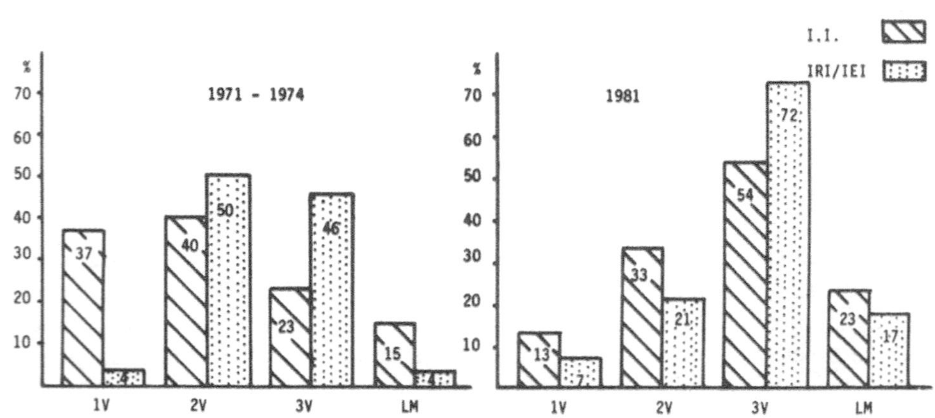

Fig. 2. Distribution of the severity of the coronary artery disease (CAD) in both study groups graded as one-vessel *(1 V)*, two-vessel *(2 V)*, or three-vessel *(3 V)* disease; patients with left main stem lesion *(LM)* are included in the 2 V or 3 V percentages. The *vertical bars* indicate percentages of patients

choice in patients with II, IRI, or IEI presenting with single vessel disease, as well as with double vessel disease in selected cases. The improved medical treatment in recent years may have influenced patient selection as well. Other differences in composition of the two population studies are evident from the age distribution and distribution of the severity of the coronary artery lesions as represented in Figs. 1 and 2. In recent years the average age of the patient population is approximately a decade higher. Fifty-four percent of the patients with II and 72% of those with IRI or IEI present with three-vessel disease including an appreciable number of patients (ca. 20%) with left main stem disease. The average number of distal anastomoses was 1.9 per patient in the early series and 4.1 per patient in 1981.

The hospital mortality for II was 1.8% (2/111) in the initial series as compared to 3.3% (1/30) in 1981, and was 0% (0/24) for IRI and IEI as compared to 3.4% (1/29) in 1981; these apparent increases in mortality should be viewed in light of the more extensive disease, higher age, etc. Of the two patients who died in 1981, the one with an IRI was over age 80, the other had to be resuscitated before the operation.

The early myocardial infarction rate was similar in both groups: 4.5% (5/111) as compared to 0% (0/30) for II, 4.2% (1/24) as compared to 6.8% (2/29) in the IRI/IEI group.

The initial series of 133 patients surviving the operation followed throughout the full 7.5 year period presented 15 dropouts: nine noncardiac deaths at a mean of 61 months follow-up, and four cardiac deaths, two in the II group at 15 months fol-

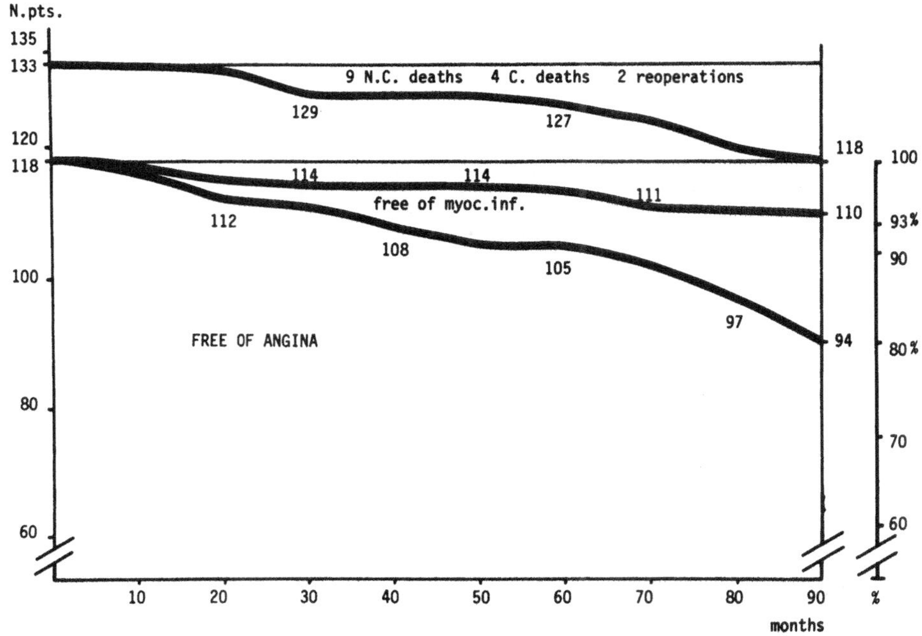

Fig. 3. Ninety-month (7.5-year) survival curve for 133 hospital survivors with an impending first or recurring infarction or an impending extension of infarction in the period 1971–1975, including two dropouts for reoperation *(upper curve)*. The *lower curve* represents the time of recurrence of myocardial infarction and angina in the 118 patients followed up for 7.5 years. *N. C.*, noncardiac; *C.*, cardiac

low-up and two in the IRI/IEI group at 42 months follow-up (Fig. 3). Two coronary reoperations for recurrent angina after 6 years of follow-up had to be performed. There were 118 patients followed throughout the 7.5 years. A total of eight myocardial infarctions recurred during the follow-up in the II group, giving a less than 2%/patient year infarction rate, including the five operative myocardial infarctions and the two probable myocardial infarctions in the cardiac deaths.

In the IRI/IEI group the late infarction rate during the follow-up was higher (4/24), including the operative myocardial infarction and two late cardiac deaths, this leads to a less than 4%/patient year myocardial reinfarction rate (7/24 or 28%/7.5 years).

The recurrence rate for angina was almost identical in the II and IRI groups (respectively 21% and 19%), although occurring earlier in the IRI group. The total group presents recurrence of angina in less than 20% of the patients at 7.5 years, or a recurrence rate of less than 3%/patient year.

Discussion

Our long-term results for urgent surgery in patients with II, IRI, or IEI have been very gratifying, with low hospital mortality and excellent long-term results in regard to late mortality, late myocardial infarction rate, or recurrence of angina.

These results should be compared to those available in different natural history studies documented with coronary angiography or with the medical candidates of randomized studies with and without surgery [1, 3, 4, 6, 8–10]. The medically treated patients in these studies showed an early mortality of approximately 3% [1, 8–10] and, exceptionally, higher rates in specific subgroups (12% for De Zwaan [11]). However, the late mortality varied according to the follow-up period and the potential medical to surgical cross-overs in studies randomized to the intention of treatment: Favaloro presents a total of 50% mortality at 4.5 years in a truly randomized study [3]; an NHLBI study give a 7% mortality in the follow-up at 2.5 years; a nonrandomized Veterans Administration study by Hultgren [6], 17% at 5 years. Gerstenblith [4] demonstrated with a recent randomized study on modern medical treatment that mortality in ideally treated patients was still 1.5% within 4 months.

With medical treatment the infarction rates appeared to be high initially (7.7% [1], 8%–10% [8–10], and 7% [6]) and high as well during the follow-up: 11% after 2.5 years [8–10], 17% after 5 years [6], 15.5% at 4 months [4].

The dominant impression is that with medical treatment an extremely high number of patients fail to become angina-free at the follow-up; the angina-free percentage varies from 20% [3] or 37% [6] at 5 years to 56% at 4 months [4]. Most of these medical studies are quite comparable to our patients of the 1971–1975 study group and include as well 7%–13% of patients with significant left main stem lesions.

In contrast to the medically treated groups, all the surgical series [3, 5–7] except one [8–10] showed a markedly lower late myocardial infarction and mortality rate. Late myocardial infarction varied from 3.3% at 3.5 years [5] to 9% at 5 years [6].

Late mortality ranged from 4.5% at 3.5 years [5], 8% at 5 years [6], and 10.7% at 4.5 years [3] to 17% ± 2% at 10 years [7].

Most series present an angina-free incidence in the range of 67% at 5 years [7], or 78% at 3.5 years [5], up to 60% at 10 years [7]. The only marked difference with our surgical experience results from the high perioperative infarction rates in the literature (13% [6] and 18% [5]) as compared to our data, although most series contain similar percentages of left main stem lesions (approximately 12%–14%), and refer to the operative experience in the time before cardioplegic myocardial preservation became a routine.

Conclusion

The urgent surgical treatment of patients with unstable angina at rest, presenting with fluctuating ST-T changes or Q waves and significant lesions at coronary angiography, with or without a previous myocardial infarction, gives excellent short- and long-term results regarding mortality, myocardial infarction rates, and recurrence or persistence of angina.

References

1. Alison HW, Russell RO Jr, Mantle JA, Kouchoukos NT, Moraski RE, Rackley CE (1978) Coronary anatomy and arteriography in patients with unstable angina pectoris. Am J Cardiol 41: 204–209
2. Ernst JMPG, Van Bemmel F, Van Mechelen R, Vermeulen FEE (1976) Late results of acute coronary surgery in patients with impending infarction. In: Stalpaert G, Suy R, Vermeulen F (eds). Late results of valvular replacement and coronary surgery. European Press, Ghent, Belgium, pp 130–134
3. Favaloro RG (1979) Direct myocardial revascularization: a ten year journey. Am J Cardiol 43: 109–130
4. Gerstenblith G, Ouyang P, Achuff SC, Bulkley BH, Becker LC, Mellits ED, Baughman KL, Weiss JL, Flaherty JT, Kallman CH, Llewellyn M, Weisfeldt ML (1982) Nifedipine in unstable angina: a double-blind, randomized trial. N Engl J Med 306: 885–889
5. Golding LAR, Loop FD, Sheldon WC, Taylor PC, Groves LK, Cosgrove DM (1978) Emergency revascularization for unstable angina. Circulation 58: 1163–1166
6. Hultgren HN, Shettigar UP, Miller DC (1982) Medical versus surgical treatment of unstable angina. Am J Cardiol 50: 663–670
7. Rahimtoola S, Nunley D, Grunkemeier G, Tepley J, Lambert L, Starr A (1983) Ten-year survival after coronary bypass surgery for unstable angina. N Engl J Med 308: 676–681
8. Russell RO, Resnekov L, Wolk M, Rosati R, Conti CR, Hutter AM, Hodges M, Schroeder J, Willman V, Kaplan E (1976) Unstable angina pectoris: National Cooperative Study Group to compare medical and surgical therapy. I. Report of protocol and patient population. Am J Cardiol 37: 896–902
9. Russell RO, Resnekov L, Wolk M, Rosati RA, Conti CR, Becker LC, Hutter AM, Biddle TL, Schroeder J, Kaplan EM, Frommer PL (1978) Unstable angina pectoris: National Cooperative Study Group to compare surgical and medical therapy. II. In-hospital experience and initial follow-up results in patients with one, two and three vessel disease. Am J Cardiol 42: 839–848
10. Russell RO, Resnekov L, Wolk M, Rosati RA, Conti CR, Hutter AM, Biddle TL, Schroeder J, Frommer PL (1980) Unstable angina pectoris: National Cooperative Study Group to compare surgical and medical therapy. III. Results in patients with S-T segment elevation during pain. Am J Cardiol 45: 819–824
11. De Zwaan C, Bär F, Wellens HJJ (1982) Characteristic electrocardiographic pattern indicating a critical stenosis high in left anterior descending coronary artery in patients admitted because of impending myocardial infarction. Am Heart J 103: 730–736

Imaging of Coronary Grafts Without Catheterization of Coronary Ostia

D. Birnbaum and D. Banzer

Selective angiography of the coronary arteries is the standard method of visualizing radiologically not only the heart vessels, but also bypass grafts. The invasive nature of this procedure, however, limits its application [1, 2].

This study deals with a new technique for radiographic angiography which compared to the conventional method is easy to apply and bears less risk of harm as it avoids selective intubation of the ostia of the vessels by means of direct contrast medium injection.

By means of digital subtraction angiography (DSA) of coronary bypasses, questions can be answered which are of interest from the surgeon's viewpoint:

1. Bypass patency rate can be evaluated.
2. Indications of suspected bypass obstruction postoperatively can be assessed, with a prospect of immediate intervention.

Methods

The principle of the DSA technique is based on photomechanical elimination of image elements which interfere and are of no interest. Since the introduction of the photosubtraction technique in 1935 [3] it has often been felt that electronic imaging with subtraction could do a far better job. The availability of high performance analog-to-digital converters and digital memory chips at acceptable prices made this technique practical for clinical use [4].

The digital image-processing equipment is shown schematically in Fig. 1.

The exposures were obtained using the Angiotron/Angioscope X-ray system (Siemens Corp.).

A 50 frames/s so-called continuous mode video signal sequence is stored on a video tape in analog form. The mask mode technique and the time interval differ-

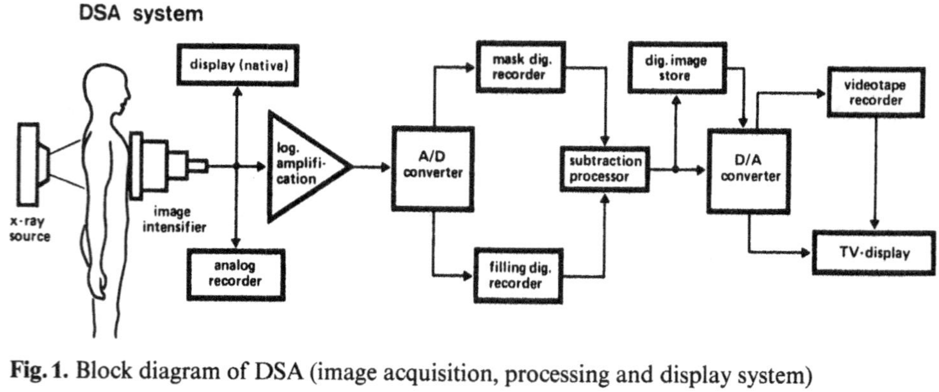

Fig. 1. Block diagram of DSA (image acquisition, processing and display system)

ence (TID) technique are used alternatively for optimal noise suppression. The TID mode is relatively insensitive to movements of the patient or the heart wall. A typical sequence utilized 60–80 KV and 10–20 mAs per frame. The interpretation of the examination is performed with a 44-cm TV monitor; for documentation a system-linked, automatic, 100-mm film-plate alternator is used.

DSA enables imaging of coronary bypass grafts by venous as well as by arterial contrast medium injection. The bypass visualization by venous injection – the indirect technique – simply requires a venous catheter (e.g., size F 5). Contrast media (30 ml; Urografin, Schering Corp.), equivalent to 350 mg iodine per ml, is injected at a flow rate of 16–18 ml/s. The direct DSA technique requires an aortic root catheter (F 5 pigtail) and an average of 20 ml dye (equivalent to 250 mg I/ml).

The venous technique was used in 26 patients, the arterial technique in 10 patients, for identification of aortocoronary bypasses 4 days to 6 months after the operation. The average time was 21 days postoperatively.

All grafts displayed by video sequence images were estimated in particular for the anastomosis-related segments, proximally and peripherally and for the course of the bypass in relation to intraoperatively obtained photographs or outlines.

Results

Figure 2 shows an example, from a patient with two bypasses, obtained by use of the venous technique. One should bear in mind that one normally looks at a video sequence recording, while this example shows only a single frame which was chosen out of the sequence. Figure 3 is an example of a triple graft implantation with an aortic root catheter in place. Since DSA is motion dependent, one must be careful to avoid misinterpretation due to double contours from heavy mobile structures such as the heart margin. Changing the plane and perhaps using the TID technique leads to a faultless RCA bypass image.

Figure 4 depicts a series of four different cases in which all implanted grafts were identified.

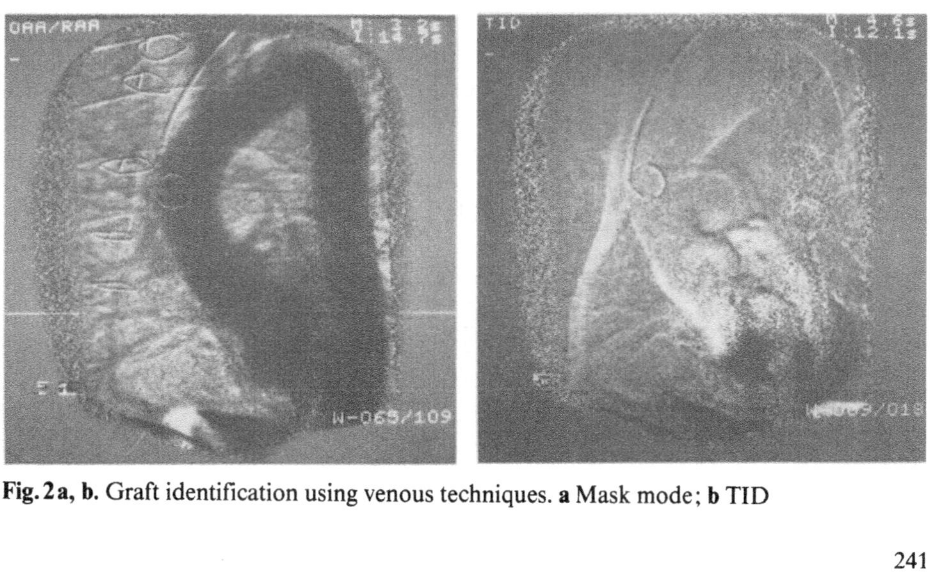

Fig. 2 a, b. Graft identification using venous techniques. **a** Mask mode; **b** TID

In Table 1 are listed the numbers of grafts identified by venous or arterial technique. Using venous DSA, only 57 of 73 bypasses could be recognized by their proximal segments, and in only 10% of all could peripheral anastomosis function whether fully open, stenosed, or obstructed be determined.

For this reason venous DSA did not meet our expectations and we abandoned this technique in favor of the arterial method, which was used for the remaining pat-

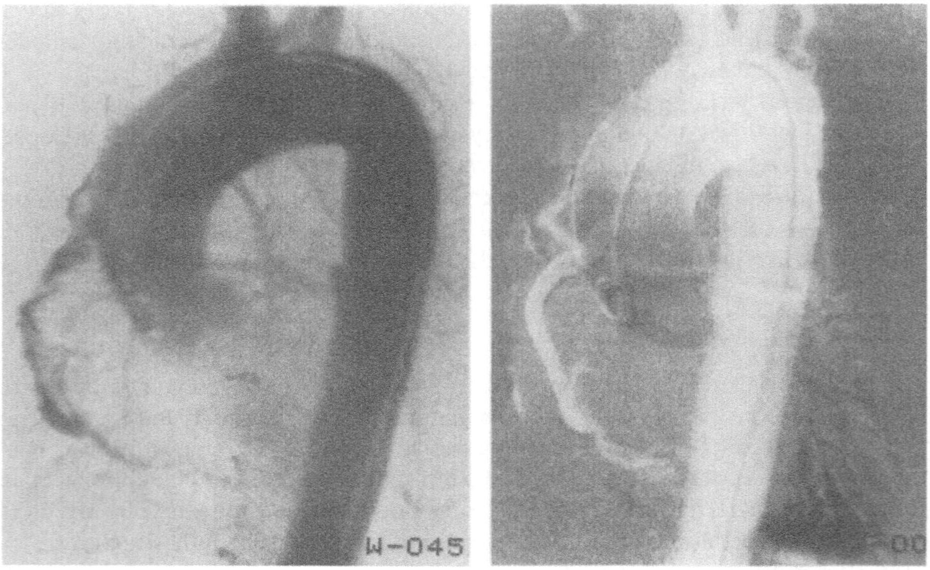

Fig. 3 a, b. Visualization of three bypasses by arterial dye injection. **a** Mask mode; **b** TID

Table 1. Grafts identified by venous or arterial technique

Grafts implanted		Grafts identified		
		Prox. segment	Course	Periph. segment
Venous DSA ($n=26$)				
ACVB	73	57	37	8
RCA	22	20	18	4
LAD	23	15	4	0
DIAG/ MARG	7	7	0	0
CX	21	15	15	4
Arterial DSA ($n=10$)				
ACVB	31	28	27	18
RCA	10	9	9	5
LAD	10	9	9	7
DIAG	2	2	2	1
MARG	7	6	6	4
CX	2	2	1	1

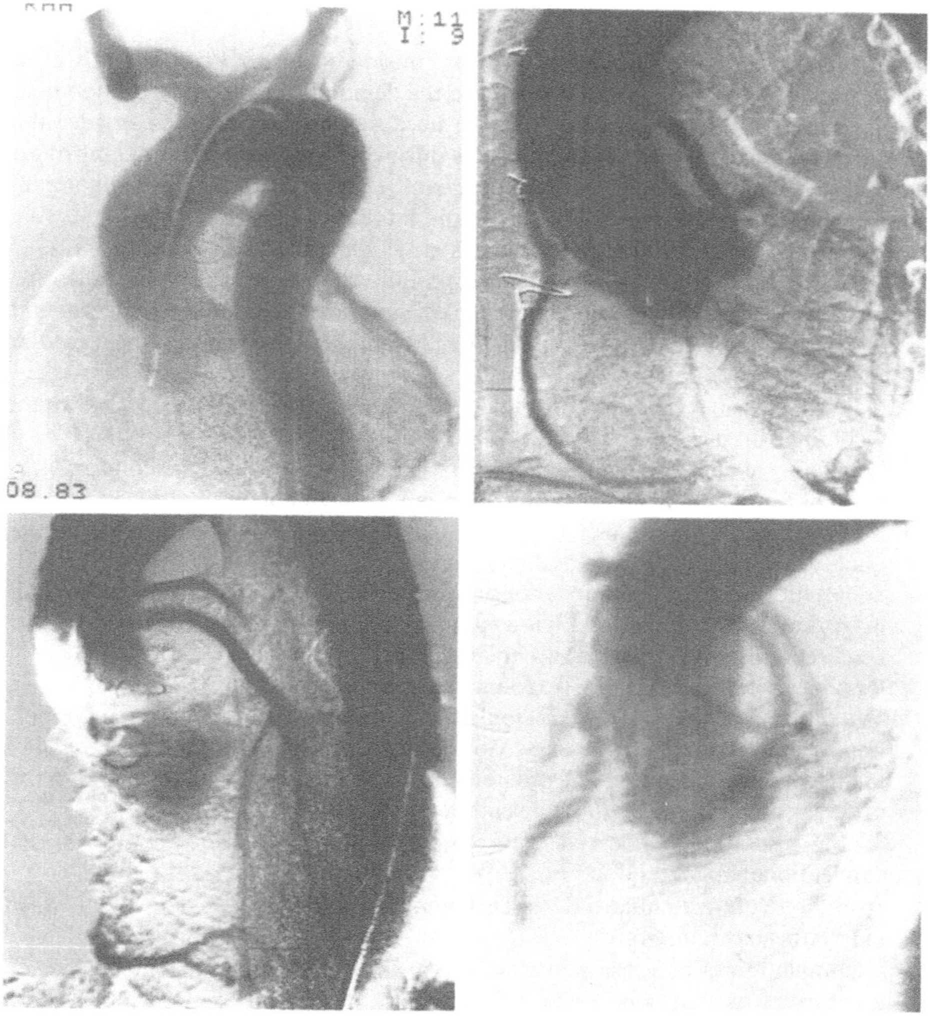

Fig. 4 a–d. Examples of images of one to four aortocoronary bypasses in four different cases

ients. Of 31 grafts, 28 could be identified (Table 1), and in more than half of the cases the peripheral anastomoses could be estimated well qualitatively.

Grafts to the right coronary artery or left circumflex artery were best visualized in their full course, while grafts to the left anterior descending artery or its lateral branches were better identified in an extracordial portion. Special notes of the surgeon as to caliber, size, or unusual lining could also be taken into account when analyzing the video-sequence recording. Interestingly, the poorest contrast was seen in eight patients with an EF < 0.35.

Discussion

At its introduction the DSA technique was considered a most favorable way of imaging the bare coronary arteries. However, the demands on spatial resolution in imaging these vessels are highly stringent, because coronary arteries smaller than 1 mm in diameter move at up to 17.5 cm/s during the cardiac cycle. Imaging of aortocoronary bypass grafts is less of a problem because of their larger diameter and because they are not subjected to such rapid motion.

Our results in identifying bypass grafts are comparable with those of Drury [5], despite the fact that direct coronary angiography could not possibly be performed in our group. Besides the particular benefit of simplicity, without the requirement of specific skills, the DSA technique has other advantages over conventional angiography:

1. It is less invasive (possible in outpatients, small-bore catheter used for arterial technique, no hazards to coronary ostia).
2. Low doses of contrast media are used (1:10; low flow, no "heat discomfort" from hyperosmotic effects, examination abundantly repeatable).
3. Real time display minimizes the period of catheterization, and better fluoroscopic quality is obtained because of digitalization.
4. Subtraction and logarithmic amplification result in elimination of shadows and overlying structures, and in high-contrast resolution.
5. Data recording is simple and archiving handy.

Possible limitations of DSA we found were:

1. The subject must be virtually motionless for subtraction to be complete. Cooperation from the patient is necessary. Motion of the object might disappear when the plane is changed. It should be possible to handle this problem if the angiographic process could be triggered by the cardiac cycle (ECG).
2. Spatial resolution is poor (as with other fluoroscopic systems) compared with conventional angiographic film.
3. Overlying contrast-enhanced vessels (such as the pulmonary veins or the mammary artery) can interfere.
4. Accumulation of contrast media may be insufficient because of low flow due to low cardiac output, poor quality of grafts and anastomoses, and/or high peripheral vascular resistance.

Differential dye flow is not considered to be a disadvantage of the method, but rather an expression of hemodynamics. In conclusion, DSA can be used to prove vein grafts open and to evaluate patency and vein quality. The method is valid for judgement of surgical results and for postoperative survey. In estimation of morphological details, however, its usefulness is restricted. Though DSA systems cannot match angiographic film resolution, functional images such as contrast medium flow properties and quantitation of myocardial flow in regions of interest combined with regional analysis of wall motion may in the future give rise to quantitation of myocardial perfusion and produce prognostic data for bypass surgery by focussing on postprocessing procedures.

References

1. Sones FM, Shirey EK (1962) Cine coronary arteriography. Mod. Concepts Cardiovasc. Dis. 31: 735
2. Judkins MP (1967) Selective coronary arteriography, part I: A percutaneous transfemoral approach. Radiology 89: 815
3. Ziedses des Plantes B (1935) Subtraktion. Eine röntgenographische Methode zur separaten Abbildung bestimmter Teile des Objekts. Fortschr Geb Röntgenstr Nuklearmed 52: 69–79
4. Meaney FF, Weinstein MA, Buonocare E, Pavlicek W, Borkowski GP, Gallagher JH, Safka B, Macintyre W (1980) Digital subtraction angiography of the human cardiovascular system. AJR 135: 1153–1160
5. Drury JK, Gray R, Diamond GA, Whiting J, Pfaff M, Vas R, Wheeler W, Nathan M, Forrester JS, Swan HJC, Nivatpumin T (1982) Computer enhanced digital angiography visualizes coronary bypass grafts without need for selective injection. Abstracts of the 55th scientific sessions of the American Heart Association, no. 917

Assisted Circulation 2

Editor: **F. Unger**
1984. Approx. 250 figures. Approx. 500 pages.
ISBN 3-540-13055-1

Atherosclerosis VI

Proceedings of the Sixth International Symposium

Editors: **F. G. Schettler, A. M. Gotto, G. Middelhoff, A. J. R. Habenicht, K. R. Jurutka**
1983. 264 figures, 214 tables. XXVIII, 982 pages
ISBN 3-540-11450-5

Clinical Diagnosis of Atherosclerosis

Quantitative Methods of Evaluation

Editors: **M. G. Bond, W. Insull, Jr., S. Glagov, A. B. Chandler, J. F. Cornhill**
1983. 103 figures, XVIII, 585 pages. ISBN 3-540-90780-7

Coronary Artery Diseases

Diagnostic and Therapeutic Imaging Approaches

By **M. Amiel, A. Maseri, H. Petitier, N. Vasile**
1984. 175 figures, 15 tables. Approx. 250 pages.
ISBN 3-540-13209-0

Coronary Heart Surgery

A Rehabilitation Measure

Editors: **H. Roskamm, M. Schmuziger**
1979. 203 figures, 104 tables. XI, 394 pages
ISBN 3-540-09345-1

B. J. Harlan, A. Starr, F. M. Harwin

Manual of Cardiac Surgery

Volume 1

1980. 193 figures (183 in full color), 8 tables. XV, 204 pages
(Comprehensive Manuals of Surgical Specialties)
ISBN 3-540-90393-3

B. J. Harlan, A. Starr, F. M. Harwin

Manual of Cardiac Surgery

Volume 2

1981. 130 figures in full color. XV, 143 pages. (Comprehensive Manuals of Surgical Specialties). ISBN 3-540-90563-4

Springer-Verlag
Berlin
Heidelberg
New York
Tokyo

GPSR Compliance

The European Union's (EU) General Product Safety Regulation (GPSR) is a set of rules that requires consumer products to be safe and our obligations to ensure this.

If you have any concerns about our products, you can contact us on ProductSafety@springernature.com

In case Publisher is established outside the EU, the EU authorized representative is:

Springer Nature Customer Service Center GmbH
Europaplatz 3
69115 Heidelberg, Germany

Batch number: 10704763

Printed by Printforce, the Netherlands